Eating Spring Rice

Eating Spring Rice

The Cultural Politics of AIDS in Southwest China

Sandra Teresa Hyde

UNIVERSITY OF CALIFORNIA PRESS
Berkeley · Los Angeles · London

University of California Press, one of the most distinguished university presses in the United States, enriches lives around the world by advancing scholarship in the humanities, social sciences, and natural sciences. Its activities are supported by the UC Press Foundation and by philanthropic contributions from individuals and institutions. For more information, visit www.ucpress.edu.

University of California Press
Berkeley and Los Angeles, California

University of California Press, Ltd.
London, England

Library of Congress Cataloging-in-Publication Data

Hyde, Sandra Teresa.
   Eating spring rice : the cultural politics of AIDS in Southwest China / Sandra Teresa Hyde.
      p.   cm.
   Includes bibliographical references and index.

   ISBN-13: 978-0-520-24715-4 (pbk. : alk. paper)

   1. AIDS (Disease)—China—Yunnan Sheng.   2.
AIDS (Disease)—Government policy—China—Yunnan
Sheng.   3. AIDS (Disease)—Social aspects—China—
Yunnan Sheng.   I. Title.

RA643.86.C62H93   2007
362.196'97920095135—dc22   2006009345

Manufactured in the United States of America

15   14   13   12   11   10
10   9   8   7   6   5   4   3   2

The paper used in this publication meets the minimum requirements of ANSI/NISO Z39.48–1992 (R 1997) (*Permanence of Paper*).

For my parents, June and George Hyde,
and in memory of Wang Zhusheng

Contents

Illustrations

Tables

Acknowledgments

Conducting ethnographic fieldwork on the emergence of HIV/AIDS in China, prior to the Chinese government's official acknowledgment that the country even has an epidemic, was difficult at best, and at times virtually impossible. As an AIDS activist in the United States, when I first set out to conduct this research, I was told by many that it could not be done. Nevertheless, the research was completed, due to the perseverance of many individuals and institutions that taught me it is "small drops of water on a stone that create an indentation." Over the past ten years, I have incurred many intellectual and personal debts, and I wish to extend my deepest gratitude and appreciation to the following people and institutions. Beginning in China, my heartfelt thanks go to everyone who offered me hospitality, generosity, and invaluable resources and assistance while I conducted fieldwork. My primary debt is to my informants—all those unnamed souls who provided bottomless glasses of mango juice and cups of Yunnan tea and who opened their homes and shared their lives with me. With the exception of a few public figures, I honor their confidentiality. I have tremendous gratitude and respect for my informants at the "New Wind Hair Salon," the Drug Treatment Centers in Jinghong and Kunming, and the denizens of Menglian and Jinghong, for without them this ethnography would never have been written.

For their incredible support and courage, I acknowledge the following professors in China: Lin Chaomin, the Vice President of and History

Professor at Yunnan University; Wang Zhusheng, Professor in his own newly organized Visual Anthropology Program at Yunnan University; and his wife, anthropologist Yang Hui. Professor Wang completed his doctorate at the State University of New York, Stonybrook, and had the deftness to delicately balance two systems: the American doctoral research requirements for fieldwork, and the Chinese government's demands to protect its interests in avoiding misrepresentations of the epidemic and the people it affected. He showed me just where and how the Chinese system was flexible in the postreform era, and how to work successfully on such a sensitive and controversial topic, and for this, I am eternally thankful. Tragically, Professor Wang passed away in March 1999, and in reverence for his work in Chinese anthropology and as a graduate student of his, I dedicate this book to him. *Ganxie.*

In public health and international development, I wish to thank Allen Beasey, Neil Boisen, Odilon Couzin, Emile Fox, Rob Gray, Nagib Hussein, Libo, Li Guozhi, Wylie Liu, Mayu, Ann Mehaffey, Panyi, Angela Savage, Sun Gung, Audrey Swift, Tan Laiyong, Kate Wedgwood, Kellie Wilson, Yang Haiyu, Zhang Miaoyun, and the staffs of their organizations for their willingness to assist an anthropologist in the midst of their busy work on HIV/AIDS prevention in China. I also extend my sincere gratitude to physicians Cheng Hehe, Li Jianhua, Li Xiaoliang, and Yang Fang for sharing with me not only their insights into the AIDS epidemic but also their humor, patience, and contacts.

As for personal contributions, first and foremost I have my parents, George Hyde and June Brady, to thank in more ways than I can count. As physician-researchers whose work spans five continents and includes long stints in three countries in Africa, they demonstrated the joys of learning from other cultures' experience, provided constant encouragement and support, and encouraged me to "push doors marked 'Pull.'" Whatever words I use to thank them will never be enough. I also thank my sister Wendy and her family in California for providing shelter and company for one month while I put the final touches on the manuscript. I thank my sister Karen and her family in Colorado for providing respite from work and great ski days. Without the love and support of Sean Brotherton, Francesca Dal Lago, and Avery Rifkin on the East Coast, and Nancy Goldman, Tim Kingston, and Lisa D. Moore on the West Coast, I would never have finished this book. Each of them has been indispensable to me in her or his own way, and I thank them for their friendship and, most of all, for keeping my heart and mind on fire. During the research phase in China, I thank the Armijo-Hussein family, especially Jackie, who extended her warm hospitality and intellectual curiosity and shared the love of her two daughters, Annamaria and Amira. I am indebted to Nagib Hussein, one of the key pioneers in HIV/AIDS prevention in China, for his willingness to teach me about HIV/AIDS in Yunnan and for providing many contacts in the midst of a very demanding work schedule.

In the academy, I gratefully acknowledge my dissertation cochairs for their untiring support and incisive comments. Lawrence Cohen has been an inspiration, a joy to work with, and a perceptive critic since my early days in the Medical Anthropology Program at the University of California, Berkeley. Sharon Kaufman was a true role model, providing careful readings of my dissertation drafts, challenging me to strengthen my arguments, and heartening me to write something I could give my family to read. My two other committee members provided unflagging academic and financial support, as well as encouragement when I felt defeat. Nancy Scheper-Hughes provided me with her own wonderful ethnographies for inspiration, and loving care throughout my graduate career. Without Tom Gold's unceasing encouragement and his introductions to contacts at Yunnan University, this project would never have gotten started. I would also like to thank Aihwa Ong for her careful and discerning readings of my original grant proposals and for her comments on early chapter drafts. I send a special heartfelt aloha to Angela Davies, whose marvelous British wit and keen intellect kept me from despair at many points along the road and who, at the very end, painstakingly read and commented on every chapter in the book before it went to press. Because of these academics, I am happy to call myself an anthropologist.

As colleagues and comrades in arms who read and commented on parts of the manuscript, muddled through my prose, and helped push my work in new directions, I extend my utmost gratitude to Blaine Chaisson, Nancy Chapman, Nancy Chen, Connie Clark, Virginia Cornue, Deborah Davis, Sara Davis, Jay Dautcher, David Eaton, Glen Etter, Suzanne Gottschang, Rebecca Hardin, Stevan Harrell, Gail Hershatter, Liz Herskovits, Lisa Hoffman, Lyn Jeffrey, Sarah Jessup, Jing Jun, Joan Kaufman, Robyn Kliger, Matthew Kohrman, Gedis Lankauskas, Margery Lazarus, John Leedom, Johann Lindquist, Kelly McKinney, Vinh-kim Nguyen, Mariella Pandolfi, Elizabeth Remick, Susan Rhodes, Lisa Rofel, Ann Russ, Jillian Sandell, Louisa Schein, Chris Smith, Kimberly Theidon, Eileen Rose Walsh, Bill Watkins, Tim Weston, Bob White, Anne Williams, Liu Xin, Mayfair Yang, Paola Zamperini, and Zhang Li.

My writing benefited from productive discussion and dissection in the dissertation-writing seminars of Stanley Brandes, Aihwa Ong, Sharon Kaufman, and Nancy Scheper-Hughes (1998 and 1999) and in David Szanton's Engendering Social Science workshops at Westerbecke Ranch in Sonoma, California (1998–1999). I also benefited from the personal and academic support from my Boston writing group (2000–2001): Chris Walley, Sara Friedman, Ann Marie Leshkowich, and Tuulikki Pietila. For my two-year sojourn in Boston, I give enormous thanks and gratitude to Byron Good and Mary-Jo DelVecchio Good, who took me on as a postdoctoral fellow (1999–2001) in the Department of Social Medicine at Harvard Medical School. To my delight, we ended up as colleagues and dear friends. I especially appreciate Mary-Jo for reading the entire final book draft before it went to press. I thank Arthur Kleinman for many opportunities to discuss and debate modern China and for his Anthropology Graduate Seminar at Harvard, "Deep China," which helped refine my thinking. I also thank the following members of the Department of Social Medicine at Harvard for their advice and comments when I started rewriting my dissertation as a book: João Biehl, Patricia Case, Doris Chang, Martha Fuller, Corina Salas Gros, Andrew Lakoff, Amaro Laria, and Karen-Sue Taussig. My new colleagues in the Departments of Anthropology, Social Studies of Medicine, and East Asian Studies at McGill University have been a consistent source of intellectual companionship and a wonderful group of people to work with. In particular, I am grateful to Margaret Lock and Allan Young for the opportunity to present parts of this research in the McGill Social Studies of Medicine lecture series, and to Kristin Norget and Michael Bisson for their wonderful mentorship.

In the final phase of a manuscript's development are the many facets of editing. I graciously thank Reed Malcolm and his staff at the University of California Press, who touched me with their patience and impeccable skill throughout the editorial process. For helping me to revise the entire manuscript from top to bottom, I sincerely thank Ralph Litzinger for believing in this project, for his invaluable editorial advice, and for getting me to refine many of the theoretical ideas expressed here. I also extend my gratitude to two anonymous reviewers for UC Press for helping to make the manuscript a better piece of writing. For editorial work in English, I thank Catherine Young and Patrick McDonagh. For editorial work in Chinese, I thank my three trilingual research assistants: Karen Tsang, Sandra Lee, and He Xiao. Some materials in this book have already been published in the following publications. "Selling Sex and Sidestepping the State: Prostitutes, Condoms, and HIV/AIDS Prevention in Southwest China," *East Asia: An International Quarterly* (Special Issue on East Asian Sexualities), 2000, Vol. 18, no. 4, winter. "The Cultural Politics of HIV/AIDS and the Chinese State in Late-Twentieth Century Yunnan," *Tsantsa* (The Review of the Swiss Society of Ethnology), 2002, winter, no. 7. "When Riding a Tiger It Is Difficult to Dismount: STIs and HIV/AIDS in Contemporary China," *The Yale Journal of Chinese Health,* 2003, no. 2, autumn. My thanks to the editors of these three journals and to Duke University Press for allowing me to publish these bits and pieces in this book.

My original fieldwork (1995–1996, 1997) was generously supported by several grants and foundations: the Fulbright-Hays Doctoral Research Abroad Fellowship; the Wenner-Gren Foundation; the Center for HIV/AIDS Prevention Studies at the University of California, San Francisco; two Foreign Language and Area Studies Grants and a Regent's Fellowship from UC Berkeley's Center for Chinese Studies; and the Lowie Award from UC Berkeley's Anthropology Department. Follow-up fieldwork research during the summers of 2000 and 2002 and writing time were made possible, first, by a National Institutes of Mental Health Postdoctoral Training Fellowship at Harvard Medical School and, second, by grants from the Social Science and Humanities Research Council of Canada and the Research and Development Fund for new faculty at McGill University.

As we move well into the twenty-first century, I wish for a world without AIDS.

Notes on Transliteration

Interviews in this book were conducted in Mandarin Chinese or English. Although I am not a linguist, I want to emphasize that in writing about the Tai people in China, one is faced with several choices in terms of transliteration. Just as there is neocolonial slippage between "Sipsong-panna," the current word used by the Tais of that place, and the Mandarin transliteration of Xishuangbanna (or in the local vernacular, just "Banna"), there are also two different linguistic terms for the same ethnic population, "Tai-Lüe" and "Dai-le." In referring to the Tai, I use "Dai" only when it is used in official Mandarin place names, and "Tai" or "Tai-Lüe" in all other cases.

I rely on pseudonyms for the majority of informants, and in cases requiring confidentiality, I have disguised identities and added characteristics that would make it difficult to identify persons. To further protect informants' identities, I have given them only one name instead of the usual two metonyms used to denote respect in China. In addition, some of the descriptions of persons are composites. I found these measures were crucial given the sensitivity of HIV/AIDS as a topic of inquiry and the legal issues involved in working with people who are ostensibly outside the law and thus potentially subject to prosecution. In the few cases where proper names are common knowledge and thus already published in newspapers, medical journals, government reports, or conference proceedings, I use people's given names.

All references to the Chinese yuan refer to the exchange rate of 1 U.S. dollar = 8.3 yuan (the average rate from 1997 to 2002).

The Cultural Politics of AIDS in Postreform China

PATTERN THREE: THE "NEW" ASIAN EPIDEMICS

Despite "the fact that AIDS had appeared simultaneously in disparate cultures and apparently unconnected places around the globe," by the late 1980s, the World Health Organization had carved up the world based on epidemiologic maps of HIV/AIDS (Patton 2002: xi–xii). The pattern of incidence associated with North America and Europe, where cases were concentrated among homosexual men and injection drug users, was called Pattern One.[1] This was followed by African cases, which were initially found among heterosexuals who were non–injection drug users, and labeled Pattern Two. The World Health Organization now warns that Asian AIDS will be the next large epicenter for the pandemic.[2] Epidemiological risk group categories of homosexuals, drug addicts, or heterosexual "sex workers" defined Patterns One and Two,[3] but geography and time define Pattern Three. In moving beyond the narrow nomenclatures that "pattern thinking" leaves us with, the public health world has been slow to explore new infections that lie in countries such as China, places outside the purview of the predominant focus on AIDS in Africa and North America. Yet Asian AIDS cases, predominantly driven by HIV in India, China, Thailand, Cambodia, and Vietnam, are placing Asia firmly on these global maps of disease.[4]

Cindy Patton (2002) notes that pattern thinking emerged out of the Global Program on AIDS (GPA) and its early divisions of the world into six different administrative regions.[5] Within these divisions, developing countries in Asia were strangely aligned with Japan and Australia. The World Health Organization's (WHO's) official story read: "Researchers believe that the virus was present in isolated population groups years before the epidemic began. Then the situation changed: people moved more often and traveled more; they settled in big cities; and lifestyles changed, including patterns of sexual behavior. It became easier for HIV to spread, through sexual intercourse and contaminated blood. As the virus spread, the isolated disease already existing became a new epidemic" (WHO 1989 in Patton 2002: 60–61). As Patton so eloquently points out, this common tale meant there was a tension between the actual disease and its translocation. Confusing time and geography, it is a tale about a virus and a description of the particular bodies that might transmit it.

China is facing a revolution in massive population migration from its rural enclaves to its cosmopolitan centers. A mobile force of some 140 million people, roughly 10 percent of the population, migrate both within and across provinces from county towns to large cities such as Chengdu, Beijing, and Shanghai. This mobility has been both theoretically and empirically associated with a rise in urban poverty and crime, risky behaviors, epidemics in drug use and sexually transmitted infections, and now, HIV/AIDS.[6] This book describes how diseases map onto certain places and people more readily than onto others and how HIV/AIDS becomes embedded in political and economic relations, embodied practices, and cultural imaginations. As a disease of postmodernity, HIV/AIDS becomes culturally inhabited at each site where it appears on the map. How representatives of the Chinese state first responded to the epidemic points toward what is particularly unique about the Chinese approach to infectious diseases and what is also shared globally and transnationally.[7]

Yunnan Province was ground zero of the epidemic, where heroin users were first identified as infected in the late 1980s and early 1990s. However—and this is key to the China story—any analysis complicates the singular idea that it was only translocal bodies, and not also government neglect or state-condoned unsafe blood-banking practices, that dispersed Chinese HIV. Therefore, as a quiet and very deadly epidemic was emerging in Henan in the late 1980s and early 1990s in villages where officials were complicit in using local poor peasants as economic canon fodder in blood and plasma collection schemes, the epidemiological emphasis was still on the counties in rural minority Yunnan (Zhang Feng 2004; Chan

2001). Since the first AIDS case was reported in 1985, China has moved into second place for the fastest-growing epidemic in Asia, behind India, and had declared close to one million infections by the end of 2004 (Bloom et al. 2004; Micollier 2004a; Hunter 2005).[8] In contrast, health experts estimate that at least one million poor farmers were infected in these "botched" blood-selling schemes in central China (Reuters 2005).[9]

REMAPPING, RECONFIGURING, AND RETHINKING THE STUDY OF EPIDEMICS

One of the major goals of this book is to approach HIV/AIDS less in terms of a study of a bounded minority prefecture and more in terms of the circulation and movement of conceptualizations of the disease across various boundaries, boundaries that require different kinds of anthropological thinking and methods. This work is *not* a definitive ethnographic account of the nascent HIV/AIDS epidemic in Yunnan Province, but an investigation into what I call *everyday AIDS practices*. It begins in the early days of the Chinese epidemic before it was seen as a major public health problem.[10] In the mid-1990s, HIV/AIDS in China was considered a minority problem; minority prefectures in Yunnan revealed the highest number of cases. However, beyond the racial dichotomy of white and nonwhite bodies—or in much of the world, white and black bodies—comes the more nuanced and regionally rooted issue of Han and non-Han bodies. Such ethnic distinctions differentiate an anthropology of epidemiology from cultural studies of disease, straight epidemiology, or a political economy of health. Toward these ends, my lines of inquiry throughout this book demonstrate that understanding transmission of HIV/AIDS requires attention simultaneously to the rise of science and public health in postreform China and to the stories of lives touched by public health in China's borderlands. In doing so, I focus on both the discursive and the material dimensions of the epidemic.

. . .

1985

At spring festival, preparing for a two-day train ride heading west, I sat on top of my backpack at Guilin train station. I joined the cacophony of hundreds of families yelling train numbers and mingled with peasants carrying shoulder poles, their goods swaddled like

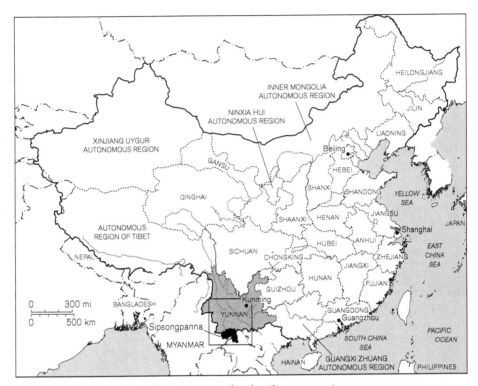

Map 1. People's Republic of China, 2005 (for detail, see map 2)

infants and tied at the two ends. Before arriving, we would travel by train, airplane, bus, and minivan to reach our destination of Xishuangbanna, the former Tai tributary kingdom of Sipsongpanna in Southwest China [see map 1].[11] I was part of a delegation of American and Chinese English teachers, colleagues from the Ministry of Mining and Metallurgy, departing for vacation following the end of our annual meeting. On a packed-dirt road in front of the state-run Xishuangbanna Hotel, known as the Banna Bingguan, sat a corner shop with one small bare lightbulb hanging down on an electric wire. The proprietor laughed when we asked, "Where is the Mekong?" He knew only the local name, the Lancang River. In the early morning hours in the town of Jinghong, the former Tai kingdom capital of Tsen Hung, we watched smoke rise from small cook fires at the local Buddhist temple. Young Tai boys performed their morning rituals dressed in the long saffron robes that mark their

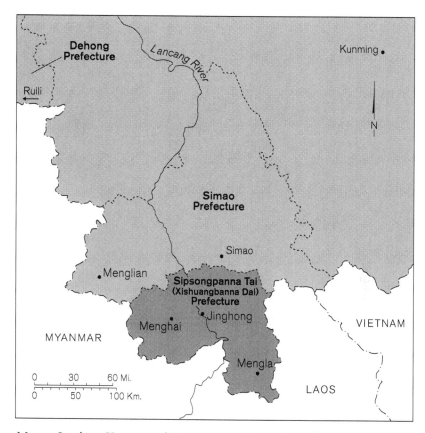

Map 2. Southern Yunnan and Sipsongpanna Tai (Xishuangbanna Dai) Autonomous Prefecture

traineeship in Buddhism. With their chants we rose to greet the day. Over the next three days, our delegation traveled down roads that roamed between rubber trees and rice paddies through the tropical jungle. Greeting the wide expanse of the river, we followed the sounds of water flowing into the black night, where we heard crickets and saw twinkling stars in the sky.

1995

Ten years pass and Jinghong is no longer a sleepy town on the Lancang River. Hawkers yell, bicycle bells ring, cars race, and tourists wake to begin another day in the life of the city. Travelers discuss with their guides where to venture for the next few hours, and decisions are made before the stifling afternoon heat drives everyone indoors into the privacy of their air-conditioned hotel rooms. Motorcycles race past shops, hair salons, brothels, karaoke bars, the beer hall, the large department store, and the government buildings crowned by a single red star. The new national bird, the construction crane, dominates the Jinghong skyline as it does in every other Chinese city. Along with these cranes are numerous construction sites decorated with an intricate latticework of bamboo poles. Rather than tending their rice fields, Han migrant workers balance gracefully on these fragile slippery scaffoldings. Money and capital are the dreams and desires of the city in postreform China.

.   .   .

After a ten-year hiatus, in May 1995, I returned to China and to Yunnan Province in the southwest. This time I was no longer a teacher of English as a second language but a graduate student hoping to conduct field research in ground zero of the Chinese AIDS epidemic in Dehong Tai-Jingpo Nationality Autonomous Prefecture, in western Yunnan. I went to study why the Chinese public health literature ascribed high rates of the human immunodeficiency virus (HIV) that causes acquired immune deficiency syndrome (AIDS)—or in Chinese, *aizibing*—to the Tai minority in two counties in rural Yunnan. Even though Yunnan had 80 percent of the Chinese AIDS cases in 1995, on my first trip to Yunnan that year, I met few people that were HIV-positive, nor did anyone provide me with Tai prevalence rates for AIDS. What I did confront was a plethora of myths, rumors, stories, and educated guesses about why the Tai minority had high rates of HIV/AIDS. I left puzzled.

Dr. Wu, my initial contact at Kunming Medical Center in the Department of Traditional Chinese Medicine, showed me her before-and-after pictures of drug addicts incarcerated in a Ruili drug prison (in Dehong Tai-Jingpo Prefecture) whom she had treated for Kaposi's sarcoma with Chinese herbs. She, along with almost every tourist who passed through the small guesthouse where I was staying, insisted that HIV/AIDS was still a confinable disease in China. They repeated like a mantra that by containing the Tai in Dehong Tai-Jingpo and Sipsongpanna prefectures, China would not repeat the public health mistakes of neighboring Thailand. By contrast, Tai villagers just south of Jinghong scoffed at the notion that Han public health officials thought they had HIV/AIDS.

When, in November 1995, I arrived back in Kunming, the capital of Yunnan Province, for a yearlong research project, my sponsors at Yunnan University informed me I could not get permission to conduct research in Dehong Tai-Jingpo Prefecture, as it was a remote area of Yunnan and on such a politically sensitive topic. However, all was not lost; instead, my sponsors selected Jinghong, in Sipsongpanna Tai-Lüe Nationality Autonomous Prefecture, as an appropriate alternative field site due to its emergent sex tourism industry—an industry viewed by many doctors, bureaucrats, and officials in Kunming as symptomatic of Tai-Lüe cultural values. The underlying assumption was that the Tai are a loose and sexually uninhibited people (*luanjiao*) and that their sexual practices were leading to high rates of sexually transmitted infections (STIs) and now, HIV/AIDS. According to several individuals in the provincial medical community, my role, since I was a medical anthropologist and a former public health specialist in sexually transmitted infections, was to find the cultural clues that predisposed the Tai to risky sexual practices. However, these views of Sipsongpanna were not new.

In another, nineteenth-century world, William Clifton Dodd, an American Protestant missionary, described Sipsongpanna in 1838 as "a country of darkness, [as] dark as pockets, [a] darkness of ignorance, superstition, and sin" (Dodd 1923: 181). In the late 1950s, a group of ethnologists working for the Yunnan Provincial Communist Party as part of a nationwide social research project to document and catalogue China's ethnic groups, described the roads to Sipsongpanna as plagued by cerebral malaria and leprosy (Yin 1986). And now, more than forty years later, I describe the roads to Sipsongpanna as linked to sex tourism and the rise of this new infectious disease. While state socialism worked to eradicate sexually transmitted infections, market socialism and the post-1979 reforms have served as a catalyst for the re-emergence of illegal drug use and prostitution and exponential increases in STIs and AIDS (Fan 1990; Zheng Xiwan 1991; Wang N. 1991; Fox 1996; Cheng Hehe et al. 1996; Cheng Hehe, Zhang, Pan, Jia, et al. 2000).

One of the chief internists in Jinghong, working at the local Tai medical center, told me that she spent several afternoons trying to convince a Tai man that because of his HIV status, he could not possibly date, let alone marry. After reviewing my field notes from my first return trip to China, I realized that Dr. Wu's perceptions of the Chinese epidemic, while considered prejudiced and even AIDS-phobic by public health workers and AIDS activist communities in the West, had a certain logic to it. From the outset, a link between two subgroups of the Tai in two regions was assumed to account for the potentially high incidence across Yunnan: the Tai-Nüa were thought to be increasingly infected in De-hong Tai-Jingpo Prefecture because of China's heroin trade, and the Tai-Lüe were thought to be infected in Sipsongpanna due to China's newly emerging sex trade and political economic ties to Thailand.

This book is both an ethnographic account of an emerging epidemic and an attempt to understand the cultural and political complexities of that same epidemic in the prefectural capital of Jinghong in Sipsong-panna Autonomous Tai Minority Prefecture (Xishuangbanna Daizu Zizhizhou), near China's border with Laos and Burma (see map 2). Thus, I focus on AIDS less as a bounded, already emerging entity than as a series of everyday practices deployed by both government repre-sentatives and working people in Jinghong who reveal how the concept of HIV/AIDS is constantly being made and remade over time. Dis-courses, in order to remain active and alive, must be reiterated and per-formed, and I treat them here as active in constituting and making and remaking cultural, political, and public health landscapes. In thinking about modern pandemics, I consider both moral and geographic imagi-naries, a world where culture maps onto place, and place onto people, and where tidy models of border partition thinking fueled much of the early public health policies toward containment of HIV/AIDS (see map 3).

This book thus adds to the emerging literature on the anthropology of epidemics by addressing the following questions: How does Sipsong-panna respond to the rise of an infectious disease often characterized as a "radio disease"—heard but not seen? In both Sipsongpanna and Meng-lian minority autonomous prefectures in Yunnan, how does a new infec-tious disease challenge fundamental cultural systems of sexuality, gender, and ethnic relations and present challenges for representatives of the state—the prefecture's anti-epidemic stations, public security bureaus, and international nongovernmental health organizations? How have epidemiological prejudice and ethnic stigmatization affected calculated policy decisions situated within transnational discourses on HIV/AIDS, which in turn affect local prevention practices (Taylor 1990; Schoepf 1992; Sobo 1993; Farmer, Connors, and Simmons 1996; Farmer 1999; Pigg 2002)? How are sexual entertainment workers implicated in these epidemiological profiles and prevention projects, and what kinds of transactional sex are they involved in, with whom, and why?

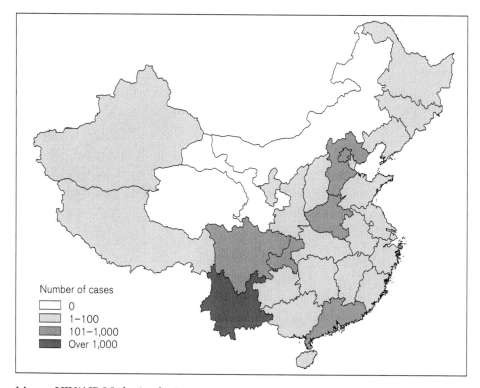

Map 3. HIV/AIDS Infection by Province, 1985–1995

Traditional ethnography presupposes that an ethnographer conducts research in one country, most likely one place, and builds on that location for understanding the larger questions about trajectories of infection. However, infectious diseases by nature are mobile and multiply; to study them requires tracing their fault lines through various epicenters as well as through the people involved in controlling them. As the epicenter of the virus in rural Yunnan was not open to investigation when I began this research, I moved my focus to tracing the actions, thoughts, and discourses of people both directly and indirectly involved in HIV. I drew not only from multiple sites for this research—a wide ethnographic map that included research trips to three countries, China, Thailand, and Hong Kong (prior to 1997)—but also on many different people. These included physicians, government officials, police officers, public health workers, and the myriad of people working in Sipsongpanna—tourist experts, shopkeepers, entertainment industry workers, sex workers, Buddhist practitioners, Tai activists, and ordinary local citizens.

ETHNOGRAPHY ACROSS SPACE AND TIME (1995–2002)

During twenty-two months, between May 1995 and August 2002, I conducted intensive multisited fieldwork in Kunming, Jinghong, Menglian, Beijing, Hong Kong, and Chiang Mai. Phase one (May 1995 to January 1996) consisted of six months of urban fieldwork in the Yunnan provincial capital of Kunming, where I worked with two nongovernmental HIV/AIDS organizations—Save the Children–Hong Kong and the Australian Red Cross—and waited patiently for government permission to go to the field. Phase two (February 1996 to August 1997) consisted of twelve months of fieldwork in Sipsongpanna (referred in the local Mandarin slang as "Banna"), Menglian, Beijing, and Hong Kong. I conducted follow-up fieldwork in the summers of 2000 and 2002 in Hong Kong and in Yunnan. In between I also attended three critical conferences—two in Chiang Mai, Thailand (one on cultural survival among the Tai, the other on HIV/AIDS in Asia and the Pacific) and Hong Kong's first big conference on HIV/AIDS. In Sipsongpanna (in 1996, 1997, 2000, and 2002), I observed patrons in video shops, hair salons, cafés, movie theaters, and karaoke bars in the city of Jinghong and made visits to Tai villages in the countryside. In the city and in the villages, I observed local cultural practices and behaviors and, more important, the representation and circulation of stories about HIV/AIDS. The practices and cultural events I observed ranged from courtship rituals between teenagers at pool tables and movie theaters, to businessmen negotiating sexual transactions with local prostitutes, to Tai villagers talking about why the Han view their sexual practices as uncivilized and backward. Due to the tremendous stigma attached to the disease, initially no one would admit to having HIV, so people with the disease in Sipsongpanna were relatively hidden.

Besides participant observation, I conducted two types of interviews. First, I interviewed twenty government officials to learn how ideas about HIV/AIDS were constructed, contested, and altered among representatives of the Chinese state. Second, I interviewed twenty migrant workers in Jinghong in order to explore individual attitudes and experiences with respect to changing ideas of sexuality, gender relations, and sexually transmitted infections. In addition, I participated in two types of behavioral surveys: a "knowledge, attitude, behavior, and practice" (KABP)[12] survey in Menglian County in 1985 and a survey in Dehong

Tai-Jingpo Prefecture in villages near the city of Ruili in summer 2002. I conducted several focus groups (each with between five and ten participants)—with villagers in Menglian in 1996, with students at the Xishuangbanna Teacher's College the same year, and with sex workers and drug addicts in Kunming in summer 2002. I also conducted archival research on the Tai-Lüe, the social history of sexually transmitted infections, and contemporary HIV/AIDS epidemiology in the archives at the University Services Center at Chinese University of Hong Kong, Yunnan University, Kunming Medical College, Countway Medical Library at Harvard Medical School, and the Asian Collection at the Kalmanovitz Medical Library at the University of California, San Francisco. In addition, I collected contemporary public health propaganda messages and the physical icons of popular sexual culture: condom boxes; sex toys; condom and sex toy advertisements; posters, pamphlets, and the other accoutrements of what is known as information, education, and communication (IEC) materials; and stories and folklore about HIV/AIDS in the popular press.

As it is now commonplace for anthropologists to position themselves within the texts they write in order to define where Western representations of the Other begin and end, I too include myself in the following narratives and stories (Marcus and Fischer 1986; Abu-Lughod 1991 & 1993; Rofel 1992 & 1999; Ebron 2002).[13] Through Save the Children–Hong Kong and the Australian Red Cross, I interviewed and interacted with government officials from Menglian to Chiang Mai who, beginning in the mid-1990s, were the pioneers in developing HIV/AIDS prevention strategies. What facilitated my access to these often tightly secured bureaucracies was my own subject-position. I was conducting dissertation research in anthropology but with a master's degree in public health and several years of work experience in HIV/AIDS, women's health, and sexually transmitted infections; I became at times a consultant. When analyzing the culture of HIV/AIDS, I was a social scientist, and when working on prevention projects, I was a public health expert. This dual positioning was a valuable asset, as my public health credentials opened many doors that an anthropologist's brief would not have; however, this also meant I had to balance and bridge the divide between public health and anthropology. The secrecy, stigma, and fear attached to the epidemic meant that many people did not want to talk about, see, or catch even the faintest breath of it, let alone share sensitive information about it with a foreign anthropologist. It also meant that my critiques of the HIV/AIDS epidemic were tainted in the sense that I often participated in studies and prevention projects, so that I was altering the very practices I was attempting to document. As Paulla Ebron (2002) notes, ethnographic interviews are another kind of performance that we ethnographer's collect and in no way are they less important than the tales and stories that informants share us with.

THE ANTHROPOLOGY OF EPIDEMICS

As anthropologist Chris Lyttleton (2000) points out, AIDS can be interpreted as an epidemic of signification (Treichler 1999), as a moral panic (Watney 1997), and following Michel Foucault (1980), as a new set of sexualities born through recurrent disciplinary responses. For Lyttleton (2000), as for myself, coming to terms with global AIDS means "laying bare aspects of the social order to calculated scrutiny and reconfiguration" (10). It is through putting a litmus test on the social orders of the Americas, and then Africa, and now Asia that anthropologists have called for a more finely tuned analysis of HIV/AIDS epidemics and the global transfer of scientific knowledge from one country to another (Farmer 1992; Biehl 2001; Carillo 2002; Eaton 2002; Nguyen 2001 & 2005).

In the process of tracking the shape and terrain of public health policies and practices around HIV/AIDS in China, I capture the transfer and circulation of scientific and technical knowledge from several different global sites—Australia, Britain, Thailand, Hong Kong, and the United States and United Nations—to China and back again. I argue that a shift in methodological thinking is essential because large public health surveys and epidemiological analytics cannot capture the subtleties of local, regional, and even national-transnational aspects of identity and sexual practice that drive this epidemic. The study of AIDS changes our thinking about just how far the Chinese state envisions the multiethnic state and also how far the state reaches into the small corners of borderland China. Cultural studies and political economy alone cannot describe the weight and tenor of epidemics such as HIV.

Much literature on epidemics in the social sciences takes either a cultural studies approach of discourse analysis, analyzing the textual and visual representations of an epidemic (Gilman 1988a & 1988b; Treichler 1991; Altman 2001; Hood 2005), or a political-economy-of-health approach, often focusing on the mechanics of how economic and political power influences where and why people get sick (Farmer 1992 &

1999; Schoepf 1992; Frankenberg 1993; Parker et al. 1993; Walby 1997; Singer 1998;).[14] I advocate building on these two sets of analytics, to be in dialogue with them, in considering an anthropology of epidemics that analyzes how people simultaneously represent, understand, and respond to epidemics through writing about practices that emerge in everyday life. My discussion of practices involves an in-depth exploration of epidemiology, the structure of certain public health practices, and the personal tales of sex workers. Thus one cannot keep either local practices or political structures as separate categories, as they are forever integrally intertwined.

I first introduce the concept of everyday AIDS practices and three main themes: socialist governmentality and epidemics, ethnicity and epidemics, and epidemics and the imagination. In addition to briefly presenting my own thoughts about how epidemics are shaped by relevant theory, I suggest how this study contributes to a better understanding of the relationships between disease and representation, the state and minority others, and the power and practice of public health in the postmodern global arena. None of these concepts is discrete; hence there is much overlap in my discussion of them.

EVERYDAY AIDS PRACTICES

HIV/AIDS, while signifying diseased bodies, also unfurls a taut canvas depicting some of the fetishes of late modernity: sexuality, desire, non-white bodies, and in this case, non-Han bodies. While Patton (2002) views epidemics from above and distinguishes between a purely epidemiological and a tropical medicine approach to understanding them, I take the view from below that advocates for the study of everyday AIDS practices.[15] I use the term "everyday AIDS practices" for two rather broad reasons. First, following Pierre Bourdieu (1977 & 1990) and Michel de Certeau (1984), I use the term "everyday practice" because it allows me to capture a whole array of practices, thoughts, policies, words, and actions involved in a discussion of HIV/AIDS.[16] I employ Bourdieu's (1977) notion that history continually mediates structures and subjective responses; that individual practices do not ignore power structures. Bringing practice theory to an epidemic allows me to bridge the variety and range of human endeavors that are involved in the social practice and discourse associated with documenting and preventing a new epidemic.

Second, in linking the very notion of Bourdieu's structured practices with Foucault's notion of discursive practice and biopower, which is much more diffuse than Bourdieu's, I move away from time-based and spatial analyses that foster a neat chronology of HIV/AIDS. I draw on what Liu Xin (2000: 24) has called the uncertainty in practice and on how practices transform themselves in the very moment when they are actualized. More important, this rubric joining practice theory and Foucault's analytics (1980) allows me to incorporate a broad range of events and activities—from the development of HIV/AIDS prevention policy to the contours of the everyday lives of HIV/AIDS bureaucrats, the medical screening of the blood supply, policies on HIV/AIDS education in middle schools, and the random surveillance and screening of prostitutes and injection drug users. As policies are subject to constant flux and change, it is the processes behind them that are important for anthropologists to document. We must situate ourselves in the creation of state public health projects and the power dynamics that accompany them. Studying public health responses to the epidemic reveals not only local state apparatuses but also a country in transition, from reform to postreform, from socialism with Chinese characteristics to something entirely new.

However, neither practice theory nor Foucault is without shortcomings. As Judith Farquhar (1994: 4) points out, "Anthropologists often express a discomfort with Bourdieu's unconcern with thought, knowledge, and intention except as epiphenomenon of unspoken bodily, spacial, and temporal practices." Farquhar advocates a study of human action in all its historical specifics, exploring the links between intention and action and, at the same time, recognizing that we do not act as we choose; we are constrained. There is also a certain slippage here between practice theory and Foucault's notion of discursive practice. The very idea of focusing on the practices of individuals is antithetical to Foucault's radically anti-humanist notion of power. Through a sort of analytical elision of Foucault's visions of power combined with Bourdieu's notion of humanistic everyday practice, I chart a unique route for studying the cultural politics of transnational infectious diseases. I focus on both representations of HIV/AIDS and the ways science created and furthered certain representations in actual scientific processes.

Anthropological scholarship on China since the Communist Revolution (1966–76) has often stressed that the state is responsible for determining identity and social relations. Although state agents and ideology have played a key role in building Chinese socialism, they have never operated with carte blanche or without local adjustments, resistances, and changes to these very narratives (Siu 1989; Zhang Li 2001; Mueggler 2001; Litzinger 2000a; Schein 2000). In an effort to understand the complexities of subjects as both influenced and changed by the state, such as the processes involved in labeling epidemics among particular ethnic groups, I present two different sets of narratives—the technical and the personal. The first discusses scientific and technical narratives of an epidemic that point toward a wide range of techniques in the collection, dissemination, and analysis of various statistical data, behavioral surveys, prevention programs, and activities that range from peer education focus groups to informational HIV/AIDS telephone hotlines. The second set discusses personal narratives of sex workers, tourists and tour guides, and small-business owners in Jinghong that reveal changing identities, political economies, and ideas about this infectious disease. In both of these sets of narratives, I move back and forth between the central government, the local government, and transnational flows of prevention capital (the AIDS industry) and between officials, outcasts, entrepreneurs, drug addicts, and prostitutes.

It would appear that I am posing two contradictory questions: First, is there or is there not an HIV epidemic in China among the Tai-Lüe? And second, how are representations of the Tai-Lüe as human vectors for HIV circulated, discussed, and repeated throughout the region? Although my fieldwork was in an area where the Save the Children Foundation found a low incidence of HIV/AIDS, members of the Kunming Anti-Epidemic Station claimed there was a much higher incidence rate.[17] Nonetheless, I am less interested in retelling epidemiological stories about the epidemic than in exploring questions around why the Chinese government represented certain areas and persons as having high rates of HIV/AIDS compared to other places and peoples.

All fieldwork accounts are partial, and mine is no exception. I had access to certain places and peoples more readily than to others. For example, I spent much time with female sex workers and very little time with their male partners and clients due to the ease of working among one's own gender in China and because of the expectations of male-female contact in this atmosphere. While I did approach several male clients, I found that their expectations were almost always different from mine. I also privilege heteronormative practices for the simple reason that homosexuality in rural China is relatively hidden and I would have had to use a very different set of research tools and methods to get at those communities. Finally, because I was working during the nascent phase of the Chinese HIV/AIDS epidemic, the stories I tell here do not concern infected and diseased bodies, as few people I came into contact with already knew they were infected or were willing to openly talk about their status.

HIV/AIDS BORDERS IN A BORDERLESS EPIDEMIC

Scholarship on HIV/AIDS has suffered not only from widespread prejudice and stigma but also from the outdated and contested official focus on epidemics as regional problems, as if they fit neatly into a post–World War I area-studies format. The way that nation-states define both regional and national boundaries is a key problem in mapping and then later developing the apparatuses of prevention. Although nongovernmental international aid organizations such as the Australian Red Cross have linked up with regional HIV/AIDS projects, such as the greater Mekong HIV/AIDS Peer Education Prevention Project, their models take the periphery as the locus of HIV/AIDS without deconstructing what exactly this periphery is.[18] Dru Gladney (1994) points out that China is often divided into a center and periphery: metropolitan areas constitute the center and rural areas the periphery. The borders in one sense define the center; the civilized metropolitan financial and political areas are bolstered by perceptions of the periphery as barbaric and exotic in comparison. The borderlands are where China's "barbarians" (*man, yi,* or *fan*) have lived since before the Yuan dynasty and where ethnic minorities live in the twenty-first century. This view of non-Han peoples as barbarians is often associated with bygone imperial China; however, it is definitely not dead (see McKhann 1995: 42).

To understand the Chinese epidemic and how it differs from epidemics in other places in Southeast Asia, such as Thailand, the center and the periphery must be investigated in relation to each another. According to the teleological view of epidemiology, HIV moved from the global northern centers of North America and Europe to the south—Africa and, more recently, Asia. However, in thinking of an epidemic in terms of borders, we miss an important point, that borders also depend on imagined other sides (see Tsing 1993). While the geographic borders of Yunnan fade into rural jungle on both sides of Laos and Burma, beyond them are imagined a whole new means of economic survival and culture. In 2000 the "go west" campaign aimed to develop China's western region by imposing several large road construction projects, the Kunming-Laos highway among them, eventually linking Yunnan with Thailand. This campaign builds on the imagined notions of increasing regional prosperity; however, in reality, rural areas along this highway sink deeper and deeper into poverty, creating even greater economic disparity between the wealthy eastern cities and the poor western countryside (Rui 2005).

The HIV/AIDS epidemic in China did not begin in Sipsongpanna; nor will it end there. It is, I reiterate, present in every province, municipality, and autonomous region. The main mode of transmission is still injection drug use; however, epidemics seldom remain within one place or one population (Yu Xiaofang et al. 2003; Wu et al. 1995). They move, grow, and terrorize other places and peoples. What is unique in China is that, in borrowing from ideas developed in early-twentieth-century colonial medicine, health officials mapped AIDS onto locations that made sense only through colonial thinking. For example, in the early 1920s and 1930s, both leprosy and malaria were prevalent in Sipsongpanna—so now, why not also HIV/AIDS? The proximity, both geographically and commercially, to Thailand, which has the largest epidemic in southeast Asia, meant that links between places on a map were set.

Cindy Patton (2002) notes in her study of global AIDS that two different twentieth-century scientific rationales of public health actually collided when it came to understanding this disease. Tropical scientific rationality argues through homology, is obsessed with geography, always views the world colonially, and spacializes disease; its goals are to map the disease, with immunity as the solution. In a different set of scientific rationales, epidemiological thinking argues through production of statistical correlation, is obsessed with transfer between bodies, abstracts or rather hides bodies in the data, temporalizes disease, defines and redefines bodies through disease categories, and has as its goal to simulate a cure solution. Alongside "tropical thinking" were also the language and the tools of "epidemiological thinking," which was less concerned with place than with specific behaviors grounded in particular bodies (Patton 2002: 27–50). These two types of scientific rationality concerning AIDS are prevalent around the world, and they reflect an incapacity to decide whether AIDS is located in bodies or in places. In my case, they are useful in thinking through how HIV/AIDS moves vectorally from minority borderlands to Han centers, and how discussions of containment lead to quarantines and police searches and seizures among prostitutes and drug addicts.

As René Sabatier (1988) points out, "Sex in nearly all human societies is surrounded by taboos. Few people discuss such a sensitive issue without making or implying moral judgments—or feeling that moral judgments are being made about them. And when people from one ethnic group discuss HIV/AIDS in another ethnic group, which inevitably involves discussing other people's sexual behavior, suspicions of racial and ethnic prejudice are easily aroused" (1). Furthermore, as Stuart Hall (1992) observes: "The question of AIDS is an extremely important terrain of struggle and contestation. How could we say that the question of AIDS is not also a question of who gets represented and who does not?" (285). Several informants (both Han and non-Han) believed that one of the main cultural characteristics of the Tai-Lüe is their high level of sexual promiscuity and, as a result, their propensity for the spread of sexually transmitted infections.[19] This belief was prevalent even in light of the rapid changes in epidemiology as more Han Chinese were registered as infected and rates among the Tai in Yunnan were proportionally decreasing.[20]

I link this sexual pathology in part to the notion that attractive sex workers in Jinghong are local Tai Lüe women.[21] In my interviews with the sex workers, I discovered that almost 90 percent were Han Chinese migrants from the adjacent provinces of Guizhou and Sichuan who came to Jinghong in search of work in the tourist industry.[22] These Han Chinese women who worked in the brothels, nightclubs, and karaoke bars of Jinghong increased their chances of receiving customers by dressing in ethnic minority clothing—that is, traditional Tai dress. While prostitutes are the current focus in the transmission of HIV/AIDS, there is also a long history of stigmatizing particular minorities in China (Harrell 1990 & 1995; Gladney 1991 & 1994; Evans 1996).[23]

Quite simply, the categories of people identified as traveling human vectors for the HIV virus in China fit rather comfortably into the larger global epidemiological narratives of disease contamination and stigma (Farmer and Kleinman 1989).[24] When I use the term "stigma," I am not talking about how Tai women are shunned on the streets of Jinghong because they are presumed to be diseased. I am talking about the larger implications of representing one ethnic group as a key vector in a ubiquitous epidemic, an epidemic that flows over the territorial and linguistic borders between Han China and non-Han China, and over national borders into Burma, Laos, and Thailand. The spread of the epidemic itself is evidence of the struggles to both resist and manifest national sovereignty along territorial borders. The transmission of HIV in China's border regions is a metaphor for the globalization of investment, trade, and cultural identity (Porter 1997).

I am not claiming that there are no Tai-Lüe with HIV/AIDS in China, but rather that there were not very many people of Tai-Lüe descent in Sipsongpanna with the disease when I conducted fieldwork in the late 1990s and early 2000s. In contrast, Dehong Tai-Jingpo Prefecture in northwestern Yunnan had high rates among the Tai Nüa, or Dehong Dai,[25] and therefore a scientific link was made that Sipsongpanna's Tai-Lüe would also have high rates. And while one can argue this is merely a function of the limits of surveillance and the hidden nature of the early epidemic, the actual numbers in Jinghong are nowhere near the numbers in the mountainous regions of northwestern Yunnan where the Tai Nüa live. This also has to do with the ethnolinguistic distinctions between the different groups of the Tai. The Tai Nüa have high rates of HIV in Dehong Tai-Jingpo Prefecture due to their proximity to Southeast Asian drug routes, with infections among injection drug users, but the Tai-Lüe near Laos and Burma in 2005 had low infection rates (Zhang Xiaobo et al. 2002; Yu Huifen 2001).

In interpreting research that points to high rates of HIV among Yunnan's minorities in the early to mid-1990s, I am not downplaying the very real lives of people with HIV, but rather questioning the beginnings of scientific inquiry into these places that are clearly crucial to continuing control of China's sovereign borders. Just what does linking minorities with AIDS do? How is this linkage interpreted? What is then done? Several interpretations are relevant here. The areas in China with high heroin trafficking, those bordering the old Burma and Silk roads, include counties with high rates of HIV such as Liangshan County in Sichuan. Recent heroin trafficking routes from China through Central Asia to Western Europe mean that drugs and AIDS affect certain kinds of people more readily than others. However, rather than looking to geography, Chinese public health and social science research studies proliferate in linking HIV to ethnic culture and its culturally specific behaviors, when actually, poverty and drug trafficking drive much of the epidemic. Part of the reason regional illegal economies, including the influence of the Asian drug trade, are ignored is a refusal to acknowledge the downsides of China's economic miracle as part of the problem. It is much easier to just define the problem as part of a small group of ethnic minorities that engage in illegal, unhealthy, and unsafe practices. Furthermore, these studies in one sense perpetuate the notion that ethnic minorities in China have been historically represented, and continue to be so, as less than ideal citizens. Johanna Hood (2005: 23), in her work on cultural representations of HIV in China, suggests that there is a new minority emerging in postreform China that she labels the *aizu* (AIDS minority). The *aizu* are people with AIDS treated as if they were all ignorant rural peasants who lack the proper scientific knowledge (for preventing AIDS) that modernity affords. Here this AIDS minority emerges without the benefit of advocacy groups that we find in much of the world, although people living with HIV/AIDS (PLHIV), and their advocates, are beginning to gain strength in China despite government interference (see Wan Yanhai 2005).[26]

SOCIALIST GOVERNMENTALITY AND EPIDEMICS

Governmentality studies abound within many disciplines and involve a wide range of engagements with Michel Foucault's (1980) thinking about power as productive versus merely repressive. His work has been applied widely in disparate studies on population and demography, civil society and development, social service industries, and the family and psychotherapy (Donzelot 1979; Elias 1982; Burchell, Gordon, and Miller 1991; Dean 1999; Rose 1999).[27] As Lisa Rofel (1999: 30) suggests in her work on women workers in a silk factory in Zhejiang, it is more useful to analyze how technologies of state power have shifted their gaze and mode of operation, and to thus move away from focusing on the amount of power citizens and states possess toward how power operates through multiple arenas, including the policing of certain borders of difference—Han/non-Han, feminine/masculine, periphery/center, and Maoist socialism/late socialism.

The tools of ethnography and the anthropological attention to details of everyday life, with all its contradictions, contestations, and multiple dimensions, are perfect for deconstructing state practices. Anthropologists have disrupted teleological thinking about both state socialism and the transition to a market economy, but they have not yet explored epidemiology in China nor epidemiological thinking and the ways it reduces the terrain of an epidemic to faceless vectors.[28] Although anthropologists working in China have produced valuable studies that examine particular populations, genders, ethnic groups, and migrants in relationship to health care and health issues, none has taken up the study of contemporary epidemics (Kleinman 1986 & 1994; Henderson and Cohen 1984; Farquhar 1991 & 1994; N. Chen 2003; Greenhalgh

1994 & 2005; Kohrman 2005). In contrast, historians have conducted studies of particular public health concerns—most important to this discussion, prostitution in late imperial and Republican China; few have talked in-depth about contemporary history (Dikötter 1995; Hershatter 1997; Sommer 2000).[29] Two key social scientists who write about the contemporary period are sociologist Pan Suiming (1992 & 1999), who is published widely in Chinese, and Elaine Jeffreys (1997 & 2004), who recently completed research on prostitution and police surveillance.[30]

To avoid reifying the state, I follow the lead of several ethnographers who focus on state actors and institutions that are far from unitary (Gupta 1995; M. Yang 1994; Zhang Li 2001). To comprehend the role of the state ethnographically means analyzing what Akhil Gupta (1995) calls "the everyday practices of bureaucracies" and the discursive construction of the state in public culture (375). He dissects the state by focusing on different bureaucracies without supposing an overall coherence or unity. My analysis is not what Gupta (1995) terms an "ethnography of the state," although it does focus on the complex relationships between state actors, public health institutions, policies, and everyday practices among the people who deal with HIV in southern Yunnan. It is difficult to separate the state from other kinds of institutions and practices, as the state does stand in for a certain kind of governance in late-socialist societies. Here I tackle the often conflicting and messy state decision-making processes attendant to ideas and policies regarding HIV/AIDS prevention.

I draw on Foucault's concept of governmentality as the "conduct of conduct." As Mitchell Dean so aptly summarizes, "the emergence of modern governmentality is identified by a regime of government that takes as its object, [first,]the population, and is coincident to the emergence of political economy, . . . and only second, its particular relationship to sovereignty and discipline" (Dean 1999: 11, 99). Discipline here is linked to biopolitics, as it is concerned with how to rationalize problems facing human beings constituted as a population, as in the organization of health, sanitation, birth rates, and race and sexuality (Foucault 1997: 73). Foucault's notions of governmentality—and by extension, biopower—are particularly useful for moving beyond the dichotomy between state and society, because in controlling and succoring an epidemic, social institutions and informal networks function within regimes of power that shape individual people's thoughts and practices. One cannot possibly study the technologies of power without also understanding the rationales that precede them (see also Petryna 2002; Kohrman 2005).

New forms of biopower technology have emerged with the regulation of bodies and diseases in the postreform era. Here I locate HIV/AIDS not only in macro-institutions but also in the interstices of biopower over local township, provincial, and national everyday practices. Foucault's concept of biopower emerges in his first volume of *The History of Sexuality* (1980) and can be defined as a matrix of relations that "brought life and its mechanisms into the realm of explicit calculations and made knowledge-power an agent in the transformation of human life" (1991: 143). Foucault resists a singular causality; rather, he pushes for an analytic of power that links technology, human beings, and their modern political and social relations. Biopower is extremely elastic in its own theoretical force as a tool for understanding power as based neither in a hierarchical sovereignty nor within particular institutions, but within the interstices, webs, networks, cracks between these grand institutions that many political scientists, economists, and I dare say, anthropologists explore. Although several have contended that Foucault ignores the role of the state in exacting biological power, in China, as Kohrman (2005) has pointed out, it is impossible to ignore its institution.

Building on previous work on the state in China, I argue that even the Chinese state is not a monolithic political entity; rather it is a multifaceted system composed of individuals whose agendas reflect the personal goals and desires of both themselves and the institutions where they work (Anagnost 1985 & 1997; Litzinger 2000a & 2000b; Zhang Li 2001).[31] While neoliberal theorists predicted that the role of the state would retreat under democratic reforms, it has done precisely the opposite; it is still present and productive.[32] Socialist governmentality is about not only control and surveillance but also resistance; it espouses local conduct and leaves space for what I call sidestepping the state.

How does the state become a social subject in the everyday life of epidemics? As Begoña Aretxaga (2003) suggests, the question of desire as well as fear becomes crucial in rethinking the kind of reality the state might be acquiring at this moment of globalization (395). Through the category of governmentality, I unfold just what is at work in the postreform socialist state and how this dynamic directs the emergence of a worldwide pandemic in the interstices of its own multiple epidemics. Understanding the epidemic in these terms means focusing on local actors and their subjectivity—party cadres who are also ethnic minority members—and exploring how the migrant population poses new challenges to the Chinese state, in particular the Ministries of Public Security and Health. The workings of a translocal institution, the Yunnan Provincial Department of Public Health, can be made visible in localized practices through their joint projects with the Australian Red Cross to develop peer education programs as a strategy for prevention among Yunnanese youth. In my interviews with state officials working on and researching the HIV/AIDS epidemic, I was struck by how strongly personal goals and desires influenced policy decisions by Chinese officials and employees of international nongovernmental organizations (NGOs). In working through the notion of governmentality, I illustrate just how the Chinese socialist state, often viewed as a monolithic category, needs to be disaggregated into everyday dynamic practice in order to fathom the logic of disease control. And I show how agents of the state in different geographic locales wed diseases to geography.

My concerns about disease and governmentality are fundamentally related to questions of the role of consumer culture in the postreform era, the cultural politics of epidemics, and what I term the processes by which an infectious disease becomes a major public health crisis. The physician-anthropologist Paul Farmer (1992) notes in his study of Haiti that HIV/AIDS appears most prevalent in areas of great poverty and despair. Poverty forced rural Haitians, held in the vice of economic hardship, to emigrate to other parts of Haiti and to other countries in search of work. Farmer argues that the Haitian epidemic is integrally bound to the United States government's development strategies in the region and thus to global economic development. I argue that it would be a mistake to view the spread of HIV/AIDS in China as simply a product of postreform economies, development, tourism, and global politics. Just the opposite may in fact be true. Closely linked to this notion of governmentality and epidemics is also the position of ethnicity and ethnic relations in the postreform era.

ETHNICITY AND EPIDEMICS

Under Mao Zedong, race *(minzu)* was understood as synonymous with class, and racial minorities in China were counted predominantly in relationship to poverty. In contemporary China this notion of race is still prevalent, but it is intersected by other conceptions of race and ethnicity. Several scholars' work on race in modern China attests to the fact that racial preferences are not just an aberration of Anglo-Saxon culture (Harrell 1991; Dikötter 1992; Diamond 1995; McKhann 1995; Mueggler 2001). These scholars used their research in the postreform era to highlight the deeply engaged relationships between the Han and the non-Han. Race in the Middle Kingdom not only was a highly contested category but was also subject to *internal colonialism*.[33] Several scholars (Goodman 1983; Schein 1997; Gladney 2002) have utilized the idea of internal colonialism, an extension of Edward Said's (1978) notion of the unequal power relations between a colonial metropole and its colony, to look internally at a country's own peripheral groups, be they the Uighur minority in Xinjiang or the Tai minority in Yunnan.

Since the late 1980s, anthropologists studying China have become increasingly concerned with cultural analyses of the market economy under late socialism and how it is socially constructed through and across time, space, place, gender, and ethnicity (Gladney 1991; Honig 1992; S. White 1993; Harrell 1995; Hansen 1999; Litzinger 2000a; Schein 2000; Mueggler 2001; Du 2002). Drawing on Ann Stoler's work (1989, 1995, & 1998) on colonial Southeast Asia, I argue that one must understand the confluences of governmentality and its attention to organizing, controlling, and succoring populations as they are simultaneously sexualized, racialized, and I emphasize, ethnicized. Rather than treating these as distinctive analytic categories, Stoler in her work on colonial Indonesia tackles the subtleties of the category of race in terms of colonial classifications—white (the colonizer) and black (the colonized)—in relationship to ethnicity and sexuality.

The key here is that the categories themselves are unstable. In modifying Stoler's analysis, I apply it to Han and non-Han ethnic groups within China. Although Stoler (1998) critiques Michel Foucault's almost exclusive focus on the nineteenth-century habit of reducing desire to something sexual, in contrast to the Freudian habit of projecting the sexual onto everything, she agrees that the practice of empire building and its attendant construction of a racial Other, influenced the discourse of sexuality in nineteenth-century Europe (28–30). The European sexual discourse was read against the rest of the world, which was understood as apart from European sensibility.

Moving away from the European colonial contexts to another Manichean division, one finds that in parts of China, defining oneself as a proper Han requires defining oneself against an uncivilized racialized other. In an extension of Stoler's thinking, it stands to reason that Han China would perceive non-Han China as a repository of pleasure, a China that is as highly sexed as it is raced. Both the Chinese state and its citizens are key players in producing and reproducing the discourses about the borderlands *(bianjiang)* with alternative ethnicities and sexualities. The state and social relationships are crucial in understanding the emerging epidemic because all prevention projects in China are filtered and regulated through layers of government ministries that are ultimately peopled by individuals with often contradictory personal and political agendas.

Across the globe much of the recent scholarship in English on sexuality and HIV/AIDS discusses why the responsibility for the transmission of the HIV virus is often squarely placed on the backs of disenfranchised others such as drug addicts and prostitutes. During the 1980s in the United States, HIV/AIDS was portrayed in the popular press as a disease of the "four H's": hemophiliacs, homosexuals, heroin addicts, and Haitians (Farmer 1992). In China, by contrast, HIV/AIDS transmission was not identified with or divided into categories of transmission: sexual, intravenous, and medical (this includes needle sticks, blood transfusions, and unsterilized medical equipment). However, by the 1990s these three modes of transmission became mapped onto the cultural disease geography of China. In China's borderlands, the public health bureaucracy began first to address the epidemic and then to blame the minority inhabitants for its spread.

In two particularly cogent studies of ethnicity, Ralph Litzinger (2000a) and Louisa Schein (2000) move away from what Liisa Malkki (1995) calls the "anthropology of sedentarism." Because anthropologists in China traditionally studied remote peoples in remote areas of the world, they often referred to people and places as if they were codetermined. It was Litzinger who pointed out that the notion of "remote" has a double significance in the Chinese imagination. It signifies geographic remoteness, the romance of the rural, and the landscape of mystical mountain peaks and colorful non-Han peoples. Inherent in this representation is also the moral construction of the stigmatized margin, the vulgar contours of backwardness, of hill tribes—in Litzinger's study, the Yao minority—and of poverty. Litzinger (2000a) focuses on how this moral framework is shaped by history as it is told by multiple actors, whereas Schein's research (2000) shows that the Miao, the fifth largest ethnic group in China, have worked to define themselves as agents in modernity, while also being cast as quaint backward rural minorities. These two studies take scholarship on ethnicity in China in new directions. As Schein (2000) says, "China's identity has to be continually crafted out of heterogeneity and . . . cultural others have played a variety of parts in this productive endeavor." She asks, "How is it that the

political systems of post socialism create, foster and organize difference" (3)? "Difference" in this case points in several directions.

Here I highlight ethnic difference because it has become a crucial
trope in the ways that HIV has been imagined in contemporary Sipsongpanna. However, a simple Han/non-Han binary is not the only division at work. Not only economic class and occupation mark ethnicity
in Sipsongpanna, but ethnic groups are also spatially divided in terms of
the lands they inhabit. While spacial division and ethnicity are discussed
in chapter 3, I want to briefly point out here that the Tai minority control the lowland wet-rice fields, the Bulang minority the middle hillsides,
the Akha the mountaintops, and the Han Chinese the townships of
Mengla, Menghai, and Jinghong. The poorest villages in Sipsongpanna
are often the minority groups that represent the smallest proportion of
the population: the Jinuo, Yao, and Wa.

By focusing on ethnic boundaries in Yunnan, I argue that ethnicity is
directly shaped by the history of Sipsongpanna as a suzerain state. This
colonizing history affects the ways public health bureaucrats aimed to
rid China of HIV/AIDS.[34] As Foucault (1980) reminds us, "We must account for the subject within a historical framework" (117). The Chinese
postreform state mirrors earlier nationalist projects to organize minority peoples in order for them to internalize governmental mechanisms of
control. Here this means defining "normal" versus "abnormal" sexual
acts (see Canguilhem 1991). This regime of control is not dissimilar to
Mao's earlier civilizing projects and the remaking of sexuality under reform, and brings us back to Patton's distinctions (2002) of "good" versus "bad" citizens (see also Cheng Sealing 2005).

In this context, HIV prevention strategies are never easy. An edifice of
state controlling practices and regulations accompanies persons placed
in these risk categories. HIV/AIDS epidemiological surveillance has been
carried out since 1995 with twice-a-year sentinel screening among the
following political targeted groups: STD patients, drug users, truck drivers, and pregnant women (UNAIDS 2002: 12). What this means is that
AIDS became more about keeping the disease contained in contaminated
bodies than about preventing the spread among healthy bodies. For example, several AIDS activists and social scientists have warned that the
containment strategy meant that many people who were also at risk did
not see themselves as such. Several heterosexual friends and acquain-
tances of mine in China believed that since AIDS was a disease of homosexual men in Europe and America and of drug addicts in China, they
had no need to worry about ever getting infected. What this leads to is

the problem of fighting an imagined disease with imaginary figures, precisely because the question of who gets tested and who is marked as a carrier has everything to do with how someone is politically labeled or geographically located, rather than how someone behaves.

Development projects in contemporary China lead to the creation of particular kinds of subjects, ones that emerge out of the chaos of the postreform era (Greenhalgh 1994 & 2005; Kohrman 2005). In understanding Chinese ethnic subjectivity, a key ideological trope reappears around HIV/AIDS and its connection to the geographic divide between center and periphery. What is unacceptable in the center, which lies in Han China, suddenly becomes pleasurable on the periphery, in non-Han China. For example, prostitution has become ubiquitous behavior for rural Han migrant women living in large metropolitan cities, but when introduced by Han migrants into rural Tai China, it becomes the locus of disease and moral decay. The reversal sharpens the association between the taboo and the pleasurable. In bringing to light the locus of disease and now sexual pleasures, I return to the notion of the imagined other side, a society free of disease and full of pleasure. Current efforts are under way by the Ministry of Health in cooperation with local and international NGOs to both control the current epidemic and reduce China's incidence rate of new cases to a level more in line with a country like Thailand. Thailand, which still has the highest prevalence in Asia, has been able to reduce its incidence rate through cooperation between active local NGOs, the government, and Buddhists who have focused on behaviors to curb transmission (Celantano et al. 1996a & 1996b). Part of this process of thinking about an imagined other side is how the imagination works to shape the course of an epidemic. I argue that it is not enough, for example, to analyze the political economy of HIV, as one must understand that it is also very much a disease of moral and geographic imaginations.

EPIDEMICS AND THE IMAGINATION

Here I want to highlight the imagination as a concept rarely addressed in discussions of epidemics (see Biehl 2005). In postmodernity we live in a plurality of imagined worlds where ordinary people deploy their imaginations in the practice of day-to-day living. Social theorists from Karl Marx to Max Weber have written about the disenchantment of modernity, in which commoditization stifles our creative imaginations and we become dupes of a grand coercive civilizing process. However, the imagination can be liberating. New consumption acts coupled with changes in the political economy can lead to new forms of agency through resistance, selective consumption, and ironic play. In the ways that the image, the imagined, and the imaginary actually influence global cultural processes, the imagination is a social practice par excellence.

The relationship between the imagination and fantasy is particularly pertinent to Sipsongpanna, as the region is seen as a paradise variously imagined by the people who live, work, and travel there. Fantasies are intentions that are not materialized in action. By fantasizing, we escape from our work lives into our imaginations (Tuan 1998). In fantasy we create nations, communities, and moral economies, including ways to receive higher wages and better working conditions. The imagination provides not only an escape from reality but also a way to re-create that reality in our own image. This is precisely the paradox I want to address in presenting Sipsongpanna as a land where imaginations run wild and at the same time are grounded in a new vision for the postreform multiethnic Chinese state.

The way the tourism industry in Sipsongpanna works to extol the exotic has everything do with the ways images of place are nurtured by social relations stretching across borders through the imagination. Borrowing from Benedict Anderson's (1992) notion of the imagined community and Cornelius Castoriadis' (1987) work on the social imaginary, I make a case that China's border region constitutes a terrain for an *imagined social community* of minority cultures for the sojourners, tourists, and immigrants who increasingly dominate the region's economy (see also Hansen and Stepputat 2001). In turn, these individuals map imaginings back onto Sipsongpanna and, in the process of seeking tourist vacations or jobs, reimagine the region through stories and tales transmitted back home.

Referring to an epidemic as "imagined" can easily be construed as creating either a misnomer or an outright deceit. How could an epidemic be linked to the imagination? When I use the term " imagination," I refer to several things at once. First, I refer to the way stories about HIV in southern Yunnan have an impact on the representation and material circumstances of the disease. In moving from Anderson's (1992) idea of the imagined community to anthropologist Lisa Rofel's (1999) idea of "imagined spaces"—in which people come together to create fantasies through re-creating their personal stories—one comes to understand the complexities of the sign of ethnicity in Sipsongpanna. In many ways, due to new media technologies, we now live simultaneously in the local and in several imagined communities. It is this imagined community that links my multiple field sites, that connects the Tai-Lüe with HIV/AIDS, and that repositions ideas about sexual transmission across time and space.[35]

Exploring Sipsongpanna as an imagined social community, or as an imagined space per Rofel, allows us to move away from the error of sedentarism and links the worlds of public health and disease prevention. If Sipsongpanna is created and re-created through the dialectical relationship between the people who imagine it (through tourism and tourist brochures) and the people who create the tourist experience, including Han entrepreneurs and Tai villagers, the imagination of HIV/AIDS also links these various peoples, places, and practices. When a male physician from Peking Union Medical College conducted one of the first public health surveys on HIV in Yunnan in Jinghong, Beijing imagined Tai actors as the site of HIV-diseased persons. However, alongside the HIV/AIDS imagination lies what I call the *Han imagination*. The Han imagination juxtaposes beautiful, rural Sipsongpanna as a tourist fantasy against another association, that of Tai-Lüe women working in the HIV/AIDS-ridden Thai sex industry and bringing an influx of disease back into China (see Tu Qiao 2000).[36]

The dominant Han imagination is a set of predispositions and ideas about ethnic groups in Yunnan. It is not just prejudice that leads the Han Chinese in the medical, HIV/AIDS, and research communities to target the Tai-Lüe as vectors for spreading infectious diseases in China, but also the difficulty of imagining ethnic relations in a remote part of China. The Chinese state officially recognizes fifty-five minority groups, but they are not all recognized equally—definitely not in Sipsongpanna. The minority project *(minzu shibie)* in the 1950s was based on the desire of the Communists to document and classify the remaining 8 percent of the Chinese population, as 92 percent of China was Han.[37]

Anthropologist Cai Hua (2001) noted in his work among the Na: "The permanent committee of the popular National Assembly of China conducted research, between 1956 and 1963, into all of the ethnic minorities in Yunnan to create an historical survey folded into a monograph on each" (25). The definition of a minority was based on Stalin's four common criteria for a nationality: territory, language, economy, and psychological nature (Fei 1980; Harrell 1995: 22–24). The Tai are an interesting case for exploring this Han imagination, because the positioning of the Tai within a local ethnic hierarchy means they are simultaneously vilified as carriers of disease and emulated and admired as the most beau-

tiful people in all of China. Many Han and non-Han informants reiterated that the Tai are the most beautiful people in Asia. This Han imagination evidences that ethnicity is just one of the intrinsic characteristics
of how a culture is perceived by its dominant Other. But of course even
these categories are unstable and change over time. Historically, the Han
imagine the Tai for the purposes of developing and capitalizing on the
agriculturally fertile and mineral-rich region near Laos and Burma.

ORGANIZATION OF THE BOOK

In illuminating the technicalities of disease prevention and their links to
individual practice, I demonstrate how the scientific-technical and personal narratives influence and play off one another in a dialectical fashion. Because my research was split between two distinct kinds of fieldwork narratives—those from a collectivity of government officials and
public health NGO workers, and those from individual residents in the
town of Jinghong—I divide the book into two distinct parts. Part I concerns official state narratives of HIV/AIDS. Part II focuses on my fieldwork in the town of Jinghong.

Part I: Narratives of the State

Chapter 1 focuses on early epidemiology and the Chinese state's capac-
ity to map the epidemic at a particular place and time and among particular peoples. I examine the first HIV/AIDS knowledge, attitude, practice, and behavior (KABP) survey, conducted in southern Yunnan's
Menglian Tai-Lahu-Wa Nationality Autonomous County, which borders Burma. The survey is significant in involving the intersection of several factors: the late-socialist Chinese state and the rising hybrid NGOs,
international survey techniques, and the aesthetics of statistical practice.
Statistics often take on a life of their own; they become part of a public
health aesthetic that relies heavily on the production of numbers and on
surveillance, both literal and figurative, of bodies. The processes associated with giving certain kinds of legitimacy to the nation-state—and by
extension, increasingly to international NGOs—has to do with recent
transnational social and scientific practices of studying and examining
smaller and smaller categories of bodies. Why was this border region a
focus for HIV/AIDS with so few reported cases? And how did the penetration of a global pandemic into China provoke representatives of the
state to survey minority autonomous counties on Yunnan's borders with
Laos and Burma, rather than other areas with higher concentrations of
HIV?

Chapter 2 focuses on the practices and subjectivities of state actors who worked in the borderlands of Yunnan Province in the early years of the epidemic (1995–2000), the years prior to the 2001 official acknowledgment that China even had an epidemic. These are actors, Communist Party members or not, who first began to police, control, and prevent the spread of HIV/AIDS from the minority borderlands into the Han interior. I first discuss the value of focusing on the concept of borderlands for understanding the intricacies of disease prevention as a goal of the Chinese state. Second, I present a brief history of the question of sovereignty in Sipsongpanna. Third, the chapter portrays four individuals who work in different locations—Beijing, Kunming, Jinghong, and Menglian—in the Ministries of Health and Public Security. It concludes with a discussion of the utility of linking borders, diseases, and the subjectivity of state actors for understanding contemporary HIV/AIDS.

Part II: Narratives of Jinghong

Chapter 3 begins Part II and shifts my focus to the small town of Jinghong, Sipsongpanna. I explore what everyday AIDS practices look like on the ground through the story of development in Jinghong. The chapter provides a sketch of the discursive links between the rise of occupations on the periphery and the emergence of sexual practices as markers of Chinese modernity and urbanity, practices that are mitigated, contested, and controlled by the state.[38] How is sex tourism imagined, proposed, assembled, and incorporated into the modern Chinese state? In Jinghong I observed how Han prostitutes construct and fulfill fantasies of the exotic Tai for Han male tourists, and how one male client observes them in return.

Chapter 4 continues the theme of prostitution by moving closer to addressing my question: why do prostitutes constitute a key focus within narrative and statistical accounts of how HIV/AIDS is spread? Currently, very little is known about sex workers' daily interactions with customers, with other business owners in Jinghong, or with the Chinese state. Although representatives of the state in Jinghong know little about the everyday lives of prostitutes and their intimate sexual practices, there is much speculation and policing of the prostitution industry due to fears about HIV.

Chapter 4 builds an ethnographic understanding of sex workers in Jinghong by focusing on the daily interactions between the women and men who worked and played in the "New Wind Hair Salon." The chapter captures the liveliness of everyday life beyond the organizational hi-erarchies in the health department and beyond the meanings of epithets such as "prostitute" *(jinü)* and "sex worker" *(xing gongzuozhe).*

Chapter 5 takes up the question of prevention and argues that when the power of the state and the power of the market compete, they col-lectively work toward opening the door for a potentially potent weapon against sexually transmitted infections and HIV/AIDS, the condom. First, to understand why prostitutes and their clients want to buy con-doms on the market, rather than receive them free of charge from the state, I open with a brief discussion of the local market. Second, to un-derstand how the state ethos of birth control changes with regard to the different locations of Chinese citizens, I turn to public health history in China and the discourse on the representations of prostitutes and their risk for HIV/AIDS. The third section of the chapter analyzes the chang-ing relationships between, on one hand, the state birth control ethos that promoted the IUD (intrauterine device), sterilization, and the rise of disease prevention and, on the other, the modern marketing of condoms. I argue that the market allows individuals to sidestep the state family planning apparatus and purchase birth control on the free market rather than in state-sanctioned hospitals and clinics.

Chapter 6, which concludes Part II, focuses on my interviews with or-dinary citizens in Jinghong. The stories of four key informants simulta-neously challenge and embrace the notion of their Sipsongpanna home-land as a place of disease and desire. I examine the connections between new-identity formation and behavioral changes, demonstrating that it is not only economic development but also a whole new way of think-ing about leisure activities that form a "new" modern Chinese sexual identity and morality that promote sex tourism. I describe the moral economy of sexuality in postreform China and build an argument for four different moral economies as ways of thinking about sexuality: the liberal market, the parochial Maoist, the Han nationalist, and the ethnic revivalist. I argue that the development project that cultural and sex tourism represents is often driven by the metamorphosis of Confu-cian and Maoist moral categories into particularly new sexual moral economies.

I conclude the book with a short epilogue bringing readers up-to-date, from summer 2002 to fall 2005, by laying out some of the current struggles and projects concerning HIV/AIDS in Yunnan in the ever evolving epidemiological, political, and cultural landscape. In the end, through the voices of my informants, I relay some suggestions about what should be done to prevent the further spread of this devastating disease.

AIZIBING AND RICE METAPHORS

With every new disease comes new terminology that allows it to be classified, labeled, and deciphered both within technical scientific worlds and among general publics that are affected by the disease. In mainland China the term for HIV/AIDS was first translated in the mid-1980s as the "love breeds sickness" (using the character for love *ai*); however, that term connoted that HIV/AIDS came from love. Later the characters were changed to a simple transliteration using the character for the Chinese medicinal herb mugwort, *ai,* to make it apparent that the three characters were not connected in meaning but were merely a translation of a foreign word. Some activists in East Asia have advocated translating AIDS as *aizhibing,* using the character for knowledge, *zhi,* in combination with the original term of love, yielding "love-knowledge-illness," thus suggesting that through knowledge and love we can overcome this disease.

Another term critical to this study, and serving as the book's title, is the popular saying used in late 1990s China that references young women and their choice of occupation: *chi qingchun fan,* or "eating spring rice." The phrase is a play on the socialist-era metaphor of having iron rice bowls *(tie fanwan),* which meant that the Chinese people would always have enough to eat, as their rice bowls would never break. The saying *qingchunfan,* "youth rice bowl" or what I have translated as "eating spring rice," plays on the earlier saying, implying that youth rice bowls do not last forever, and as girls' youth fades, they can no longer live off their youthful beauty.[39] Under late socialism, the saying expresses how young women are living off their youthful appearance and sex appeal—in this case, as female sex workers. Rice metaphors abound in discussing sexuality and modernity in China. At one of the many hair salons that were fronts for brothels, one of my informants teased me by asking, "How can you know China without tasting Chinese men?" According to her, in Sipsongpanna men taste like sticky rice *(nuomifan)*; in Thailand, where she worked briefly, they tasted like pineapple rice *(boluofan)*; and in her hometown of Guizhou, they just tasted like plain white rice *(bai fan).*

To reiterate, while AIDS signifies diseased bodies, here the study of Chinese AIDS unfurls a taut canvas painted with fetishes of late modernity: sexuality, desire, and nonwhite, non-Han bodies. This book offers a way to showcase what is unique about Chinese AIDS, but links it back to everywhere on the globe. In understanding the anthropology of epidemics by focusing on everyday AIDS practices, one captures people, institutions, and processes in order to arrive at a more nuanced and contoured analytic of a disease in motion.

PART ONE

Narratives of the State

CHAPTER 1

The Aesthetics of Statistics

One afternoon when the southern rains collected in the overgrown potholes along *Shida Lu,* I sat in Professor Guo's office translating into Chinese Mark Twain's famous quote "There are lies, damn lies and statistics."[1] Guo, a scientist by training, responded, "How can statistics lie—they are truths unto themselves?"

"TRUTHS UNTO THEMSELVES"

This chapter makes sense of the production of statistics through examining the first HIV/AIDS knowledge, attitude, practice, and behavior (KABP) survey conducted in southern Yunnan's Menglian Tai-Lahu-Wa Autonomous County, which borders Burma. The significance of this survey involves the intersection of several factors: the late-socialist Chinese state and the rise of hybrid nongovernmental organizations (NGOs), new forms of socialist governmentality, international survey techniques, and the aesthetics of statistical practice, as well as the personal (Hacking 1990; Mitchell 2002; Kohrman 2005).[2] I locate the Chinese HIV/AIDS epidemic within global standards of scientific discourse and illustrate what happens when a survey confronts social prejudice. I argue that the early stages of the Chinese HIV/AIDS epidemic and the pursuit of survey data express an "aesthetics of statistics" (Good 1995 & 2001).[3] Statistics take on a life of their own; they become part of a public health aesthetic that relies heavily on the production of numbers and on the surveillance, both literal and figurative, of bodies. As Timothy Mitchell (2002) has pointed out, the processes associated with giving certain kinds of legitimacy to the nation-state and, increasingly by extension, international NGOs, has to do with recent transnational social and scientific practices of studying and examining smaller and smaller categories of bodies. Why was this border region a focus for HIV/AIDS when it had so few reported cases? And how did the penetration of a global pandemic into China provoke representatives of the state to survey minority autonomous counties on Yunnan's borders with Burma rather than other areas with higher concentrations of HIV?

Statistics allow governments to expand their moral and material authority over their citizens (Hacking 1990). Nation-states have a fetish for numbers. Nevertheless, it is not just statistics that should concern anthropologists but also the actual processes, the subject-making of statisticians, and the microprocesses of statistical inquiry that allow us to understand the links between state regulation and statistics (see Anderson 1992; Gupta 1995; Mitchell 2002; Kohrman 2005). Georges Canguilhem (1991) argues that the normal and the pathological are not simply determined by statistical and scientific analysis; rather these concepts are steeped in political, economic, and technological imperatives. It is the processes of making scientific knowledge that are inextricably linked to the forms of power those processes legitimate and create solutions for (Petryna 2002: 10).

I begin the chapter with a discussion of how science travels to underdeveloped peripheries, then I outline some of the official Chinese narratives of HIV/AIDS, and finally I trace the movements and the ideas generated by a team of medical and public health researchers who in December 1995 conducted the first large-scale rural HIV/AIDS survey in Yunnan. The processes involved in the collection of survey data unfold a narrative of how the actual survey became the fulcrum for the dialectical relationship between the Chinese state's role in disease containment and the NGO's policies of disease prevention, reflecting once again Patton's (2002) two divergent thought styles about reservoirs of infection—tropical thinking (containing the epidemic in a place) and epidemiological thinking (containing the epidemic in specific high-risk bodies). In addition, at each stage of conducting the survey, power and ideological struggles emerge over the correct or truthful way to represent minorities, women, migrant workers, and youth in this remote border area.[4]

Rather than merely embracing Twain's cautionary note, I wish to point out how statistics in their making produce certain discourses that reveal a cascading web of ideas, alliances, convergences, and conflicts around their production. They ultimately become objects that reveal new kinds of state medical and public health interventions, or new forms of governmentality (Foucault 1991; Dean 1999). I use the term "governmentality" here as representing the exercise of the Chinese late-socialist state as articulated in the regulation of its citizens through medical, social, and political processes. Foucault alerts us to the limitations inherent in linking any subject's agency too closely to intentionality (Dean 1999). James Ferguson (1996) points out, however, that most development projects have unintended consequences, linked to the perpetuation and articulation of particular forms of power. The production of statistics by public health workers themselves reveals political agendas in these border regions that may be secondary to their original intentions.

Although I write this chapter as an analytical observer, I was also part of the survey team during the early stages of training and data collection in the four sites discussed here. Therefore, like many medical anthropologists who study development NGOs, I was producing public health data that I planned to analyze as an anthropologist (Clifford and Marcus 1986; Marcus and Fischer 1986). Given the nature of multisited ethnographic writing and the place of anthropologists who study scientific processes as not-so-distant observers, reporting of these observations presents a challenge for both authenticity and subjectivity. Whose subjectivity and whose authenticity are being written about?

"SCIENCE" TRAVELS TO UNDERDEVELOPED PERIPHERIES

Following the epidemiologists, public health projects are created to prevent the spread of HIV; these projects become sites where local, national, and global practices are articulated and disarticulated in particular geographies (see Packard and Epstein 1991; Malkki 1995; Porter 1997; Pigg 2001; Sassen 2002). Analogous to the early British cartographers in Africa, medical colonialism serves to map and name diseases as the first means of conquering them in the name of science (Fabian 2000). The process of mapping and naming creates internal social groups and reproduces certain spatial and power relations. Foreign NGOs thus become party to a form of medical neocolonialism as they work within a participatory development framework through joint projects between them and their Chinese government counterparts (see Pandolfi 2003). With the survey, representatives of NGOs (the Australian Red Cross) and local Chinese government officials (the provincial Yunnan Red Cross), like their nineteenth-century European counterparts, mapped bodies in newly emerging epidemics. Only this time, instead of malaria, sleeping sickness, and tuberculosis in native populations, they were mapping and surveying practices that might lead to HIV infection in specific minority groups—the Lahu, Wa, and Tai (see Arnold 1993; Porter 1997; L. Cohen 1998).

In the mid-1990s Chinese public health officials in Kunming, the provincial capital of Yunnan Province, reported that heterosexual transmission of HIV was on the increase in China's southern minority border regions, particularly the Dehong-Tai area in western Yunnan. Because the Dehong-Tai prefecture had high rates of HIV, there were speculations that other regions with a Tai minority would also have high rates of HIV. A cultural link was presumed. Therefore, both Sipsongpanna-Tai Autonomous Prefecture and Menglian Tai-Lahu-Wa Autonomous County in Simao were targets for preliminary research and interventions for HIV/AIDS. Yunnan's public health practitioners accounted for new HIV infections by pointing to changing sexual behavior, increased heroin use, and the medical use of unsterilized syringes, but other factors remained veiled (Wang N. 1991; V. Li et al. 1992; Sun Xinhua, Nan, and Guo 1994; Cheng Hehe et al. 1996; Cheng Hehe, Zhang, Pan, Jia, et al. 2000).

Although the Chinese epidemic may be transmitted and experienced by local bodies, many Chinese view HIV/AIDS as not only a foreign disease but also a "barbaric" one. As I noted in the introduction, the notion of the disease as "barbarian" has to do with the way that HIV/AIDS first appeared in the minority prefectures along the Burmese and Laotian borders, in the heart of the Golden Triangle. The idea of blaming Others for dangerous infectious diseases is well documented the world over (Sabatier 1988; Farmer 1992). In the case of China, some Chinese public health officials presented such strong prejudices against people with HIV that in May 1999, Chengdu city in Sichuan Province enacted a law that prohibited anyone who tested positive for HIV from applying for a marriage license (96 percent of the adult population in China marries (see Di Ya 1989 in Kohrman 2005: 177). A group of deputies is currently lobbying the People's National Congress in Beijing to make it a lifetime criminal offense for a prostitute to transmit HIV/AIDS, while their male customers will face sentences of seven to fifteen years (*Yunnan Ribao* 2004). In Jinghong city in late 1996, Dr. Zhuang, one of the chief internists working at the Jinghong Tai hospital, told me that she spent several afternoons convincing the few locals with HIV that due to their confirmed positive status, they could not possibly date, let alone marry.[5] Dr. Zhuang's rationale was that HIV is a deadly disease and no amount of education would change behavior. Her perceptions had as much to do with the limited resources available for HIV/AIDS medical education as it did with the local geography, prejudice, and fear of infectious diseases.[6]

Although 80 percent of China's HIV/AIDS cases were detected in Yunnan Province in the early 1990s, by the mid-1990s the epidemic democratized into all of China's thirty provinces, municipalities, and autonomous regions (Zheng Xiwan 1993; Cheng Hehe et al. 1996). By the Third International Conference on HIV/AIDS in Asia and the Pacific in Chiang-Mai, Thailand, in September 1995, reports circulated that a seroprevalence survey of the Chinese blood supply revealed that not one province, municipality, or autonomous region was free of HIV (Cheng Hehe et al. 1996; Liao et al. 1997).

Historians note that Yunnan has a long history of tropical diseases, such as cerebral malaria, leprosy, and now HIV/AIDS, that have been attributed to remote barbarian regions and to barbarian peoples (see Armijo-Hussein 1997; Benedict 1996; Hsieh 1995; Yin 1986). Historian Jacqueline Armijo-Hussein (1996) points out that rural Yunnan is unique in that it has for centuries represented to Han China a place of exoticism and promiscuity, the land of exotic minority women who have unusual sexual practices (see also Chow 1987; Gladney 1994; Harrell 1995; Schein 2000). In the early 1830s, American Protestant missionaries considered Xishuangbanna ripe for Christian proselytizing because it was full of heathens engaged in superstitious folk practices, perpetuating unhealthy habits and sin (Dodd 1923). Contemporary physicians working in the area suggest that while HIV/AIDS receives maximum global attention and resources, the rise in other infectious diseases—namely cerebral malaria, tuberculosis, and hepatitis B—is almost ignored.[7]

This process of exoticization lives on in public health and the resurgence in Christian missionary activity in Yunnan (see Hyde 2001). The story of missionary activity in Yunnan would be the subject for an entire book. I concentrate here on the links between proselytizing, the arrival of public health NGOs, and their impact on local practice. Contemporary missionaries in Jinghong note that Protestant missionaries from the United States came to Sipsongpanna in the 1920s and 1930s, both to proselytize and to provide medical care for those with leprosy. The mission houses and church were built of river stones from the Lancang and are still standing in the city of Jinghong. The mission school itself was actually converted into a school of Mao Zedong Thought during the Cultural Revolution (1966–76), and faint lines of paint still show traces of former Maoist slogans. The degree of success of these historical missions varies according to whom one talks to. Several Tai informants told me that only one village withstood the test of time and still considered itself Christian in 2000. However, those Christians were stigmatized by other Tai village leaders and were forced to move their village from near Ganlanba to the present site further south.[8]

The return of missionary activity beginning in the early 1990s suggests that Yunnan Province is still viewed as the land of barbarians who need converting into good Christians and good public health citizens. With increasing economic and religious ties to greater Southeast Asia—Burma, Thailand, and Laos in particular—and to indigenous groups that defy national boundaries, Yunnan is within China but not *of* China.[9] Here several anxieties converge: stigma about barbarians and pathologies, the rise of HIV/AIDS, gender as expressed through minority women, nationalism and colonialism, the leitmotifs that link nineteenth- and twenty-first-century health practices, and finally, globalization and transnationalism in the form of global HIV/AIDS discourses and the international NGOs that deliver them.

GUARDING THE BORDERS AGAINST GLOBAL PANDEMICS

Shortly after the first case of HIV/AIDS in Kunming was reported in 1985, the Ministry of Health in Beijing set up a working group for the prevention of HIV/AIDS. By 1995 the State Council established a Co-ordinating Conference for the Prevention and Treatment of Sexually Transmitted Diseases and HIV/AIDS and provided special funding for three regional centers in Guangdong, Jiangsu, and Yunnan. Dr. Li was appointed the head of this government HIV/AIDS center in Yunnan, as he was instrumental in its establishment.[10] I met Dr. Li at a Red Cross meeting in 1996 that had been called to discuss the Yunnan provincial disease control plan. That year the Yunnan provincial government was to invest close to 500 million yuan (roughly 60 million U.S. dollars) to build a disease-prevention zone along its border and, in the following four years, to set up an elaborate border HIV/AIDS control surveillance network (*China Daily,* April 1996).

The notion of the border is complicated here because, for a regional HIV/AIDS center based in Kunming, border patrols would be adequate to determine who came into China and who did not. The local notions of a border are much more porous because, in the South Asian tropical climate of southern Yunnan, migrants from several countries, particularly Burma and Laos, come in and out of China without proper documentation or visas on a daily basis. While I was conducting fieldwork in Jinghong, on several occasions boat owners offered me rides to Thailand down the Lancang River (the local name for the Mekong), hidden and disguised in the hull of their boats—no visas or passports required. As of 2005 any foreign citizen applying for Chinese residency permits for longer than six months was screened and tested for HIV, and those found positive would either have their permits reduced or revoked (Zhang Min, Li, and Zhang 2005).

The goals of the HIV/AIDS prevention directive in 1996 was to tighten security and health controls along the Yunnanese border, to erect multiple new guard posts, and to test people coming back and forth across the border for a variety of infectious diseases, including HIV/AIDS. Another local health official told me: "The biggest problem in the Sipsongpanna is its freedom, its openness. What we need to do is secure our borders." I questioned him: "If HIV/AIDS knows no borders, and the locals know where to cross in the jungle, trying to place an iron-clad HIV/AIDS prevention belt around Yunnan just doesn't make sense epidemiologically." Again he repeated, "As a public health measure, we need this disease prevention belt around the province." I asked, "What about the sex industry in places like Jinghong? What about putting HIV/AIDS prevention announcements on all the flights, and free condoms in hotel rooms?" He replied, "That would be impossible." As a final point, I question why an epidemiologist would treat HIV/AIDS as a problem for the border police rather than one of behavioral practice.

Yunnan had a population of 44,152,000 in 2003, including twenty-five of China's fifty-five officially recognized ethnic minority groups (Yunnan Provincial Bureau of Statistics 2005a). The Greater Mekong Subregional (GMS) development area—comprising Cambodia, the Lao People's Democratic Republic (Lao PDR), Myanmar, Thailand, Vietnam, and southern Yunnan Province—became critical for understanding the traveling vectors for HIV/AIDS, in what was often reduced to the "Golden Quadrangle," leaving out Vietnam and Cambodia. With development and globalization have come unequal levels of development and wealth, and large-scale migrations of peoples, goods, and services, and epidemics across geographic borders.[11] In the early 1990s, in contrast to the coastal cities of Shanghai and Xiamen, landlocked Yunnan, in the far southwest, was not targeted as a special economic zone or as an area deserving special attention for foreign investment and economic development. In 1994 foreign investment trickled into China from twenty-four countries and regions, yet Yunnan remained one of China's poorest regions. Seventy-three of Yunnan's 127 counties are designated as poor, and 75 percent of the seven million people living below the poverty line are members of ethnic minorities.

Ultimately, in the mid-1990s, representatives of the Yunnan provincial health department maintained an ongoing discourse of the border. Although this will be discussed in more depth in chapter 2, here I point out that this discourse led toward deconstructing just what constituted the center and the periphery, and that it became tangled in the ways by which the definition of the border served different ideological, social, or political purposes, depending on different subjects' positions (see Berdahl 1999; Lindquist 2005). China's borders are defined by military and political strategists in Beijing, and Yunnan's official border, while reflecting the political boundaries set by Beijing, also reflects a more sociological understanding of who uses these borders and for what purpose.

China must also constantly strive to reinscribe its borders, especially as its border regions are semiautonomous political entities, the majority of whose citizens have allegiances to other neighboring states and people. For example, the Tai-Lüe ethnic group in Sipsongpanna can also be found in three other nation-states: Burma, Thailand, and Laos. When seeking funding for rebuilding Buddhist temples torn down during the Cultural Revolution, for the revival of local Buddhist religious practices, the Tai-Lüe in Sipsongpanna see themselves as very much a part of greater Southeast Asia.[12] The Chinese state, then, must constantly seek relegitimation in these semiautonomous governing regions because they also receive political and economic support from Thailand and Burma. The rapid changes brought about in the late 1990s in Yunnan have meant that several new anxieties emerge at the edges of these provincial borderlands. Borders evoke images of lawlessness and imply the permeability of both diseases and the state. Through public health surveys the Chinese state continues to intervene in everyday village life, maintaining and controlling a healthy body politic and overcoming the permeability of these borders. I argue that state intervention actually goes hand in hand with public health methods: to count bodies scientifically is also about control and surveillance (Foucault 1991, Hacking 1986). However, counting bodily behavior, or rather what people actually say about their behavior, presents only a partial view of an individual's history.[13]

Although international NGOs describe HIV/AIDS as "knowing no borders," the provincial health departments locate the epicenter of the epidemic on the borders in Dehong, Simao, and Xishuangbanna, in the remote prefectures and counties of Yunnan Province. This is where HIV/AIDS is attributed to the global high-risk categories of injection drug users *(xiduzhe)* and prostitutes *(jinü)*. Understanding this story of AIDS requires that we actually first understand the official state epidemiological narratives on HIV/AIDS. In this endeavor, it appears that instead of writing a critique of statistical narratives, I am fetishizing them. This close reading of the official epidemiology is important, however, as it provides a launching point into just where and when the Chinese government began to take up HIV/AIDS as a major threat to the health of its citizens.

THE "OFFICIAL" EPIDEMIOLOGY OF HIV/AIDS IN CHINA

In the early 1990s, China was beginning to look like other countries in Southeast Asia—like Thailand, where the earliest Asian HIV/AIDS epidemic was attributed to the rise in injection drug use and prostitution (Cheng Hehe et al. 1996). By April 2000 Liu Baoying reported in the *Renmin Ribao* (the *People's Daily*—the central government newspaper) that the incidence of HIV in China had increased by 20 to 30 percent over each previous year (Liu Baoying 2001). By 2003 China ranked second to India among Asian nations and fourteenth in the world in the number of HIV-infected people (UNAIDS 2004).

According to Dr. Zhang Konglai (2001) of Peking Union Medical College's Epidemiology Department, China's HIV/AIDS epidemic has gone through four distinct phases. The first phase is marked by the first index case, an Argentinian tourist from the United States who died in a Beijing hospital on June 6, 1985, and continues through 1988 with only sporadic cases of HIV. The second phase, from 1989 to 1993, centers on four counties in Yunnan province. The third phase, 1994–2000, marks the arrival of HIV/AIDS in every province, municipality, and autonomous region, with registered cases of both HIV-positive persons and full-blown cases of AIDS. The fourth phase begins in August 2001, when the central government estimated that between 600,000 and 800,000 people were infected with HIV and that 6 percent of them were infected with AIDS through blood transfusions (see figure 1).

China first began its national HIV/AIDS surveillance program in 1984, and by the end of 1994 had selectively screened and tested more than five million people, reporting 1,173 HIV-positive people and sixty-five people with full-blown HIV/AIDS.[14] At that time, injection drug

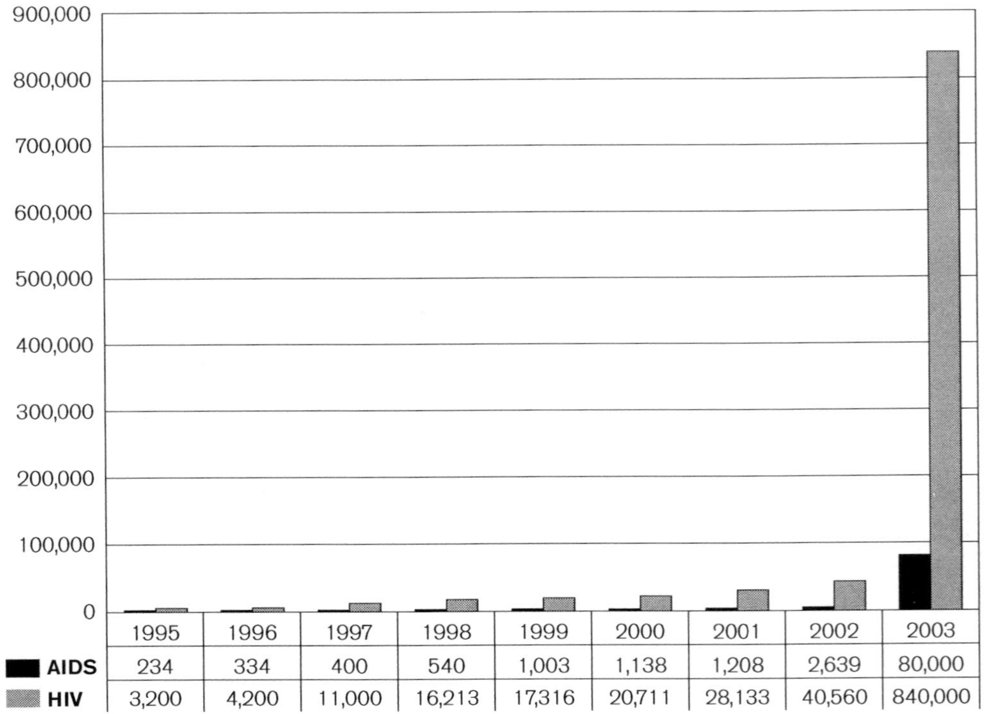

	1995	1996	1997	1998	1999	2000	2001	2002	2003
AIDS	234	334	400	540	1,003	1,138	1,208	2,639	80,000
HIV	3,200	4,200	11,000	16,213	17,316	20,711	28,133	40,560	840,000

Figure 1. Annual Reported Cases of HIV/AIDS in China, 1995–2003. (Data from Chinese Ministry of Health AIDS Office)

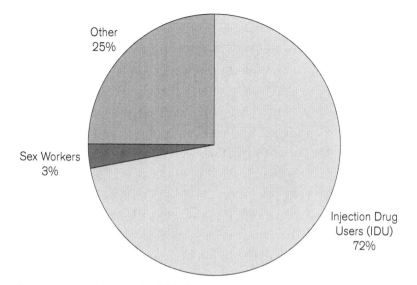

Figure 2. HIV Infections by Risk Group, 2002. (Data from Chinese Ministry of Health)

users from Yunnan Province made up 78 percent of the total number of people with HIV (Zheng Xiaoyun and Yu 1995), as compared to 2004, when they made up 41 percent (UNAIDS December 2004). By global comparison, in September 2000, China was considered a low-prevalence country with respect to HIV. However, Zhang warned, if HIV was not addressed in widespread prevention campaigns, China could have upwards of ten million cases by 2010 (Liu Xin 2000; Zhang Konglai 2001).[15]

In 2002, injection drug users (IDUs) made up 72 percent of reported infections, and "sex workers" 3 percent (UNAIDS 2002; see figure 2). However, by the end of 2004, the numbers again were beginning to look completely different, with IDUs reduced to 45 percent of all infections (see figure 3). It is necessary here to deconstruct the referents to these particular categories. The debate around the appropriateness of using risk behaviors versus risky groups of people dates to the beginning of the epidemic. Many western AIDS activists in North America and Europe have criticized the reliance on the idea of risky people, precisely because of the stigma attached to AIDS-related infections and also because of its presumption that if you are not one of these risk groups, you have nothing to worry about (Watney 1994; Altman 2001; Patton 2002). The idea of targeting or lumping together a wide range of occupations asso-

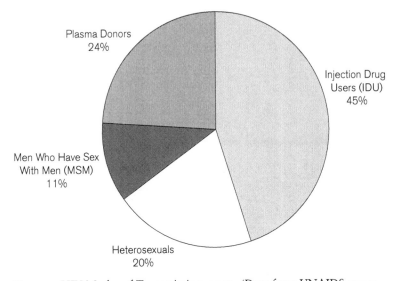

Figure 3. HIV Modes of Transmission, 2003. (Data from UNAIDS 2004; Kaufman 2005)

ciated with what is labeled "sex work" creates much confusion over just who is at risk. But more to my point, these categories are important for my argument as to how HIV/AIDS in the early stages in China was understood as a disease of political categories. According to Chinese sexologist Pan Suiming (2000), other factors that contribute to an increase in local epidemics include the large migration of people from the countryside into the cities *(liudong renkou)*, the increase in the number of men who have sex with men (MSM), the widespread use of blood and blood products for illness treatment, inadequate screening of blood in medical settings, and mother-to-child transmission. The inadequate screening for HIV/AIDS was just the tip of the iceberg.[16]

As an NGO China AIDS Survey cited, "Gao Qiang, the Executive Minister of Health, while addressing the HIV/AIDS high-level meeting of the UN General Assembly on September 22, 2003, reported that China has 840,000 people living with HIV, and 80,000 with AIDS symptoms," with an overall prevalence rate of around 0.1 percent (Settle 2003: 2; *Wuhan Ribao* 2004). This dramatic increase in just one year was attributed to new surveillance techniques carried out jointly by the Ministry of Health (MOH) and the World Health Organization (WHO), so that by early 2004 the Chinese Centers for Disease Control and Prevention reissued the figures. Unofficial estimates from several sources, including

UNAIDS and WHO, suggest that more accurate rates remained closer to 1.5 million to 2 million. Many claim there has been drastic underreporting of HIV/AIDS nationally. The difference between the official and unofficial estimates results from partial and incomplete reporting in rural and remote areas, widespread fear of HIV/AIDS and the stigmatization often associated with an HIV diagnosis, the expense of confirmation tests, and the relative inaccessibility or unavailability of antiretroviral drug therapies (see Dechamp and Couzin 2004). As in many countries across the globe, from central Beijing to the Yunnan periphery, bureaucratic action at the local level is often stymied and mired in politics, geography, and notions of blame (Sabatier 1988).

Despite the actual low prevalence (less than 1 percent), Dr. Zeng Yi of the Chinese Academy of Sciences stunned a Beijing conference audience in January 2002 by stating that China could soon have one of the highest number of HIV/AIDS infections in the world. According to the Chinese Academy of Preventive Medicine, HIV/AIDS would grow to six million by 2005, from the estimate of 840,000 in 2003 (Settle 2003). Still, these statistics were contradicted in other official reports. Dr. Shen Jie, the deputy director in the Division of AIDS and STIs in the Ministry of Health, speaking at a Beijing HIV/AIDS conference in January 2001, estimated that over one million people were probably already infected with HIV in one province due to illegal blood banks; but the rate of six million has not been confirmed. Others have reported that HIV has unduly affected ethnic minorities, representing 9 percent of the overall population of China and almost 75 percent of the people with AIDS-related symptoms (Kaufman and Jing 2002). Rural Han residents of eastern-central China who were commercial blood donors and were increasingly being infected with HIV were ignored, and in turn, there was a singular focus on the four counties in Yunnan that happened to have large percentages of minority populations. This meant that in early surveillance efforts, there was a preference for testing the non-Han minority population, or rather testing for minorities only.

Currently, some counties, such as Liangshan in Sichuan, have high rates of infection in minority areas that are attributed to injection drug use, while other counties that are predominately Han, such as Shangcai county in Henan, have high rates of infections due to illegal blood pooling. The illegal commercial blood banks, believing they were preventing anemia and fortifying the donors to repeatedly give blood, thus securing their market, were spinning down the plasma and returning the intermediary cells to the donor. The key route to infection was that inter-

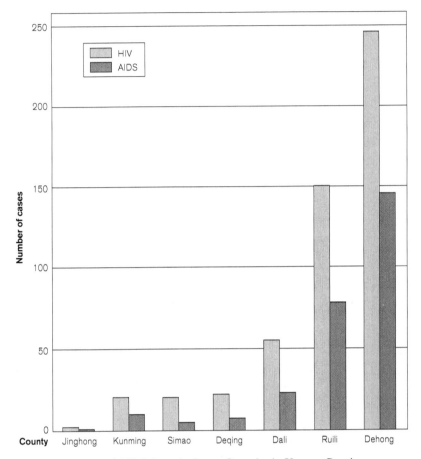

Figure 4. HIV+ and AIDS Cases in Seven Counties in Yunnan Province, 1997. (Data from Yunnan Provincial Anti-Epidemic Station)

mediary cells were not put back into the person donating them, but rather were distributed to several people with the same blood type—a practice called blood pooling. This meant that if one donor had HIV, then all donors of the same blood type, and later their wives and often children, became HIV-positive. Experts estimate that through blood pooling, over one million Henanese villagers may have HIV, a number that compares with the entire rates for the rest of China combined. In Wenlou village in Shangcai County, over 60 percent of the population is HIV positive (Settle 2003: 3).

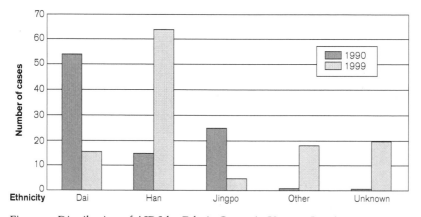

Figure 5. Distribution of AIDS by Ethnic Group in Yunnan Province, 1990 and 1999. (Data from Yunnan Provincial Anti-Epidemic Station)

Although Yunnan no longer has higher rates among minority populations than among the Han, in the epidemic's early days the figures presented the opposite because of the surveillance activity in minority areas and the fact that these were the early epicenters (UNAIDS 2002; see figures 4 and 5). Currently, epidemiologists note that China has not one but several epidemics that occur simultaneously, including the large epidemics in central China, due to the illegal blood bank activity in the early to mid-1990s.

By August 2000 the *Renmin Ribao (People's Daily)* reported that while it took five to six years for Yunnan Province to accumulate 70 percent of its HIV infections, due to injection drug use, in Xinjiang Province (in northwestern China) it took only two to three years to reach a similar rate of infection. The epicenters in 2004 for the epidemic were concentrated in Yunnan, Xinjiang, Sichuan (just north of Yunnan), and Henan (in south central China) provinces and coastal enclaves in Guangdong, Fujian, and Hebei provinces. After compiling three years of surveillance data, researchers at the National HIV/AIDS Prevention and Control Center in Beijing identified eight subtypes of HIV-1 virus in China—A, B, B1, C, D, E, F, and G (Beyrer et al. 2000).[17] In terms of my argument, this means that the Chinese HIV/AIDS epidemic is truly an example of the globalization of infectious diseases. China not only has distinct subtypes of HIV but also has absorbed subtypes from neighboring countries in Southeast Asia, including B, Thai B, C strains, and circulating recombinant strains of C and B (Yu Xiaofang et al. 2003;

Yang Rongge et al. 2002; Beyrer et al. 2000).[18] According to Beyrer and colleagues (2000), by 2000 four outbreaks of HIV-1 among injecting drug users appeared to follow drug trafficking routes through South and Southeast Asia: from Burma's eastern border to Yunnan, subtype B and then C; then going north and west to Xinjiang Province with B, C, and a recombinant B-C; then from Burma and Laos through Vietnam into Guangxi Province, subtype E; and finally, Western Burma across the Indian border to Manipur with C, B, and E. These recent strains demonstrate that the Chinese AIDS epidemic is truly an example of how a global pandemic has penetrated greater China (Beyrer et al. 2000).

As this AIDS epidemic began to democratize beyond Yunnan, it was discovered that in Henan Province in central China, entire villages had infection rates close to 60 percent due to unsanitary practices at illegal blood collection centers (UNAIDS 2002).[19] From 1992 to 1996, the majority of these blood banks targeted poor peasants, the victims of China's economic reforms, by giving them money in exchange for selling their blood and plasma.[20] It was a big business. According to Dr. Gao Yaojie, the winner of the 2001 Jonathan Mann Award for her work among AIDS orphans in Henan, covert studies give the rural villages of Henan some of the highest local rates of HIV infection in the world (Rosenthal 2000). By September 2003, HIV infections from former commercial blood and plasma donation centers were reported in all provinces, autonomous regions, and municipalities, with the exception of Tibet. While the overall national average prevalence rate was 2.7 percent, there were wide variations in these rural villages in Henan (UNAIDS December 2004: 6).[21] All of these illegal blood banks have been closed, and many officials jailed and fined for putting so many peoples' lives at risk. Obtaining blood is still a problem in China because of beliefs about the body and about the strength of blood, and because there are relatively few legal blood collection centers in rural areas.

In sum, the border region is marked traditionally through epidemiological surveillance methods, historically as a minority region, economically by the drug trade, and politically by recent concerns about infectious diseases jumping borders and penetrating China. In addition, a number of new actors are actively pursuing AIDS surveillance and prevention, namely the Chinese government health departments and local, national, and international NGOs. In Yunnan in the mid-1990s—the early days of the epidemic—economic liberalization combined with a rise in HIV opened the floodgates for international and national NGOs to enter China as registered organizations to work on AIDS prevention. The

World Health Organization (WHO) initially came to China in 1988 at the request of the People's Republic of China (PRC) government to assess the epidemiological surveillance for AIDS, assist in the development of sentinel surveillance systems, and assess assistance for prevention and control programs. At that time, the data confirmed an extremely low prevalence for HIV but also a rapidly growing epidemic (R. Chen 1988). In building my argument concerning stigma and anxieties about borders and border populations, I turn now to public health NGOs.

SOCIALIST GOVERNMENTALITY AND PUBLIC HEALTH NGOS

With the changes brought on by the introduction of a socialist market economy in the late 1980s, foreign NGOs benefited and initially operated as hybrid institutions of the Chinese state—they were neither entirely independent nor entirely subject to state regulation. The Chinese government, in conjunction with international public health NGOs (such as the International Red Cross, Save the Children Foundation, and Médicins Sans Frontières), conducted the first epidemiological HIV behavioral surveys in Yunnan. In 1993, at their Regional Congress in Beijing, the Red Cross/Red Crescent Societies committed themselves to addressing the regional HIV/AIDS epidemic in accordance with their mandate to provide health and humanitarian aid in Southeast Asia, and an Asian task force was established. During this congress, the China Red Cross made a public statement about its commitment to develop responses to AIDS, and by April 1994 the Australian Red Cross contacted its China counterpart to discuss the situation.

In November 1994 the first delegate from the Australian Red Cross, an international NGO, arrived in the provincial capital of Kunming to assist Chinese public health workers with the first steps in combating their own HIV/AIDS epidemic. Yunnan was selected as the most appropriate place to begin because it had the highest numbers of people who were HIV-positive in the mid-1990s (Armijo-Hussein and Beesey 1996: 3). After discussions between the Australian Red Cross (ARC), the Yunnan Red Cross (YRC), and the AIDS Office in Yunnan, it was decided that the first phase of the HIV/AIDS prevention project would be a knowledge, attitude, behavior, and practice (KABP) survey, as it was considered part of the standard global HIV/AIDS armamentarium.[22]

According to health education logic, in order to develop health prevention policies and programs, HIV/AIDS prevention strategies first require mapping the kinds of risky behaviors in a given population. Al-

though any of the seventeen counties in Yunnan would have sufficed for
a large-scale survey, the border minority regions were given top priority,
thus illustrating what I call the provincial government's focus on as-
signing geographic blame. The ARC was interested in carrying out the
rural section of a comparative HIV/AIDS knowledge survey in Ruili, in
Dehong Prefecture, the county with the highest rate of HIV; however,
permission was not granted.[23] Nor was it granted in Jinghong, the prefecture capital of Sipsongpanna, a place suspected of a growing prostitution and sex tourism industry. The methodology that ARC personnel
used to mark the locations for possible survey sites became equally
problematic. Since many counties in Yunnan did not want to be associated with HIV/AIDS for fear of being stigmatized and losing local revenue, selecting survey sites was a politically sensitive issue. While the
ARC provided financial backing and survey tools, the Yunnan Red
Cross selected the Menglian site as a third alternative rural survey site
on the grounds that it was a border town where the vice-director of the
anti-epidemic station and the police were eager to conduct such a survey. Menglian is located in the far southwestern corner of Yunnan, close
to Burma's northern border and the former territory of Burmese drug
lord Khun Sa (Armijo-Hussein and Beesey 1998).

In designing health education programs to prevent HIV/AIDS, public
health researchers seek to understand what their target audience already
knows about HIV. It is common practice in international public health
research to use a standard KABP survey and interview tool. A KABP
survey captures on paper what people think they know, or what they
report they do; however, KABP surveys often end up regurgitating an
endless list of possible, probable, and also actual behaviors. After these
surveys are completed, what will be done then? In the process of conducting surveys, health workers are reduced to public health archaeolo-
gists whose microstructural concerns sacrifice political-economic and
cultural factors to the goal of identifying risk behaviors in the "at-risk"
population. Producing an HIV/AIDS behavioral survey meant that so-
ciocultural and political-economic nuances were often dismissed, and, I
argue, sometimes misrepresented, in favor of epidemiological statistical
accounts that presented HIV/AIDS as certain: one either knew about
HIV or one did not, one either practiced prevention or did not, and one
was either a prostitute or not, an injection user or not. If behavioral
change is the goal, in the context of deadly sexually transmitted diseases, surveys may take us astray, or even lead us under rose-trellised ar-
bors to avoid getting pricked by the thorns. To complicate my skepti-

cism, I have myself engaged in and encouraged public health surveys in China, including this one.

Looking for HIV/AIDS in this part of China was similar to playing hide-and-seek—as if the disease were in motion, eluding researchers. I am speaking here of a discursive materiality: the survey actually grounded the local discourse on HIV/AIDS. I am by no means suggesting that HIV/AIDS did not exist; rather, I am pointing to two different orders of analysis, the discursive and the material, and the chasm between the discursive linking of HIV/AIDS and border bodies, on one hand, and the materiality of these same persons' bodily practices, on the other. Although the survey was completed and its attempts at quantification were used to address these matters, it yielded data that in effect were unreliable and noncomparative. In other words, both Mark Twain's "damn lies" and the actual dimensions of an epidemic are hard to assess.

WHY MENGLIAN WAS IDEAL FOR A KABP SURVEY

According to Cheng Hehe, one of the leading infectious disease epidemiologists in Yunnan, the early cases of HIV were detected in Dehong Tai-Jingpo Minority Prefecture, along the Burma border. In 1989, almost 70 percent of all HIV/AIDS cases in Yunnan were detected among persons living in Dehong-Tai (Cheng Hehe et al. 1996). In cumulative data from 1989 through 1993, 56 percent of HIV-positive persons were Tai, 24 percent Jingpo (Kachin), and 17 percent Han. However, by 1995, when I began my research, 30 percent of the HIV-positives were among the Tai, and over 50 percent were among the Han, with another 5 percent attributed to the Jingpo minority. In 1995, Dehong Prefecture and the city of Ruili had 73 percent of the cases in Yunnan, or 92 persons who were infected with HIV, compared to Simao County (the county Menglian is governed by), which had only two people who were HIV-positive (Cheng Hehe et al. 1996). From 1986 through 1993, 147,330 persons were tested for HIV-1 in Yunnan Province, with 977 positive results, or less than 1 percent. There were also a few cases reported outside of Dehong Prefecture, where nineteen HIV-positive persons were identified in the capital city of Kunming and another fifteen persons in Simao County, which includes Menglian prefecture.[24]

While the Anti-Epidemic Station in Kunming began collecting data as early as 1985, statisticians report that reliable data were collected only from 1989 forward. In early surveillance reports, categories of persons at risk for HIV were prioritized in a hierarchy beginning with drug users *(xiduzhe)* and proceeding to spouses of drug users *(peiou xiduzhe)*, persons with blood and blood-related illnesses *(xue you binghuanzhe)*, persons crossing the border *(chuguo jiuguo renyuan)*, sexually transmitted disease patients *(xing chuanran binghuanzhe)*, overseas Chinese *(haiwai huaren)*, and finally, foreigners *(waiguoren)* (Zhang Wenjian 2000; Holder 1995). These categories parallel earlier risk categories and prejudice used in the United States in the early 1980s: the four H's that marked risky individuals—homosexuals, heroin addicts, hemophiliacs, and Haitians (Farmer, Connors, and Simmons 1996). In many ways, the American category of Haitian mirrors the Chinese categories of persons crossing the border, overseas Chinese, and foreigners. As Farmer, Connors, and Simmons point out, these categories of people were targeted because of stigma attached to alleged practices rather than their actual behavior. Similarly, a woman crossing the border into Thailand was presumed to be working as a prostitute.

A 1996 report on HIV surveillance in Yunnan noted that ten HIV-positive women worked as "sex workers": one in Kunming, another in Simao, and the other eight in Thailand or Burma (Cheng Hehe et al. 1996). Another category marked as high-risk included nine women who returned from working in Thailand and tested positive for HIV. These women were presumed to be sex workers; however, as Dr. Cheng and colleagues note, "Although some women in the study are categorized as prostitutes, they may not have been involved in sex work before leaving China, and may not continue to exchange sex for money when they return." The report revealed no direct correlation between working in Thailand and ethnic status. Dr. Cheng stated, "Although commercial sex work in Yunnan was limited, it was crucial that researchers examined whether the same behavioral and social conditions that had contributed to widespread transmission of HIV in Thailand were also present in Yunnan."[25] In addition, the actual figures for the number of women working in Thailand are dubious at best, due to the temporary nature of the work of many women sex workers. If few persons, let alone sex workers or the Tai, Lahu, or Wa minority, were linked to HIV/AIDS in Menglian, why the focus on Menglian in the first place? Before moving forward into an ethnographic analysis of the survey logistics, I summarize what has been established thus far: Yunnan was selected for a KAPB survey because of high prevalence rates. Menglian was selected because of its border nature and the fact that public health officials there were both eager and willing to conduct such a survey. And women crossing the border into Thailand were considered one of the most suspect and vulnerable groups to be studied.

PRODUCING THE SURVEY

In December 1995 I joined a team of twelve representatives from the Yunnan Red Cross, the Kunming City Anti-Drug Institute, Kunming Medical College, the Provincial Anti-Epidemic Station, the Women's Cadre Training School, and the Australian Red Cross; we interviewed 387 residents in nine villages, in the town nighttime market, and the county drug prison.[26] These local residents were from four ethnic groups: the Tai, Lahu, Wa, and Han. Our purpose was to conduct the first-ever large informal survey of people's attitudes toward, beliefs about, and behaviors around HIV/AIDS in Menglian and, based on this information, to establish health policy guidelines for prevention. The first draft of the survey contained over seventy questions that addressed basic demographic information, knowledge and attitudes about HIV/AIDS and other sexually transmitted infections, and attitudes about sexual behavior. Another three small sections were gender specific and highly judgmental. Women who were suspected of engaging in sex work were asked detailed questions about their sexual partners, and men who might have frequented brothels were asked specific questions about their partners, as well; finally, drug users interviewed at a drug treatment center were interrogated about injection drug behaviors.

Approximately thirty-five people were to be interviewed in each village, and another hundred at the Menglian drug rehabilitation center and the town night market. As this project would reach across four ethnic groups and four different language groups, interpreters were selected by the local anti-epidemic station using the following criteria: equal numbers of men and women, and two from each minority group. The result was seven local interpreters, two Lahu, two Wa, and three Tai. Initially, there was some controversy about whether people could be interviewed at the local drug center in light of the expectation that the local public security bureau would not approve a survey on HIV/AIDS-related topics, certainly not one conducted by foreigners. In the event, the public security bureau was more than complicit in conducting the survey, because it too was concerned about the rapid transmission of HIV/AIDS. The survey, when interpreted, demonstrates the cascading layers of international, national, local, and police and medical positions on HIV/AIDS prevention in China.

The research survey began with a flight to Simao, the county seat, where Mr. Guo, the Hani mayor of Simao,[27] met the members of the team for dinner. A jovial man, rotund and full of the local rice liquor (*baijiu*), Guo kept repeating, as he chain smoked and the smile lines on his face moved in waves: "Your research is very secretive and sensitive; you must be careful and cautious in what you do and say . . . but your biggest obstacle will be getting people to use condoms." This was said directly to me, since I was acting as an additional interpreter for the representative of the ARC, Mark Bester, who did not speak Mandarin. At lunch the next day we met with the deputy magistrate, a Lahu Red Cross worker, and a man from the anti-epidemic station in Lancang, the second largest city in Simao County, to discuss the survey. Madam Wu (the designated leader and the deputy secretary of the Yunnan Red Cross), who had recently returned from an "exposure" trip to Thailand,[28] had a very specific goal in mind: to prevent a Thailand-like epidemic in Yunnan. As the highest-ranking official in our group, she greased the wheels for entry permits and permissions and attempted to alleviate the fears of local officials. At this she was extremely effective.

This was not the ARC's first trip to Menglian. Shen, the vice-director at the local anti-epidemic station, a freckled-faced woman with boundless energy, was desperately trying to get the Kunming Provincial Health Bureau to pay attention to her county's needs, as she had invited the ARC to Menglian as early as the summer of 1995. A brave and audacious woman, Shen had recently been criticized for permitting a Beijing-based television production team to videotape people with HIV/AIDS in Simao County. The governor was upset and, as Shen explained, wanted, like many others, to believe that HIV/AIDS comes from somewhere else, not from Menglian. Prior to our arrival in Menglian, there were rumors of a rise in HIV/AIDS cases, especially among Tai minority women who were crossing the border to work in the Thai sex industry.[29] Shen had recently returned from a visit to a village where a mother (a former Thai prostitute) and her one-year-old child were HIV-positive. She considered the scope of her work to include alerting people to the dangers of transmission in an area where few dared to venture. Again, I wondered about the accuracy of the seroprevalence data, as the actual numbers on the incidence rates of HIV/AIDS in Simao County and Menglian were sketchy at best.

Menglian is not a tourist town, and little health education information, if any, was available about this strange new deadly disease. Shen wanted to invite the three young women who tested positive for HIV to attend the "HIV/AIDS 101 training" as anonymous participants.[30] They all declined, as it was risky to be exposed publicly due to the local stigma attached to an HIV diagnosis in an area where few even knew HIV existed. Shen welcomed us warmly and worked hard; the days began sharply at eight in the morning and often finished well past midnight.

Menglian County is situated in the southwest of Yunnan Province and borders Lancang County to the east, Ximeng County to the north, and Burma to the west and south.[31] Menglian County town, designated a provincial-level "open port," is an important gateway to Southeast Asia, although mountains blanket much of the county. The county administration governs two townships *(zhen)*—Menglian and Mengma—and five areas equivalent to a township *(xiang)*—Jingxin, Nanya, Fuyan, Gongxin, and Lalei. There are a total of thirty-nine village committees and one Street Office. By the end of 2000, the total population of the county was 123,500, of whom 89,300 (72 percent) were agriculturally based and 34,200 (28 percent) were nonagricultural workers. At that time, six ethnic minority groups accounted for 80 percent of the total population—Lahu (31 percent); Wa (25 percent); Tai (22 percent); and the Hani, Jingpo, and Lishu (less than 3 percent). The remaining 20 percent are Han Chinese (Simao Prefecture Party Committee 2004). Bordering Burma by land and water, Menglian was historically an important port on the ancient "Tea and Horse Trade Route" linking China and Southeast Asia. There are currently two main roads spanning the ninety-eight kilometers between Menglian town and Jindong in northeastern Burma, making these roads among the most convenient land routes from China to Burma, Thailand, and other Central and South Peninsula countries.[32]

Menglian town is a small, dusty, ramshackle town with a population of less than fifty thousand. It has one main paved road, a sports stadium, a theater, and the Communist Party headquarters. Most buildings are one or two stories; the exceptions are the Communist Party headquarters and the one fancy hotel, both of which are four stories tall. The hotel housed a large conference delegation in town to discuss cross-border transportation between Burma and China. The government building houses all government officials, including those from the Anti-Epidemic Station, the Health Department, and the Women's Federation *(fulian)*. The only other large building in town is the primary school. For secondary school, students move to the town of Lancang or Simao, the county seat. Our Red Cross delegation first stayed in the police hostel, a cozy but basic dormitory barracks; after profuse apologies from the

governor, we were moved to the main hotel. The standards there were
hardly what one would expect for a standard, meaning top grade, room
(biaozhun fangjian). Despite the designation, there was no hot water
and often no running water at all. In the town itself were many signs of
trade with Burma and Thailand—colorful batiks (locals use the Burmese
term longyi), Burmese jade, herbal remedies from Burma, packages of
Thai medicine and candy in the small shops. There was a small marketplace in the middle of town where people gathered at night. There were
twenty small video theaters and sixteen bars where karaoke and bar
girls were available. According to the local anti-epidemic station staff,
many of these women, from the adjacent county of Lancang, exchange
money for sexual services. Menglian was a frontier town where street
fistfights were common. I observed two in the space of one day, angry
brawls resulting in bloody faces and noses.[33]

AIDS 101: TRAINING SURVEY WORKERS

At the first meeting of the survey team, Dr. Su, the director from the
Menglian Anti-Epidemic Station, presented two local case profiles of
people with HIV. Though the profiles were presented, no definitive incidence or prevalence rates for HIV/AIDS in Menglian were given, due in
part to the probable lack of significant HIV antibody testing. Test kits, I
was told, were difficult to import and, if available, difficult to process. In
1995 the ELISA and Western blot tests for HIV, the international stan-
dardized tests to document HIV seroprevalence, were often available in
China only in large metropolitan areas. One woman who worked at the
anti-epidemic station explained that the government required refrigerated trucks be supplied to the county, and only then, when completed test
kits could be driven refrigerated to Simao County for processing, would
the station be able to estimate the incidence of HIV. The original plan was
to train local people to conduct the survey; however, after recognizing the
challenges of translating the questions into three or four languages, it was
decided that public health employees from a variety of institutions and
work units in Kunming would instead conduct the survey through local
interpreters when necessary. The ARC then insisted that the local community, especially local interpreters, would participate in a one-day
workshop on the basics about HIV/AIDS, covering everything from the
biology of the virus to prevention and surveillance. The Menglian survey
itself was preceded by this one-day HIV/AIDS training course (known as

"HIV/AIDS 101 training" in the United States), conducted jointly by the ARC and the Yunnan Red Cross (YRC). The topics covered included an explanation of HIV/AIDS, modes of transmission, and condom demonstrations on bananas, and small groups discussed local myths about HIV/AIDS.[34] The training itself revealed the interplay between three very different agendas: the local, regional, and global perspectives on HIV/AIDS prevention. Madam Wu was the secretary general of the YRC, Wu Zhi was from the Menglian County government, and Mark Bester was the project director from ARC's Greater Mekong Regional HIV/AIDS Prevention Project.

The training began with a speech from Madam Wu:[35]

> In China in 1985 the first case of HIV/AIDS was identified in an American tourist, and now there are 2,038 people who are HIV-positive in China. This year alone six hundred people were identified as having the HIV virus. At the Beijing meeting [referring to the first all-China HIV/AIDS conference, in December 1995], they estimated the more likely figures at 50,000 and 100,000 *aizibing ganranzhe* [roughly, "people with HIV/AIDS"]. In comparison to Thailand, where we discovered the first case in 1984, in Menglian the first case was discovered in 1994. We need to learn from the Thai example because we are also developing rapidly. In Thailand there are 800,000 HIV-positive people and 108,000 people with AIDS, including women, children, and teenagers. Right now China needs about 20 million RMB [2.5 million U.S. dollars] to prevent HIV/AIDS . . . the importance is paying attention to prevent China from becoming another Thailand. The problem in China is now extremely important and of grave concern because we have the ability to prevent a future crisis.
>
> In order to deal with this problem and China's economic development, China must pay attention to HIV/AIDS prevention. The HIV/AIDS problem in China includes injection drug users in Dehong and prostitutes everywhere. The most important method to prevent HIV/AIDS is education. [The] most difficult situation is in Africa, and in Yunnan it is a problem of importation *(jinkou de wenti)*.
>
> I hope that everyone can assist in preventing HIV/AIDS; we must especially get leaders to help because the health departments cannot conquer HIV/AIDS alone. I implore leaders to provide assistance and give them thanks in advance for this assistance. Not only is HIV/AIDS related to economic development and health, but also our youth are our country's hope for the future, and therefore preventing HIV/AIDS is extremely serious.
>
> It is important to understand that we are not investigating how many people are ill or carriers in this survey, but trying to understand people's attitudes, beliefs, and practices that may lead them to contract HIV/AIDS. There are problems that arise in dealing with ill people; as for the police, physicians, and government officials who cannot help at this time, we need to find a way to get them involved in dealing with this grave problem.

Wu Chi, a woman and the local county vice-head, said in response to
Madame Lu:

> We must realize this is a problem of the entire country and not put all the
> pressure on one county, but at the same time recognize that this is a prob-
> lem for Menglian County. The problem is even graver outside Menglian
> County. In the seventeen counties in Yunnan, only one, Wenshan, does not
> have a reported case of HIV/AIDS.

Madam Wu then replied:

> It is a necessity to understand that if people can understand materials and
> read, and are not illiterate, that activities can be planned for prevention of
> HIV/AIDS on the radio, TV, and through the print media in Simao County.
> In our survey we don't need people's addresses, phone numbers, or names;
> these won't be printed anywhere. Again I ask for your help and the help
> from the village leaders in carrying out our survey.

Mark Bester, from ARC, added a few words in English that were
translated into Mandarin:

> Our original plans were to train young people here to conduct the survey,
> but we decided to use those youth already trained in survey techniques
> from Kunming. Interpreters will work with HIV/AIDS trainers and will re-
> ceive one day of HIV/AIDS 101 training. . . . In 1996 the education and
> prevention phase of the project will begin. This is a crucial time to work
> in Yunnan to avoid the HIV/AIDS problems of other countries. There
> has been good collaboration and cooperation to prevent HIV/AIDS in
> Menglian and Simao, and these instances provide other counties in Yunnan
> with good examples.

Of these three persons' opening remarks, Madam Wu's represents the
provincial perspective. She understood HIV/AIDS in Yunnan as a problem of importation *(jinkou de wenti)*, as she linked her genealogy of
HIV/AIDS to the first case in the American tourist in 1985, and then
through the internal vectors of injection drug users and prostitutes in
Yunnan's minority prefectures. Of greatest import to her was preventing China from becoming another Thailand. Wu Chi took a more local
position to avoid stigma and to alert the Red Cross that it must realize
HIV/AIDS is a problem for the entire country: the Yunnan Red Cross
could not possibly place all the pressure on Menglian County! She said
the problem of HIV/AIDS was even graver outside Menglian, where out
of Yunnan's seventeen counties, only one, Wenshan, did not have a reported case of HIV/AIDS. Finally, Mark Bester took the Western international aid and scientific perspective. He presented his concerns with

the survey methodology and later stated that the original plans were to train local people in Menglian to conduct their local survey, but that for the purpose of expediency, peer educators from Kunming were employed. Later Mark Bester explained, "This was a problem because scientific survey methods were not being adhered to."

These three vantage points are not independent of one another but are interlocking positions in which international interests directly influenced local practices. Combined, these three positions actually had the effect of stigmatizing local bodies. In Menglian County, the aim was to focus on the minority villages; in Kunming the aim was to deflect the epidemic out of the city, or to target the internal Other; and in Australia the aim was to take the armamentarium of HIV/AIDS prevention and peer education and map it onto China. All three positions point to how the local and global became mired in one another at the site of the survey.

Although the three main voices may seem at odds with one another, they actually interacted in a dialectical tour de force. The vice-director of the Menglian Anti-Epidemic Station began to understand why arresting people and forcing them to get tested was not a prevention method supported by international NGOs. Mark Bester understood that certain notions of statistical accuracy would have to be modified to meet the needs of the local county. And Wu Zhi began to see her county as a stellar example and a leader in HIV/AIDS prevention, rather than just a place stigmatized as the target of an HIV/AIDS survey.

QUESTIONS OF LANGUAGE AND TRANSLATION

Whereas the local staff openly discussed the presence of HIV/AIDS in Menglian, the research team embraced larger concerns with border bodies and why these were identified as the Other. At the beginning of the survey, Dr. Pang, a YRC employee and an epidemiologist by training, asked, "Do minorities live together before marriage?" Yanghu, a Lahu interpreter, laughed and, glancing in the direction of the two foreigners, said, "We Lahu are like you foreigners—we live together before marriage." Dr. Li, a professor of Medicine from Kunming, said that the idea of who lives together, sleeps together, and eats together may be established differently among different minority groups and could pose a problem for data collection.

Bi Wei, the Wa interpreter, suggested there was no equivalent for HIV/AIDS in the Wa language, so what should he call it? Lao Ai, who

spoke both Tai and Lahu, said they didn't have words for sex in Lahu.
A woman interpreter in her early fifties chimed in to say that she
couldn't possibly ask questions about sexuality; they were culturally inappropriate. Many Lahu and Wa respondents knew nothing about the
HIV/AIDS pandemic and thus did not even have the term "HIV/AIDS"
in their lexicon. These are just some of the many examples of how
counting HIV/AIDS bodies in China is mired in problematic assertions
and languages that do not carry well across cultural divides.

If researchers such as Dr. Pang saw HIV/AIDS as located among the
internal Other—the local minority peoples—and if the minority persons
themselves, such as Bi Wei, could not even locate HIV/AIDS within a
common language, what would the survey show? To understand why
the Menglian County survey was important for assessing the knowledge
base of people in the county, one also needs to know how the survey was
conducted. The actual collection of survey data reveals exactly what is
problematic about the collection of these kinds of soft statistics: namely,
that they can be highly subjective, not only in their collection but also in
their interpretation.

In the following pages, I discuss interviews with four different
women who participated in the survey. The story of these interviews dis-
closes how researchers attempt to produce fixed statistics that can be relied on to build future projects for prevention of HIV/AIDS transmission
in the region. Yet instead of providing a neat set of statistical certainties,
the interviews tell a very different tale, one that cannot be tied to identities or fixed places and certainly cannot provide the kind of *avidity of
statistics* that HIV/AIDS researchers rely on.[36] However, Menglian was
not the only center of activity for this survey. There were also the outlying villages and hamlets along the border with Burma, such as the village of Sanya. Once again, there was little to justify the means of intervention when collecting statistics for KABP surveys in these outlying
border regions with few HIV/AIDS index cases: we were dragging almost three hundred peasants out of their fields for the sake of research
on a disease for which they barely even knew the name.

In four settings—Sanya, the hilltop village of Meng Ting, the night
market, and the drug prison—I interviewed a total of ten women.[37] In
the following analysis of interviews with four young women,[38] I aim to
show how the survey tried to quantify and reduce these women's personal profiles to a neatly formulaic statistical profile, one that could then
be easily translated into data for epidemiological processing by using an
American software program called EpiInfo.

THE VILLAGE OF SANYA

The team was introduced to the village of Sanya through several case studies, including the profile of an HIV-positive man whose wife infected him after she returned from working in Thailand. "Working in Thailand" had become a euphemism for engaging in prostitution. When I asked about what efforts were being made to prevent future infection, it became clear that, apart from Shen's visits to the villages, no systematic prevention information was given to anybody, including women returning from Thailand. It was pointed out that the translators should not be acquainted with too many people in the village of Sanya, where they were working as translators.[39] The Australian Red Cross was trying to uphold its own social scientific standards of separating the researchers from their subjects to avoid a kind of selection and answer bias. Shen said that "off-season planting will make it difficult to interview young people during the day; we may have to work at night." Five interviewers would work at one time: four people for each village (two men and two women), with one person remaining in Menglian town. Shen stressed we should approach the village headman for any advice about certain customs and special behaviors to avoid. Women could interview women and, in a bind, men as well, but men should interview only other men. And Dr. Su, the director of the anti-epidemic station, would not be allowed to oversee interviews, as he was wont to do, as this would breach confidentiality.

After walking for about a quarter of a mile to the Tai village of Sanya, on the southern perimeter of Menglian town, to interview Tai youth, we were first invited to the village headman's house. After he received permission from his superiors, he graciously offered us tea, cigarettes, and liquor. When I refused to drink, he insisted that I must return to drink some of their local rice liquor.[40] We then went in search of the village physician who works in the small public health clinic to ask for her assistance in locating the best places to find young people. We were looking for youth in a rather wide age range, from sixteen to forty years old, and since that covered most of the people in the village, with the exception of the elderly and children, it turned out that there was really no need to bother the physician. Her clinic was a small room next to the village's storage rooms; her walls were washed a dull green, the tattered remains of old public health posters still sticking to them.

When women's lives and stories are reduced to the larger global concerns of proposed HIV/AIDS prevention projects, the real challenges and demands of these women's lives are erased. Questions included "Do you know anyone who has had premarital sexual relations?" and "Do you know what a condom is?" And for women and men suspected of engaging in commercial sex, the following questions were asked: "How many sexual partners have you had in the last three months?" "Have you ever used condoms?" "Have you ever had a STD?" Men were questioned, "Do you know anyone who has had sex with prostitutes?" and "Did they use a condom?"

Shen was so enthusiastic that, although we were all exhausted, she wanted the team to continue conducting interviews well past midnight. What emerged from the interviews was that people's knowledge of HIV/AIDS varied greatly: one hotel worker knew how it was transmitted and how to protect herself, whereas a customs worker who knew nothing of either claimed to know everything. However, unlike residents of the villages, most of the participants at the night market did know something about HIV/AIDS. I now turn to interviews in three of the sites—Sanya, the night market in Menglian, and Meng Ting. With these three sites as a backdrop, I profile four young women whom I call Yufang, Li, Xiao An, and Xiao Zhu.

"Yufang," a divorced Tai woman of thirty-five, said she worked independently in Chiang Mai, Thailand, but had not been to Burma. She said she knew a lot about HIV/AIDS and had acquired this knowledge while working in Thailand. She kept repeating "Ni baohu ziji, mei you wenti" (If you take care of yourself, there is no problem). Shen had encouraged her to get tested for HIV, but she had refused. She was also threatened with police arrest if she didn't get tested, but these dire measures had not yet been taken.

Yufang lived with her six-year-old daughter and her mother in the village of Sanya, in a modest two-story Tai house on stilts whose walls were lined with new travel posters from Thailand. She was wearing strings of beautiful twenty-four-karat yellow-gold Thai jewelry. The family lived around a large courtyard with an abundance of green flowering plants and a few scrawny chickens running around. Her mother could speak Mandarin, and Yufang exchanged a few words in central Thai with Mark. Yufang said, "The main reason so many men get HIV/AIDS in Thailand is that they use their mouths and lips (kouzui). To prevent getting HIV/AIDS and to baohu ziji (take care of yourself), you cannot cut your customer's fingernails or their hair, you cannot puncture their skin, nor tattoo their arms, and of course, you cannot not use public swimming pools." Yufang had heard all this in Thailand, not in

Menglian or Sanya. After we discussed how one couldn't get HIV/AIDS from cutting people's hair or fingernails, but only through exchanging bodily fluids, she expressed concern and asked me a litany of questions.

I gave her literature on HIV/AIDS prevention and would also have given her condoms, but Xiao Yu, the investigator from the Kunming Anti-Drug Institute, brought the poorest-quality condoms, a brand from Tianjin.[41] They had a picture of a happy white couple on the box and were four mao each (about five U.S. cents), as compared to higher-quality condoms that cost from two to ten yuan each. Yufang mentioned that condom use was acceptable in Thailand, but that most men in China wouldn't use them. We also had a longer discussion about what to call her work. She said she didn't work for anyone but herself, wasn't an independent businessperson (*getihu*), and couldn't really call herself a professional or a service worker. She worked for herself ("wo dui ziji gongzuo") in the nightclubs in Chiang Mai and Chiang Rai entertaining men. I took her to be a part-time bar hostess, although she did not use the term herself.

Li, also Tai, was thirty-six years old and lived in Sanya with her mother and two small children by her Han husband. Unfortunately, Li said, with a pained expression on her face, her husband was now in Zhejiang Province (near Shanghai) living with another woman. Li commented on the bitter lives of women with no husbands. She said her husband fooled around, but she didn't, and she didn't know very much about sexual disease prevention. She said most women used the coil for birth control and, after giving birth to two children, were sterilized. According to state family planning policies, the coil and sterilization are the only sanctioned methods of birth control, although that is changing with the re-emergence of sexually transmitted diseases and HIV/AIDS. Li said she knew little about HIV/AIDS and certainly did not consider herself at risk. And why were we asking her all these questions? She had spent a short time in Thailand and was suspected of being HIV-positive.

While Yufang is marked in three ways—as a Tai woman, as someone who crossed the border and worked in Thailand, and by her presumed HIV status—Li represented women without husbands whose fate was isolation and infection. Here crossing the border presupposed engaging in prostitution, the political and gendered category compounding the specific ways that the survey marked certain individuals and their alleged practices, recalling Patton's comment about risk categories. Individuals who engaged in prostitution would likely not admit to their illegal activity, but the less forthcoming the women are about their activities, the quicker public health workers jump to their own conclusions. One of the goals of the survey was to determine what ordinary people actually knew, as opposed to what they were supposed to know. Li also substantiated the general perception among the survey team that local women in Menglian knew very little about HIV/AIDS.

THE NIGHT MARKET IN MENGLIAN

Shen was eager to get young people at the night market to participate in the survey; she encouraged them in a polite and persistent manner, suggesting that I had come all the way from "Old Golden Mountain" (*Jiu Jin Shan*, Mandarin for San Francisco) just to interview them. Off the main street, the night market differed from a day market only in that the lighting and many of the activities were different, as most people were there for relaxation and enjoyment rather than to purchase goods for daily use. The youthful crowd was seated in a poorly lit, flat area with tiny narrow benches and low tables. They ate small fried potatoes smothered in hot peppers and barbecued beef cooked Tai-style on long thin wooden sticks, like Thai satay. The low lighting and candles created an ambience suggesting that people did not want to be seen. The night market did not appear very inviting, but it was incredibly easygoing compared to fast-paced Kunming. Shen said this area was where most young people hang out in Menglian at night, flirting in the marketplace and visiting the one movie theater in town. Besides young couples, there were many very drunk young men with red faces and *baijiu* bottles next to their squat tables; many of the habitués looked Burmese rather than Han.

My first interview at the night market was with Xiao An, a young Han woman from Lancang city who was fourteen years old and from a poor family. She couldn't read, so she ended up working at a night stall as the boss's assistant (*xiao gong*). She knew nothing about HIV/AIDS. My second interview was with a twenty-three-year-old woman I call Xiao Zhu who was from the Bulang minority. "I am not married yet," she said, "so I cannot answer any questions about sexual behavior." As a survey worker, I felt I was being asked by the survey's instructors to judge her based on my knowledge and her customs. On the other hand, after engaging in polite conversation, she said that, after all, she knew lots about HIV/AIDS from her boyfriend's mother's his grandmother (*po po*). In fact, she still was not quite clear about how HIV/AIDS is transmitted. She said, "The three ways not to get HIV/AIDS were not to swim in the public swimming pool, not to get a tattoo, and not to share toothbrushes." She greatly assisted me in answering the questions and asked her own questions in return.

Since the goal of the survey was to represent both urban and rural communities in Menglian County, a rural village site was included in the overall survey. This final interview site was a couple of hours drive from the town of Menglian: the hilltop village of Meng Ting.

THE VILLAGE OF MENG TING

Driving into the hills surrounding Menglian town, we went up a long winding dirt road lined with electrical power lines. Small children ran to the side of the road and waved as the jeep drove by. Cows ran through the village of Meng Ting, which surrounded a large man-made fishpond. People were friendly and smiled a lot. Mali, a Red Cross trainer, was to interview a woman who had just tested positive for HIV. My interviews here were conducted with the assistance of Yishui, a Tai interpreter, and we often had to ask the same question several times, first in Mandarin, then Tai, and then again in Mandarin and Tai—a tedious process. To myself, I continually questioned the merits of the survey: Does it exclude people who are not literate? Without pictures as visual aids and condoms for show, are we making any sense?

The houses in the village were built in the traditional Tai style of bamboo on stilts. The village headman's house was the largest, and many people filled its interior. He appeared to be about thirty-five and was surrounded by older men and women. We were invited to a generous lunch at his house after we finished interviewing. During the interviews I noticed men fishing in the pond, and when lunch appeared to consist entirely of fish dishes, I realized they had gone fishing on our account. They refused to accept payment for lunch and said it was their duty to treat guests from the government! The village headman said to us, "Our conditions are poor but our hospitality is bountiful."[42]

I interviewed four women, all in their early twenties. While most didn't know the first thing about HIV, it is difficult to say whether this was a consequence of our translation dance from Mandarin to Tai and back to Mandarin over and over again, or a matter of an actual lack of knowledge. Often Yishui and I interviewed people in front of their houses. One woman who had just had a baby spoke to us from the balcony of her house but still within earshot of her husband. Another woman didn't want to answer questions because she was in the middle of tending her fields. I kept having to remind Dr. Su, the director of the Menglian Anti-Epidemic Station, that we were using scientific research methods (a term I felt he would respect) and that meant he couldn't stand over Xiao Yu's shoulder listening to informant responses. He kept saying it was so interesting, and later I surmised that my adamant rule against eavesdropping may not have been such an important requirement here. After all, I was the one imposing my own public health standards on him.

LOCAL CUSTOMS INTERRUPTED

After the morning interviews, lunch appeared with a flourish: fish soup, fish heads, cow's blood, sticky rice, and lots of alcohol, mainly local *baijiu*. All the men I noticed had tattoos on their lower arms, and when I asked about these, they just said it was a Tai custom. All the women were dressed in traditional Tai clothing—tight-fitting long-sleeve short top and Chinese exercise pants, covered with a a sarong *(longyi)*. The women rolled up their sarongs, exposing their exercise pants when working in the fields and at the afternoon brick-making site. I refused to drink the alcohol that was offered, saying that in the United States lunchtime on a workday was not a time for drinking. In truth, I would have fallen asleep in the boiling noonday sun had I drunk anything stronger than tea. The headman complained that in China things are different and we should all enjoy ourselves. I relented a little and said, of course, they could drink as long as our driver, Dr. Su, stayed sober (another cultural impediment—I had seen too many car crashes on jungle roads); otherwise, I told him, I would walk home! The winding, badly tattered roads were no place to be driving drunk. Mali chimed in her agreement. Dr. Su said it was too far for us to walk; he wouldn't drink. After that, the village headmen referred to me as the boss *(laoban)* and kept teasing me about my antidrinking policy. All the older men in the village came to the lunch, and we had two tables' full of food that the headman's mother and wife served.

The village headman maneuvered easily between four languages— Wa, Lahu, Tai, and Chinese. He discussed several important local customs, saying, for instance, "Men marry young here, and preferably to fifteen- or sixteen-year-old girls." He accompanied us to the afternoon survey site in order to facilitate interviewing. He also suggested that the brick-making site outside the village would be a good place to conduct interviews, as long as people who weren't being interviewed continued to work. Although the ARC's Mark Bester insisted on not having village headmen pick our candidates, in the end this method proved to be the most efficient. After lunch, we took a fifteen-minute drive by jeep out to a house-building site where young people from the village were making bricks in the scorching heat. The headman asked the young men to participate in our survey (most of the morning interviews in the village had been with young women).

The work site smelled of dirt, dust, gas from the tractor engine, and smoke from their small fire. We saw many tractors on the village road but only one gasoline truck. There were thirteen workers in all, five men and the rest women. The women carried the finished bricks on poles to dry in the sun, while the men ran the machines and made sure everything ran smoothly. This is another example of a sexual division of labor, whereby Tai women often do the hard work while men sit on the sidelines watching.

The only large mechanical machinery was a tractor whose engine was rigged to a machine that forms and cuts equal-size bricks. It costs about two or three fen per brick (ten fen equals one mao), and RMB 30,000 (about 3,700 U.S. dollars) to build an entire house. Everybody in the village comes together in a house-building project, and when a family's turn comes for a house, everyone else repays the favor—a gift exchange of sorts. This house was to be built on the edge of the road in front of the village's wet rice paddies. As the afternoon interviews were mainly with men, I sat and watched while talking to Shen and Mali.

MULTIPLE MEANINGS OF AIDS

At the end of the day, the survey results showed that 75 percent of the locals in this region knew some of the basic ways that HIV is transmitted: through blood and blood products, sexual intercourse, and injection drug use. Sixty-five percent responded that they knew where to buy condoms (Armijo-Hussein and Beesey 1998). Also noteworthy was the percentage of people who saw HIV as transmitted by sharing toothbrushes or food, hugging an infected person, using toilets, getting a haircut, donating blood (few reports about blood donations and HIV were heard of at the time), and getting a mosquito bite. According to the authors of the final ARC report, Jacqueline Armijo-Hussein and Allan Beesey (1998), the most startling finding was that 60 percent of the respondents said they would avoid someone with HIV and that only a very few thought men having sex with other men would transmit HIV.

The latter belief may be due to the fact that homosexuality is stigmatized in rural Yunnan and therefore rarely discussed in terms of health prevention in any context.[43]

The majority of respondents (80 percent) were farmers, or rather rural peasants. The most knowledgeable of the three ethnic groups were the Tai-Lüe (Armijo-Hussein and Beesey 1998). The Tai are also the group with the highest socioeconomic status in the county, compared to such ethnic groups as the Lahu, who had both the lowest income levels and the lowest knowledge about HIV/AIDS. This division accords with Paul Farmer's argument (1992) that HIV/AIDS follows a society's fault lines, so that those with less education have less access to information on prevention.

In reference to HIV prevention, Doug Porter (1997) points out: "There is a tendency to presume categories of persons in a way that occludes the fluidity of identities and perpetuates essentializing and stigmatizing risk groups rather than risky behaviors or situations." In other words, what was at stake in the small villages and towns surrounding Menglian where women such as Yufang lived was the production of knowledge, of disease, and of prejudice, all of which seemed to go hand in hand. Here women such as Yufang and Li were marked for working in Thailand, for not having husbands, and for crossing the border, rather than for their direct behaviors. Also, Yufang and Li needed more than just condom handouts and a survey to document their knowledge about HIV; they needed jobs, a livelihood, and a partner to help them with the work in their rice paddies. Referencing Porter's work, Leonore Manderson and Margaret Jolly (1997: 20) suggest that "constructing epicenters of core transmitters [of HIV/AIDS] provides an illusory cartographic certainty in what is actually a very fluid and turbulent terrain."

While Yufang may have worked in Thailand for a short time, there was no guarantee she would return, nor any indication that she was a prostitute. However, even in the final report of the Menglian survey, she is identified as a woman who engages in transactional sex. The survey team fit her into the neat categories of risk transmission when in fact her identity was fluid, as she worked one month in Thailand and the next back in the village of Sanya, tending her rice paddies. Here the two thought styles about reservoirs of infection converge in one woman. Tropical thinking linked Yufang to a specific place of infection, Thailand, while epidemiological thinking tallied her as a "sex worker"; she had worked in Thailand and thus was in a high-risk group.

As Ferguson (1996) aptly points out: "If unintended effects of a project end up having political uses, even seeming to be instruments of some larger political deployment, this is not some kind of conspiracy; it really does just happen to be the way things work out" (256). Although the Menglian survey was the fulcrum for public health intervention into villagers lives, it also points to several layers of anxiety about these borders: notions of former barbarian pathologies, gender as expressed through minority sex workers (those women working in Thailand), former colonial and continuing missionary activity, and global health discourses that arrive in the form of a survey from an Australian NGO to reform China's methods of collecting surveillance data. Surveys are part of elementary public health data collection, but what I show is that the survey itself cannot be separated from other political, cultural and economic, and ethnic concerns. Surveys in one sense reflect the larger political agendas in the region—the concerns over migrants moving into and out of Chinese sovereign territory for work and, possibly, for drug trafficking, the root ideas behind marking migrants as reservoirs of infection.

Several different competing discourses also operated here, bringing the analysis back to the three perspectives with which this chapter began: the local folk categories of HIV/AIDS, the national government's ideological categories, and the global HIV/AIDS discourses. HIV/AIDS in this region is ideologically linked to the global risk behavior categories of injection drug use and prostitution, and now equally to the researchers who were carrying knowledge about HIV/AIDS into Menglian with their survey tools and the power of their words. As a kind of symbiotic relationship exists between the local, provincial, and global prevention goals for disciplining diseased bodies within the Chinese nation, there are also incredible disconnects, such as competing notions about protection and prevention promoted by the police versus public health workers. Here "international projects of development and national projects of modern governance are both major channels through which publics on the periphery encounter technoscience, [which now moves] as a truly translocal bundle of practices, meanings, and technologies" (Pigg 2001: 526).

Under socialist forms of governmentality, adopting and modifying western scientific tools, even in the form of a KABP survey, not only produce problematic results but also reinforce ways of the state. Surveys also become another avenue for the state to maintain and control a healthy body politic and to overcome the permeability of the border. HIV/AIDS statistics are problematic in their production and their methods of dissemination; in the selection of appropriate categories, data collection methods, and types of analysis; and in their effects on the implementation of future public health prevention programs. Surveys operate as research tools but also as ways of demonstrating proper hygiene and behavior; they hint at behaviors considered unhealthy, such as not using condoms, and encourage healthy behaviors, such as not going to Thailand to work, or rather not trading sex for money. But what they do not show is the intricacies of people's lives, the very lived challenges that people face in light of economic hardship and easy access to border communities and jobs outside China. On one hand, citizens are encouraged to be entrepreneurs and be creative in finding new kinds of livelihoods; on the other, they are stigmatized for doing just that, because the jobs are deemed risky and unhealthy.

Because Chinese officials have anxieties about the border areas due to their histories and their proximity to the Golden Quadrangle and the drug trade, they map HIV/AIDS anxieties onto those borders. Rather than having no borders, as the international HIV/AIDS lingo suggests, HIV/AIDS in China is an integral part of the border. Mapping HIV/AIDS onto borderland bodies maps the disease onto the borders of China, where prejudice and stigma are key (see Farmer and Kleinman 1989; Kleinman, Das, and Lock 1997; Jing 2004). Here state encroachment actually goes hand in hand with public health methods: to scientifically count bodies is also to control them. Counting bodies in the HIV/AIDS epidemic means that the *aesthetics of statistics* leaves out other key narratives. The process of controlling borderland bodies, those whose borders are threatened by tourism, drugs, and development, unveils the state's goal of reifying China's borders and re-imagining its integrity in a period of economic and political reform.[44] While local and international medical practitioners are keen to measure and quantify the Chinese HIV/AIDS epidemic, research methods, borrowed from abroad, often go beyond the implicit purpose of counting borderland bodies in an epidemic. While it may be jejune to say that statistics lie, they do tell a very different story than a cursory reading would show.

CHAPTER 2

Everyday AIDS Practices

Risky Bodies and Contested Borders

In one strike-hard campaign *(yanda yundong)*, we rounded
up 120 drug addicts in one night! Where are we going to
place all these young people? Does the government think
about that? We fine them six hundred yuan [two months'
local salary], hold them for the night, and release them in the
morning. Prostitution is the same. Like a poisonous weed, it
keeps growing back. AIDS is just another problem attached
to a long list of problems we face as a border region. Illegal
car smuggling and border drug smuggling are much more
pressing problems for the police than AIDS.

Policeman, Jinghong, June 1996

MIGRATIONS OF PEOPLE, GOODS, AND VIRUSES

When this policeman downplays HIV/AIDS, he is not ignoring the emergence of the epidemic; rather, he reflects a recurrent discourse around
HIV/AIDS that emphasizes policing and surveillance of the border regions. Borders here provide a liminal space where many transactions
occur and where the spread of HIV/AIDS in Xishuangbanna, an autonomous minority prefecture bordering Laos and Burma, symbolizes
what Arjun Appadurai (1996) characterizes as late-twentieth-century
cross-border mass migrations of peoples, goods, services, and, I would
add, viruses, all coloring a moving transnational canvas. This chapter focuses on the late-socialist Chinese state and untangles the actions of certain actors, such as the policeman quoted above, as the state first began
to police, control, and prevent the spread of HIV/AIDS from minority
borderlands into the Han interior. It traces the actions, institutions, and
multiple positions and interests the state had in defining and transform-

ing what I term "everyday AIDS practices." All over the globe, associations involving diseases get mapped onto certain places and peoples more readily than onto others, and I argue that the identity of a disease gets spatialized through the discursive construction of diseases and borders by these state actors.

My intellectual terrain in this chapter is wide. I first discuss the value of focusing on the concept of borderlands for understanding the intricacies of disease prevention as a goal of the state. Second, I present a brief history of the question of sovereignty in Xishuangbanna. Third, I turn to my ethnography and explore four narratives that draw on the everyday AIDS practices of state actors. Following Bourdieu (1977 & 1990), I use the term "practice" to discuss an array of words, customary actions, and measures by state actors in the prevention of HIV.[1] I conclude with a discussion of the utility of linking borders, diseases, and the subjectivity of state actors for understanding contemporary Chinese HIV/AIDS. I focus on the practices and subjectivities of state actors that worked in the borderlands of Yunnan Province in the early years of the epidemic (1995–2000), prior to the 2001 official acknowledgment that China even had an epidemic.

INFECTIOUS DISEASES AND THE POSTREFORM STATE

Armed with international and local public health intervention and health education prevention strategies, China by the mid-1980s embraced the idea of risk groups for HIV/AIDS. Similar to many countries around the globe, China defined HIV/AIDS through epidemiological categories that linked groups rather than individual behaviors to HIV. For while the categories of injection drug user, prostitute, migrant, and foreigner are perceived as having higher rates of HIV than the general population, it is not membership in a group but actual individual behaviors such as sharing dirty needles and having unprotected sex that put people at risk. Furthermore, on the prevention front in the late 1990s, surveillance of "risky bodies" was intensified in the name of preventing the spread of HIV/AIDS. In chapter 1, I discuss how these risky bodies are also ethnic bodies (see also Hyde 2000; 2001; 2002).

In this chapter, I discuss these broad categories that designate bodies as risky not only in terms of their ethnicity but also in terms of their location. As I emphasized in chapter 1, according to central government reports and interviews with government officials, it is borderland peoples who shoot drugs, engage in unsafe sex, and travel to Thailand to work (see Gilman 1988a & 1988b; Arnold 1993; Porter 1997). Here, I emphasize that the strategies of defining risky people rather than risky behaviors brings with it a whole edifice of state control practices and regulations. This edifice is not without historical precedents. Chinese historians note that on the eve of liberation in 1953, the Sipsongpanna borderland was perceived as a desolate wasteland of malaria- and leprosy-infested jungles, full of barbarians (Yin 1986; Wang Lianfang 1993).

Given these conditions, we need to think about the nature of states and how state actors in the post-1979 reform period, often referred to as late socialism, address the emergence of a socialist civil society (see Jing 1996; Yan 1996; Liu Baoying 2000; Zhang Li 2001). Litzinger (2000a), in his work on the Yao minority in Yunnan, argues that the state is not merely a static or singular structure, but a series of processes whose social intertextures reveal how the state is reproduced through cultural milieu, ethnicity, and local histories (see also Shue 1988; Mueggler 2001). Anagnost (1997) was one of the first scholars to study the state as a series of processes mired in historically messy and contested decisions that regulate disruptive and unruly bodies. Nancy Chen (2003), in her work in Beijing mental hospitals, points to the late-socialist state's medicalization of certain martial arts and spiritual practices in order to keep tight controls over public order and space. I build on the work of these scholars and of other scholars of late socialism and the postreform state who have rejected this notion of the unitary state.

Postreform China offers an excellent counterexample to the empirical problem of what political science calls the demarcation between civil society and the state. China does so precisely because the state ushered in many of the international NGOs that in the mid-1990s begin to work on HIV/AIDS prevention. At the same time, these NGOs were not independent; rather, all were hybrid organizations of the Chinese government in the sense that every foreign NGO had a government counterpart.[2] Having recognized this state–civil society distinction as spurious in China, we can more clearly address the centrality of the borderlands to the construction of individual AIDS practices and the state's regulation of risky subjects. Provincial government officials are the vanguard; they create new HIV/AIDS policies, as they are themselves simultaneously subjected to the larger regimes of power within postreform China.[3] HIV/AIDS policies evolve from a state apparatus that unites multiple discourses and techniques of power that are never straightforward and that create different kinds of political subjectivities and contradictions.[4]

These include efforts to survey and police the minority borderlands in the name of disease prevention and sovereignty, as well as cultural ideas about minority gender relations. All of this leads back to the problem of fighting an imagined disease with imaginary figures; who is tested for HIV or marked as an HIV/AIDS-carrying person has everything to do with how one is imagined both epidemiologically and geographically, rather than strictly how one behaves. Before proceeding to questions of sovereignty, I want to explore the notion of the borderlands.

BORDERLANDS AND BORDERS

As Thongchai Winichakul (1994: 15) so powerfully argues, modern nations arrive through the very act of imposing boundaries around borders, whether those boundaries are geographic or are categories not yet labeled as such in the case of new, previously unrecognized peoples and spaces. Furthermore, according to the imagined-community approach to modern state building, the Chinese state's definition of its borders and boundaries allows it to exist as one continuous geopolitical space because China is historically perceived and rhetorically revered as having been around for thousands of years (Anderson 1992 in Gladney 2002: 1). In another sense, studying the borderlands of a nation-state, one sees just what the central state considers the essential terrain of government control, including biological control over everyday life.

Whereas anthropologists such as Van Gennup (1960) studied cultural boundaries and their creation as a way to understand social and cultural expression and identity, recent work in anthropology on borders and boundaries moves away from the notion that they simply divide states, peoples, villages, and communities into two distinct entities—what is inside and what is outside, what is sacred and what is profane. Gloria Anzaldúa (1999) instigated a wave of research and writing on how women, mestizas in particular, were divided between two borders and often two cultures of Mexico and the United States. What is crucial about her work for my argument is that she instantiates the idea that borders are not just geographic; borders become embodied through the people identified with them. Building on Anzaldúa's work, Daphne Berdahl (1999) argues, in her research in a village on the former border between East and West Germany: "Boundaries are symbols through which state, nations and localities define themselves" and their distinct territory and cultural limits (3). The idea of the borderlands allows new possibilities for theorizing subjectivity and actions of the state, the relationship between the center and border, and how center and periphery influence each another in a dialectical dance.

Furthermore, as Akhil Gupta and James Ferguson (1992) point out, "the borderlands are just such a place of incommensurable contradictions," and rather than dismissing them as insignificant or marginal, they, and I, want to conceptualize the borderlands as a "normal" locale of modernity (Berdahl 1999: 6). As Berdahl emphasizes, a borderlands approach highlights the processural, fluid, and multidimensional aspects of identity and the ways these identities in turn are constantly remade as the notion of the border shifts within larger political and social projects. Individuals and the state negotiate borderlands in specific ways.

The narratives of the individuals I write about are in one sense state narratives; these individuals are the embodiment of the Chinese state through their jobs and their Communist Party affiliations. As a very real geographic border here dictates much of the discourse on the disordering effects of HIV/AIDS on this chaotic and lawless territory, China's geopolitical borders with Laos and Burma must not get lost in this argument (see Lyttleton and Amarapibal 2002; Lee 2003). In the eyes of the central government in Beijing, the illegal trade in cars, drugs, and sex represents the disorders of this border region. If drug use and sex are two of the key routes to HIV, controlling the borderlands must be part of state efforts to limit the spread of these very disorders. As Foucault (1977) pointed out, forms of state surveillance and control are never straightforward; they are remade, reinforced, and contested throughout history (see also Burchell, Gordon, and Miller 1991). Here I draw on the colonial notions of the borderlands as places of barbarian diseases, places that, prior to colonization by the Chinese, were cesspools of tropical infection and, in the 1990s, were local sites for the spread of the most recognized disease of the twenty-first century, HIV/AIDS.

SIPSONGPANNA AND CONTESTATIONS OF SOVEREIGNTY

The question of borderlands and central state sovereignty is key in contending with the complicated relationship of the central Chinese state to its minority borderlands. As I show in the introduction, Sipsongpanna, a former independent state of the Lan Na kingdom of Thailand, was rechristened as Xishuangbanna Dai Nationality Autonomous Prefecture (Xishuangbanna Daizu Zizhizhou) by the Chinese Communists in January 1953 (Hsieh 1995). Prior to its integration into China, Sipsongpanna had a long history of patronage to Burma and to Qing China. Although many scholars disagree about the strength of Burma and China as the two suzerain states of Xishuangbanna, they do agree that after the Communists took over in 1953, the kingdom finally lost any semblance of independent status and became part of China's multiethnic frontier (Sethakul 2000).

Instead of a unified singular Chinese state that transformed and erased the feudal aspects of Tai Buddhist religious practices after 1953, what emerged in the late 1990s was a Tai cultural renaissance that manifests itself in social practices that capitalize equally on the rising market economy and what I call a moral economy of cultural revival. While many Tai citizens of Sipsongpanna complain about the presence of the Han Chinese and their selfish and greedy ways, the Tai themselves have benefited enormously from the rise in economic markets, markets for their religious beliefs, organizational links to kinship groups in Laos and Thailand, and the resurgence in temple building and preservation, to name a few developments (Borchert 2005).

During previous regimes the religious and cultural habits of the Tai were suspect and suppressed as backward and feudal. Today the shift toward tolerance for ethnic difference occurs in the search for new markets, in this case ethnic tourism. For example, restrictions have been loosened and religious practices encouraged, as through rebuilding Buddhist temples torn down during the Cultural Revolution. A burgeoning network of Tai religious organizations throughout Southeast Asia may in the future assist in training young monks, teaching the Tai language, and preserving Buddhist palm leaf scriptures (see Davis 1999 & 2005). These cultural exchanges often point toward contradictory goals: a Han state intent on raising revenues for tourism, and the Tai minority using tourism to revive and repair aspects of its cultural heritage after the violent suppression of the Cultural Revolution (1966–76).

The prefectural capital of Jinghong was the capital (called Yunjinghong) of the Tai-Lüe kingdom for over eight hundred years. By the late 1980s it became a tourist destination for Chinese who could afford vacations (see chapters 3 and 4 for in-depth discussions of sex tourism). Understanding Jinghong's ethnic tourism involves acknowledging its allure as a tropical paradise and exploring its linkage, simultaneously, through the rise in sexually transmitted infections to sexual pathology and an urban erotic subculture. The dominant Chinese ethnic group, the Han, believe one of the cultural characteristics of the Tai ethnic group is a high level of sexual promiscuity, and this belief leads the Han to assume that the Tai are particularly susceptible to sexually transmitted infections. These cultural prejudices aside, there are real grounds for concern, as Jinghong has a cosmopolitan sex industry that feeds the tourism market. Based on my fieldwork (1996–2002), I found this sexual pathology linked to the notion that beautiful sex workers were local Tai minority women. During my fieldwork I discovered that 80 to 90 percent of the sex workers were Han Chinese female migrants from neighboring provinces of Guangxi and Sichuan (Hyde 1999; 2001; 2004). As sexual transmission is now seen as the next wave for the Chinese HIV/AIDS epidemic, female entertainment workers are currently viewed as the infectious bridge population to the general population through their male clients (see also Porter 1997; Jeffrey 2002; Gregory 2003; Xia Guomei 2004). Therefore, interpretations of sexual risk become highly gendered and are accompanied by notions of blame in terms of ethnic identification and territorial social space.

THE STATE IN FOUR NARRATIVES

The government office is a banquet of bareness. Green paint is strategically mopped up the side of the walls just high enough for a ten-year-old to stand and point with her thumb to a dividing line where whitewash rises to the ceiling. Scattered on a desk marked with ink splatters and small knife holes lie yellowing *People's Daily (Renmin Ribao)* newspapers, beneath teacups made of recycled glass jars. There's a poster of Deng Xiaoping and a large map of China. A quiet smoldering hiss from the fluorescent lights disturbs the ticking of a clock.

This quiet hiss evokes images of government offices in the Communist era; today these same offices and the bureaucrats who work within them have changed with the growing market economy. During my fieldwork between 1995 and 2002 in Beijing, Menglian, Jinghong, and Kunming, I observed the often shifting and conflicting positions that professionals took in response to local understandings of HIV/AIDS. Their positions filtered down into the intimate personal connections *(guanxi)* between professionals and their charges, and often were politically motivated and contested.[5] Because promoting prevention strategies is never easy, China's initial focus on demographic and geographic categories, as opposed to risky behaviors, ensured an edifice of state practices and regulations over certain groups.

How do individuals who work in the anti-epidemic stations in Menglian and Kunming and in a high-security drug prison in the hills outside Jinghong react in the face of what seems to be a borderlands epidemic? The impact of what state workers say and do is crucial to understanding the decisions the state makes and how ideas about HIV/AIDS are created and disseminated through these people's everyday practices. Narratives of four different state employees—Dr. Hui, an epidemiologist and physician; Dr. Jing, a psychiatrist; Chen, a health worker; and Lao Yan, a policeman—illustrate how preventing HIV/AIDS involves the interplay between the pressures of prestige, political maneuvering, personal ethics, public health, and geography. These accounts of HIV/AIDS prevention practices illustrate key tropes about how HIV/AIDS was understood, contested, and controlled in the mid- to late 1990s in China's borderlands. As Clifford Geertz (1977) has remarked, people often know what they do and why they do it, but they do not know the consequences of what they do.

The individuals I introduce here often occupy multiple positions: their social and professional roles intersect with other institutional roles. One might be a physician, a government-employed health worker, an academic researcher, and a state official all rolled into one. In the first two narratives, I explore the larger social and cultural context of HIV/AIDS prevention from the point of view of two people at the forefront of HIV/AIDS prevention in Beijing and Kunming, Dr. Hui and Dr. Jing. The diametrically opposed views of HIV/AIDS revealed in these two physicians' everyday AIDS practices point toward the contradictory ways that HIV/AIDS prevention strategies have emerged and how the border regions were perceived.

Dr. Hui and an HIV/AIDS Hotline

I met Dr. Hui, a tall, wiry man with thick glasses, in Thailand in 1995, at one of the first international HIV/AIDS conferences that Chinese delegates attended. We were both delegates with Save the Children Foundation based in Kunming. Later in Beijing, Dr. Hui invited me to his offices in the north of the city. Dr. Hui had a considerable amount of printed material on HIV/AIDS prevention, and as of August 1996, he operated the only nationwide HIV/AIDS hotline staffed by volunteers with medical training. These volunteers worked a four-hour shift every two weeks, from four to eight in the evening Monday through Saturday. The funding for the hotline came directly from the Chinese Ministry of Health, although much of the health education material was initially funded by international donor organizations including the World Health Organization and UNAIDS. Dr. Hui explained that most callers just wanted to know where they could get tested for antibodies to HIV. In Beijing confidential but not anonymous testing was conducted at the anti-epidemic stations for fifty yuan (about six U.S. dollars) per test. The results were returned one week later. As for the treatments available for opportunistic infections, Dr. Hui mentioned that drug trials were being conducted at Peking Union Medical Center and that the patients in the research trials were also given AZT free of charge. Dr. Hui explained, "There is relatively little outreach and information gathering for this hotline, and we do not receive many calls unless there is a program on television or the radio on HIV/AIDS." He also kept reiterating, in reference to ethnic groups and their particular subcultures, that "the Tai in Thailand are wild," meaning they engage in too much sex, and "that is why we have so much HIV/AIDS in places like Xishuangbanna."

As I wanted to observe the fine workings of the hotline, I simply asked Dr. Hui if that would be possible. He suggested instead that since I was the expert, I should be the one to answer hotline calls rather than him. I assumed his invitation had more to do with his not wanting to be observed, or rather criticized, than with wanting to assist me in my own research. I answered two telephone calls on the hotline. The first call was from a young man who was terrified he had contracted HIV/AIDS from kissing a foreign male at a gay nightclub in Guangzhou. The second was from a man who had unprotected sex with a prostitute while traveling south on vacation. The fear in both their voices was palpable; however, I found the first caller compelling, as being a closeted gay male in China was extremely difficult. At the end of the telephone line I heard the small mild-mannered voice of a young man slowly speaking Mandarin with a clipped Guangdong accent. He explained his recent encounter at a disco and bar: "A foreign male, an exchange student from the University of Wisconsin, kissed me and he used his tongue *(shetou)*, and I got some of his saliva *(tuoye)* in me. He didn't only kiss me, but he used his teeth and he bit my tongue, and I am so scared; I am too young to get sick and die. My mother is sick and I am worried about leaving her with an ill son."

At first, I suggested that if he thought he caught an STI, he should see a doctor who could treat him. But as his story unfolded, it became apparent that his was a case of misinformation, indicative of the fact that there is limited access to accurate information about HIV/AIDS. He was afraid of getting HIV/AIDS from kissing an American student on the floor of a Guangzhou disco. I kept saying there are only three ways to transmit HIV/AIDS and that exchanging saliva and biting someone's tongue posed little risk of transmission. He reported having had a fever, though it had subsided by the time of his hotline call. I began to understand the problems associated with trying to explain one's fears about contracting HIV/AIDS without admitting homoerotic activity to a stranger. He was also concerned about getting a test for HIV. Dr. Hui pointed me to the telephone number for the anti-epidemic station in Guangzhou, where anyone could be tested for fifty to one hundred yuan, and I told the caller he would receive the results in one week. Again, the young man reiterated, "We didn't have intercourse, we just kissed."

Dr. Hui explained that the majority of calls are made when their hotline numbers are actually advertised in Beijing, Fujian, Hainan, Zhejiang, and Guangzhou newspapers. All these cities and provinces have individual hotlines and materials provided by Dr. Hui, if they have not already developed their own location-specific materials. "Unlike your country," Dr. Hui said, "in China we cannot promote condoms for certain segments of the population, such as prostitutes, who should abstain from having sex; students, who should abstain; farmers, who would be too embarrassed to even read the information; and migrants, who are too ignorant to read it." He also commented on the immorality of prostitution and how it must be stamped out as it was under Mao in the early 1950s. According to representatives at the United Nations HIV/AIDS (UNAIDS) Office, plenty of money was available for innovative programs, yet Dr. Hui kept reiterating that to prevent HIV/AIDS, he needed more money. The early information, education, and communication (IEC) brochures he developed in 1996 offered questionable depictions of what he deemed both risky bodies and risky behaviors, and provided little education for the public about prevention other than abstaining from sex.

Dr. Hui represents one attitude in China about HIV/AIDS prevention—that HIV/AIDS is caused by immoral people, a view that parallels those of many Christian groups in the West. Dr. Hui had developed some of the first IEC material in China on HIV/AIDS prevention, but at the same time, he did not include information on condom use for fear of offending people. Rumors also circulated that much of his international funding was from the Reverend Sun Moon. One may view this narrative as that of someone struggling with the notions of a changed China, a China no longer under the hold of Maoism and the kind of moralizing that stigmatized, imprisoned, and killed people for not upholding the moral fervor of the state. Dr. Hui was born into the generation of Chinese that came of age after the revolution, in the 1950s, and many of his ideas reflect some of his generation's enthusiasm for the Mao period.

Although the state's everyday AIDS practices are carried out at the local level—for example, the multiple local AIDS hotlines—they are funded by a variety of international donor agencies such as those that supported Dr. Hui's institute. As William Fisher (1997) contends, one way to assess the work of NGOs is to fathom what they do rather than simply how they are organized. I would add that knowing what NGOs say and what sorts of discourse they encourage also helps in assessing their work. At the same time that Dr. Hui dedicates his life to alleviating suffering from HIV/AIDS by reducing the numbers of cases through his health education hotline, he comes down extremely hard on anyone who already has HIV, especially if he or she is a drug addict, a prostitute, a migrant, or someone with multiple sexual partners. Thus Dr. Hui's individual goodwill coincides with his personal moral stance that denigrates "immoral" people. Both of his subject positions influence the political will of the state and remake what HIV/AIDS prevention means according to the central government in Beijing. Dr. Hui embodies the local, national, and global perspectives on HIV in his roles as a physician and health educator. Through the hotline, Dr. Hui devised his own folk categories for HIV/AIDS prevention that incorporated the dangers of promoting condoms. Though a government employee working in a national institute with support from the Ministry of Health, he is of a generation whose personal moral views reflect socialist ideas about putting one's country first and one's private desires second. These views came into direct conflict with some of the international NGOs working on AIDS in China. He channels a parochial morality originating in Confucian and Maoist notions of the good citizen, according to which prostitutes and drug addicts are not casualties of marketization but bad citizens who must be punished.

Dr. Jing and Drug Use Prevention

I first met Dr. Jing, a young psychiatrist, on my first research trip to Menglian County in 1995 and then on several subsequent occasions in Kunming. Dr. Jing works on the front lines of HIV/AIDS prevention through the Yunnan Institute of Drug Abuse and with two NGOs that funded the early HIV/AIDS prevention programs in Yunnan, the Australian Red Cross and Save the Children. She also conducts research on drug use and teaches psychiatry at a medical college in Yunnan. Although my interviews and interactions with her covered many conversations and topics, I focus here on her comments on the rise of STIs and HIV/AIDS and the challenges facing prevention.

As in the rest of the world at that time, the HIV/AIDS epidemic in Yunnan was first seen as a disease of others—foreigners—then as a disease of the internal Other—minorities. More recently, as I argue, it was framed as a question of geography. Dr. Jing said: "Sexual promiscuity *(luanjiao)* may be more prevalent among the Lahu minority than the Tai. HIV/AIDS is also a problem of the floating population [people moving from place to place] and perhaps more of an issue for demographers than for epidemiologists." "As for those who link HIV/AIDS to the Tai, it has more to do with geography and the tourist trade in Xishuangbanna than with cultural ideas." Dr. Jing added: "While both the Tai and Lahu are more sexually open than, say, the Akha or Wa, and they are culturally more open to sexual variations, that does not mean they are conduits for HIV/AIDS."

In reference to the kinds of people presenting for STIs in the small health clinics, Dr. Jing declared that it is those people with multiple partners who are at risk: prostitutes, their clients, drug addicts, and others who trade in sex and drugs. She also pointed out, "if you test for a disease like hepatitis, you may get some idea of the spread of HIV, as there are similar routes to infection." "In 1990 Yunnan," she said, "only 30 percent had hepatitis and now [1996] it is 88 percent. We still test for three cardinal STIs at marriage [syphilis, gonorrhea, and hepatitis B] but not HIV."

Since the beginning of the millennium, sexual transmission through drug use has become a key focus for organizations like Jing's Institute of Drug Abuse. She argued that people are now using heroin more than ever before, and even though she agreed in part with the basic premise of harm reduction, she was not sure if the public security bureaus would agree to handing out free needles. "While they give people methadone for free for a period of three months, it is too expensive to give it out for much longer periods." "Getting tested for HIV/AIDS costs one hundred yuan but can be made free for people without means. This means that those who frequent all these clinics are often those with funds, and those without money must face the humiliation of the public hospital."[6] "Drug rehabilitation is a new concept and it will take time to do anything along the lines of exchanging needles as in the United States and

Europe." She further explained the difficulties of trying to institute a program of harm reduction using needles, noting how this difficulty is exacerbated by the complicated authority structures among work units.

Perhaps one of the biggest challenges is the bureaucracy itself. She said, "The relationship of my work unit *(danwei)* to the Public Health Bureau is only marginal because the provincial level *(ting)* is under the National Public Health Bureau *(weishengbu)* and the high-security drug center *(qiangjiedusuo)* is part of the *bu* [National Public Security Bureau]. To complicate matters, my work unit is also organizationally related to the provincial public security bureau *(gonganting)*, the bureau for capturing prostitutes, and the army [see Li Xuezhong 1996]. So, for example, if my work unit wanted to plan a needle exchange program, we would need the permission from officials in different ministries—Public Health, Public Security, and the army."

Dr. Jing identified some of the problems associated with health education programs and condom use: "[The] problem with prostitutes and condoms is that the number of condoms women have on them often measures the legal evidence of prostitution. I have been trying to enlighten hotels in Kunming to distribute condoms to customers through informal networks—for instance, sending agents to the Holiday Inn at eight in the evening when most girls start working. Another avenue is an official network, getting health educators to distribute condoms in hotel rooms themselves, . . . but we must convince the managers of the hotels first before we can educate their customers." Dr. Jing here provides a wonderful example of how certain notions of what the state declares as unclean get embodied. The idea that nice, clean Chinese women do not carry condoms leads to just the sort of laws that embody difference.

In February 2004 the Yunnan Standing Party Committee passed a broad-ranging HIV/AIDS Prevention and Control Law that required public places—hotels, inns, guesthouses, and commercial entertainment establishments—to provide condoms free of charge, or at the very least for purchase (Zhang Zizhuo 2004). By March 2005 another law was enacted that forced all persons working in these establishments to be tested for HIV and then fired if they tested positive (Zhou 2005). Policies regarding HIV prevention are erected and then made virtually impossible to implement because they compromise both the health and the livelihood of those working in entertainment establishments. If one acknowledges that one works in a nightclub or massage parlor, one must submit to being tested and risk being fired. However, the same occurs if one carries condoms to protect oneself and one's customers, because carrying condoms also risks one's being searched and fined or, perhaps worse, locked up in a prison for prostitutes.

According to Dr. Jing, early prevention projects in the border minority region of the Dehong Tai-Jingpo Nationality Autonomous Prefecture, in northwestern Yunnan, meant that in the villages with active HIV/AIDS prevention messages, there have been few new cases. She said, "The biggest problem is finding appropriate materials that will reach out to the non-school-going population, those who don't read or cannot read either Dehong-Dai or Mandarin.[7] I think peer education programs *(tongban jiaoyu)* are the wave of the future in HIV/AIDS prevention."

She discussed the role of the economy in the spread of HIV/AIDS and STIs: "In places like Xishuangbanna, with development has come the tourism industry, and with tourism has also come the sex industry. Although there is no clear direct connection between development and the sex industry, my colleagues and I do know that certain select places in Yunnan, Ruili, Xishuangbanna, and Menglian attract people from the border countries who come for sex. With sex tourism also comes prostitution, and some prostitutes buy drugs to keep on working."

In these narratives, Dr. Jing's position is that of a modern scientist; she embraces the latest international drug prevention techniques of harm reduction rather than incarceration and forced detoxification— the methods currently operative in much of China. Her ideas and interests clearly contrast with those of Dr. Hui; in fact, one may say they are diametrically opposed. Her suggestions for prevention are also on the cutting edge of what was imaginable in Kunming in the late 1990s; her idea to promote condom use in commercial sex followed often widely circulated international discourses, particularly that in Thailand, with its 100 percent–safer sex condom use policy for all commercial sex establishments. In fact, Dr. Jing asked me to find her more materials on harm reduction, and while cautious about the identification of the seven counties in Yunnan with high rates of HIV/AIDS and their location in minority prefectures, she also believed that minority women had a certain predilection to sexual habits that were unlike those of Han women. Also, Dr. Jing belongs to a generation that came of age well after the revolution, and was a small child during the Cultural Revolution. She embraced modernity and science as the hallmarks of international medical development and economic advancement.

In her wonderful description of the difficulties of implementing harm reduction in Yunnan, we see precisely the intricate web of government bureaucracy that makes new ideas and new methods extremely difficult to initiate. Dr. Jing's political position as both a physician and an employee of a state work unit meant she channeled certain contradictory beliefs in her own mind: culturally, she thought minority women were more prone to promiscuity; at the same time, she questioned the value of the state's dominant position on minorities and HIV/AIDS, a view of minority women stemming from perceived ideas about Tai culture and history. Contemporary Tai culture, according to the Tai themselves, allows for open alliances between unmarried men and women and for more fluidly defined sexual and gender roles. For example, in several Tai villages in Sipsongpanna, I saw men who remained at home taking care of babies while the women worked the rice fields. On the other hand, when translating or interpreting long-held cultural practices by simply mapping them onto current disease categories, we get the distinction that the Tai are more prone to HIV because of their cultural beliefs about sexuality and gender.[8]

Although Dr. Jing held prominent positions in the Provincial Department of Health and in her research institute, she was somewhat removed from the front line of the epidemic. The agencies involved in on-the-ground decisions about HIV/AIDS were the anti-epidemic stations and the public security bureaus. Each prefecture, county, and city in China is affiliated with a designated anti-epidemic station and public security bureau; these two government ministries fulfill the dual purpose of public health: to survey and control bodies through disease prevention, and to maintain order and security. In my third and fourth narratives, I explain the second set of prevention processes that revolve around questions of securing the borders.

In the following narratives, I explore how HIV/AIDS was perceived and regulated from within the minority border prefectures themselves. Through their everyday AIDS practices, we see just how government officials, or rather employees of the state, treated minority infections, how they choose to represent themselves and the Han majority's risk for HIV, and how in turn their own subject positions then marked and actually influenced state policy at the local level. Just how were these border regions, in particular Menglian Prefecture and the capital tourist city of Jinghong in Xishuangbanna Dai Prefecture, perceived and then targeted for early surveys and later health interventions? In working through the final two narratives, I begin by introducing the health department structure at the provincial level, because without having a clear understanding of the bureaucracy, the two agencies I discuss, the Menglian Anti-

Epidemic Station and the Jinghong Public Security Bureau, appear to be completely disparate institutions, when in fact they are linked in the prevention of HIV.

In 1995 the HIV/AIDS office of the Yunnan Provincial Department of Public Health established twelve departments within the Provincial Anti-Epidemic Station in the provincial capital of Kunming. In 1995 early HIV/AIDS prevention policy involved directives discouraging behavior, namely, using drugs and sleeping with multiple sexual partners. The mention of condoms for prevention was considered to be too sensitive a topic. Dr. Yao, a preventative medicine specialist in Kunming, said that difficulties surrounding the use of condoms for HIV/AIDS prevention reflected the Chinese saying *"Zhiqi ran, bu zhiqi suoyi ran"* (One knows what something is but does not understand its purpose). In other words, people may recognize that HIV/AIDS exists but not know how it is transmitted or understand the infectious nature of the disease. Furthermore, the market-oriented health prevention policy has prompted local health stations to move toward financial independence by generating income rather than relying on the state for full subsidies. Thus in practice there was no way to assist behavioral change because the local anti-epidemic stations did not have the money or the personnel to carry out their tasks. Dr. Yao further stated: "The other major problem in dealing with HIV/AIDS is the paralysis or constraint placed on structural response by the anti-epidemic stations themselves. The idea of building anti-epidemic stations at the local level was a health tactic inherited from the Russians. The problem now is that since 1992 we are losing control of the epidemic because individual units under economic reforms are being made financially accountable. They must make money."

For local anti-epidemic stations, the only recourse is to increase activities that generate income: selling vaccines, tests for HIV, and hygiene exams for employees in the food industry. Several informants reported, using the local vernacular, that the anti-epidemic stations now "kick their problems to another court" or "merely put out fires"; they have little time and even fewer resources to devote to prevention. In many communities the anti-epidemic stations are simply testing agencies that have been stripped of their roles as public health educators. These agencies barely keep their heads above water in terms of surviving economically, let alone meeting policy and prevention objectives of the Beijing-based Ministry of Health.

Some anti-epidemic stations, such as the one in Menglian (the county due west of Xishuangbanna), have some money for testing certain high-risk populations; but their main work is limited to providing health education classes or nurse aides to people who are dying. In a tourist region such as Xishuangbanna, these agencies consider it extremely important to maintain an image of a healthy local community. For example, as mentioned previously, the HIV/AIDS prevention messages in Jinghong are found only in back alleys, not on the main streets. Friends I have asked about this reply, "We don't want tourists to disappear." The notion of barbarians and barbarian diseases is revealed not only in historical accounts of northerners' conceptions of southerners' diseases but also in the everyday speech of northern tourists traveling to Xishuangbanna (Yin 1986).[9] Many Han Chinese tourists speak of their fears of diseases, especially malaria, and would never travel to minority villages on their own, outside of an organized tour. Han tourists were not the only people caught by these fears. Han physicians, originally from the provincial capital of Kunming, who were working in these autonomous regions reflected on cultural beliefs about the wild and hot climate of the southwest contributing to the spread of HIV/AIDS. Dr. Jing's perceptions of minority women reflects nineteenth-century notions of the border regions as full of barbarians and also mirrors Patton's critique of the persistence today of colonial thinking about the tropics. In the final two narratives, I reveal how nonphysicians involved in HIV/AIDS prevention find themselves in contradictory positions vis-à-vis the institutions they work for and how this contradiction in turn reflects their own sense of subjectivity.

Shen and the Menglian Anti-Epidemic Station

Throughout the early 1990s the Yunnan Provincial Anti-Epidemic Stations were criticized for not moving fast enough in developing local HIV/AIDS prevention policies. While the criticisms came from the Ministry of Health in Beijing, the stations' paralysis can be traced to reliance on existing channels of expertise. What follows is a discussion of two people who worked on the HIV/AIDS periphery in a frontline center for prevention; they both regarded the HIV/AIDS epidemic as an insurmountable problem leading to disorder and thus, they believed, the epidemic would become a problem for the border police to solve.

In December 1995, while in Menglian as an adjunct member of the Australian-Yunnan Red Cross survey team, I met Shen, a health worker at what was then known as the Menglian Lahu-Dai-Wa Autonomous County Anti-Epidemic Station. During the survey training, she pulled me aside to explain that she had recently been criticized for permitting a Beijing-based television production team to videotape people with HIV/AIDS in Menglian. The criticism was based not so much on the validity of the coverage as on the notion that Menglian would as a result be marked as a diseased site. Shen noted that many people wanted to believe that HIV/AIDS came from somewhere else. Shen was extremely diligent and eager in collecting survey information; she was up early in the morning and had the entire team working well into the night. Her participation on the survey soon brought Shen recognition, when she was promoted to a position in the county seat.

Shen and Menglian County's public security officials were most concerned by the recent number of women (about twenty) who were crossing the Burmese border and then moving into northern Thailand to work in the "entertainment industry"—a euphemism for prostitution. The number of HIV cases had apparently risen in Menglian County, and these twenty index cases were seen as a sign of rising rates of migration linked to increasing rates of HIV in Thailand (Thailand has the highest numbers of HIV cases in Asia). When I asked what efforts were being made to prevent future infection, it was clear that, apart from Shen's visits to the villages, no systematic prevention information was being given to anybody, least of all to women returning from Thailand.

Thai agencies monitoring the presence of Chinese women in Thailand report widely varying figures on how many women are crossing the Burmese border to work. According to the National People's Congress, in 1989 and 1990 a total of 65,236 people countrywide were arrested for trafficking in women and children (Kristof and Wudunn 1994). According to the Committee for the Protection of Children's Rights and the International Organization for Migration, both based in Bangkok, every month, dozens of women cross the borders of Yunnan to work in brothels in Thailand (Feingold 1998). In Menglian, Shen reported that she knew several of these women and had tried to contact all of them on their return to China. She was also eager to work on the repatriation of young female prostitutes from Thailand to China. However, one week later, Shen confessed in secret that while she tries to encourage young women to get tested rather than call on the police to arrest them, if they balk, "I bring in the police because these women must get tested to protect their families."

Thus, although Shen was sympathetic to the women and men with HIV in her county, she was concerned about transmission to the degree that she would instruct the police to force women to get tested. She was

part of the generation of youth sent down to rural areas such as
Menglian during the Cultural Revolution. She saw her political duty
arising out of that former Maoist medical regime, which promoted prevention of major epidemics by controlling the individual in the name of
the collective. In addition, she perceived these women as polluted, unlike Han women, who were clean. Here a government health worker
was, on one hand, preventing HIV/AIDS by protecting individuals and,
on the other, protecting the community by turning over individuals to
the police—actions reflecting the contradictory nature of early practices
in HIV/AIDS prevention in Yunnan. The contradictions between Shen's
ideological position and her sanctioned prevention policy reveal the un-
easiness and inconsistency of the HIV/AIDS discourse in China. Much
of the rhetoric about HIV/AIDS in Yunnan surrounds the protection of
the family unit; Shen was merely acknowledging this in her campaign
against the spread of HIV/AIDS. An early HIV/AIDS prevention poster
in Yunnan bore the image of a happy family—mother, father, and son—
and declared that the happy family knows how to prevent HIV/AIDS.
However, Shen did not just bow to the policy makers in Simao; they criticized her invitation to the Beijing film team. Shen's own actions point
to the contradictions not only in local HIV/AIDS policy but also in how
these policies are actually mediated through political subjects who live
and work in minority prefectures such as Menglian. Shen's own subject
position reveals her as an official who felt deeply about people suffering
from HIV and, at the same, maintained central party-state political convictions that HIV/AIDS must be controlled at all costs.

My fourth narrative is about a policeman who works for the public
security bureau in Jinghong. Because HIV/AIDS was initially associated
with drug addicts and trafficking, the public security bureaus mobilized
resources to capture and incarcerate HIV-infected individuals. Due to
the early efforts of Dr. Samid, the Kunming-based Save the Children's
first HIV/AIDS adviser, things began to change. Samid pointed out that
since AIDS was considered a negative, often polluting disease, one associated with a threat to security due to its appearance in China's most
southwestern border, gaining permission to begin a prevention program
required rather difficult political and diplomatic maneuvers. Getting
permissions from both provincial and local Jinghong public security bureaus involved a circuitous route through the military, the military hospital in Jinghong, and finally a drug prison that would become the site
of a Save the Children HIV/AIDS intervention program on drug rehabilitation. In the mid-1990s, most drug addicts were left alone, caught

by the police and sent to prison, or taken care of by their families; there were no rehabilitation centers. Also, Save the Children became involved because the postreform government reduced state subsidies to the health sector. Thus the state's role in disease prevention, and now HIV/AIDS prevention, was augmented and in many instances taken over by international health NGOs working in China. One may argue that transnational NGOs and their development agents prop up the state by injecting their own international agendas into China, providing seed money for HIV/AIDS prevention projects; however, through the power of their organizations they redefine the terrain of everyday AIDS practices (see Pandolfi 2003). These seemingly foreign NGOs are not entirely independent of the state bureaucracy; they are hybrid organizations, in part state managed and politically aligned with provincial governments. In fact, to register as an NGO, an organization had to have a government counterpart. Save the Children had the army; the Australian Red Cross had the Yunnan Red Cross.

Lao Yan and the Security Drug Center

The city of Jinghong sits on the banks of the Lancang River. If one drove across the old bridge over the river, past the army hospital into the hills, past rubber plantations and rock quarries, and up long winding dirt roads peppered with potholes filled with muddy water, one arrived at the high-security drug center. Vines covered the high red-brick walls, an old Beijing jeep lay in a heap by the side of the road, mangy mongrel dogs barked, and a few inmates and guards squatted in the sun, smoking tobacco from long water pipes. It was here that I first met Lao Yan, a member of the local Tai minority and one of the guards, in his thirties; he welcomed me by showing off his small zoo. He was raising bamboo rats (which he promised tasted great), fruit trees, and a few chickens and dogs. The red-brick buildings at the center, all in various states of disrepair, were organized according to various levels of security: the prison cells where inmates were assigned when they first arrived; the medium-security rooms where inmates shared bunk beds and a courtyard; and the unlocked rooms above the prison cells in which, as a result of the Save the Children project, only female inmates were in rehabilitation. Inmates reached the prison through exasperated family members, police raids on drug addict hangouts, or individual arrests.

The high-security section of the prison had four enclosed cells, each surrounded by Cyclone fencing on all four sides about two stories high. Each cell consisted of a small outer courtyard with an opening large enough to let in the tropical sunlight, and a small room with bunk beds and a window covered by iron grating. Each cell had a water spigot with a small concrete tub in the courtyard and a few stools. About eight inmates lounged, smoking cigarettes, while others chopped wood. Xiao Tan, a nineteen-year-old woman, told me, "We are all cigarette addicts" *(yangui)*.[10] Above the old prison cells were newly built rooms. The new, low-security wing housed nine young women, including one who had only two days left in her confinement. All nine appeared to have spent time in the lower section, the Cyclone-fenced cages. Apparently, the previous week three young women had set fire to the wood platforms of their beds and burned holes in the mosquito screens, an act the guards regarded as arson.[11] As punishment they were sent back to the high-security cages.

Lao Yan euphemistically attributed the divisions in types of security among the inmates to their levels of education and their previous occupations. He said that those with more education were easier to control and less likely to become aggressive. Dr. Samid, the Save the Children Foundation HIV/AIDS adviser, pointed out that where addicts get assigned was based on prejudice and class background. Those of higher social status, despite being addicts, tended to spend less time in the high-security cages, while an old man in his sixties, a former opium smoker, would, because of his age and social status, never leave the high-security section, let alone the prison. Many of the young addicts were incarcerated for about six months and then released to their families. According to Lao Yan, 60 percent of the young women addicts worked as prostitutes to obtain enough money to buy drugs, while the others acquired drugs from friends. He said, "If one works as a successful tour guide, one can fund a habit on one's commissions." Lao Yan reported that 90 percent of the prostitutes in Jinghong had a drug problem and that, once released, most of the inmates ended up back at the center, as recidivism rates were high. This contradicted local physicians' oral reports. Most of the drugs came from Burma near Dehong, not through closer routes through Laos and Thailand. All three of the female inmates I interviewed insisted they used clean needles. Xiao Tan said: "Clean needles are cheap [one yuan each] and are easy to purchase over the counter at local pharmacies, so we wouldn't think of using other peoples' needles; they are so dirty."[12] She continued, "I know about HIV/AIDS and am worried about getting it."

On my visits to the center, the guards complained there was never enough money to make repairs, let alone to do HIV testing and counseling with their injection drug–using charges. Money was so scarce that the resident nurse hadn't received her monthly salary of three hundred yuan in two months. Lao Yan said, "We really try to economize. In fact, even Premier Li Peng encouraged us not to buy expensive foreign cars but local jeeps." Later, on reflection, I noted that it was the premier who donated 100,000 yuan (over 12,000 U.S. dollars) to build a new brass and gold-glittered gate, a facsimile of a Tai Buddhist temple gate, to mark the entrance to Jinghong's new tourist district, when the only minority technical training school in Xishuangbanna had had to close its doors for lack of money. Lao Yan recounted how the provincial public security bureau sent thirty-five midlevel police officers to northern Thailand to review highland tribal police efforts in Thailand's minority tourist belt. The business trip was followed by a trip to Phuket for rest and relaxation, and Lao Yan boasted that the trip cost hundreds of thousands of yuan. Coming of age in the generation just before Dr. Jing, Lao Yan was subject to the scarcity of material goods during the Mao years and especially during the Cultural Revolution.

I want to elaborate here on this discussion of money. In China, the practice of using money as a symbolic currency in social relations is not limited to business lunches and dinners. The practice includes circulating money in a way that benefits the individual bureaucrat at the state's expense, as by buying expensive dinners for one's employees or friends. In what the Chinese call a "market with special socialist characteristics," the practice of selling, buying, and exchanging relationships, or *guanxi,* is paramount in conducting business. What may from a global perspective be perceived as a form of corruption (e.g., trips to Thailand) can also be read as an exchange relationship, part of the cultural practice of conducting business. As Mayfair Yang (1994) argues, unpacking state bureaucrats' personal *(guanxi)* relations reveals the "arts of the weak," those particular tactics that in the end destabilize and weaken the state's smooth operations. Zhang Li (2001) observes that, in the late-socialist period, clientelist networks, or what she calls clientelist *guanxi,* also reflect these kinds of alliances (108–9). As stated earlier, postreform public health governance changed markedly with the advent of public health departments that need to raise a large portion of their funds. These funds come from a variety of sources, ranging from the police measures that force prostitutes to take HIV/AIDS tests to grant monies provided by international NGOs.

Lao Yan said that during the most recent strike-hard anticrime campaign *(yanda yundong),* which focused on pornography, prostitution, and other illegal businesses, the police had picked up 120 drug addicts

in one night. And where were they to put all these people? With the previous *yanda yundong,* the police arrested a total of two thousand drug
addicts. Although users are fined six hundred yuan per person, they
are also often held for one night before they are released. The police
now concentrate on drugs and gambling salons and are temporarily
ignoring prostitution unless it involves drugs. Lao Yan said, "The police efforts to deal with prostitution amount to literally driving women
back to Simao, but we aren't very successful because they come back
here a week later. Why would many of the prostitutes who come from
Guizhou, Sichuan, and as far away as Guangdong, want to stay in
Simao?" He said, "The worst drug addicts work as prostitutes because
they need this business to feed their habits." Then he added, "As a border region we have more pressing problems than prostitution and
HIV/AIDS. Another example is the recent black market in illegal, un-
registered cars." Lao Yan explained that smugglers drive cars from
Burma to Jinghong to avoid the Chinese government's stiff import taxes,
and then sell these same cars for exorbitant profits on the Chinese side
of the border.

Lao Yan revealed his personal views about prostitutes and drug addicts, and through his views the problems of the Chinese state: there was
little money for prevention but lots for tourism, plenty of money for expensive cars but not for nurses' salaries. Lao Yan showed a mixture of
emotions when it came to drug and HIV/AIDS prevention, emotions
that filtered into everyday practices in his state police job. In not receiving enough money or resources to do his job, he felt maligned by Beijing. He felt entitled to expensive trips to Thailand for police training.

MULTIPLE SUBJECTIVITIES OF THE STATE

These four narratives of employees of the central government, the Yunnan provincial government, and local township government—Dr. Hui,
Dr. Jing, Shen, and Lao Yan—show that as representatives of the state,
they are often placed in contradictory positions, positions that reveal
multiple subjectivities. For example, as officials they alternate between
desire for personal gain (trips to Phuket, Thailand) and duty to police
bodies (HIV testing of women who cross the border into Thailand). As
individuals they balance practices that define HIV/AIDS as a fundamentally personal and confidential matter (Chen refusing to disclose
the HIV status of women at our first training) against practices that
treat HIV/AIDS as a border disease requiring forced police intervention

(high-security prisons and forced HIV tests for prostitutes). Furthermore, when epidemiologists such as Dr. Jing try to map cultural prejudices onto risk variables, the results may reflect their own prejudices
more than anything else (see Patton 1996). In addition, these state actors are operating within different historical memories, and thus different generations. Those who are younger were more open to and perhaps
better trained for taking into consideration the international norms and
literatures concerning harm reduction and HIV, versus those of an older
generation trained under Mao who were more apt to restrict persons
with HIV.[13]

In the case of HIV/AIDS, the state reacts to the exercise of individual
power by trying to craft new sets of boundaries and borders. When geography and politics are wedded in this way, HIV/AIDS ceases to be a
disease without borders and becomes a disease with distinct borders, as
if it seeps through only at certain points on a map, with no room for the
natives to slip through. As noted throughout this book, Chinese historians argue that even on the eve of liberation in 1953, the Xishuangbanna
borderlands were perceived as malaria- and leprosy-infested jungles full
of barbarians (Wang Lianfang 1993; Yin 1986).[14] These notions about
barbarians and barbaric diseases live on in the perceptions of Kunming
physicians such as Dr. Jing and of Shen in Menglian and Lao Yan in
Jinghong. Dr. Hui is concerned with the maintenance of a parochial
morality and seeks to control high-risk behaviors among commercial
sex workers and intravenous drug users. His ways are problematic in
the eyes of public health physicians such as Dr. Jing. Even Dr. Jing, who
is knowledgeable of harm reduction techniques, maintains that ethnic
minorities are more promiscuous than Han women such as herself.

This ethnography of everyday AIDS practices illuminates the internal
contradictions of the Chinese state and exposes the differing interests of
its bureaucratic actors, those who are often devoted to competing goals
and feelings. If we understand the state as acting locally (in Menglian),
nationally (in Beijing), and internationally (with NGOs), we recognize
that HIV/AIDS policy and action does represent a uniform narrative.
HIV/AIDS policies are often both local and transnational, negotiated by
actors who engage in relationships that span the local and transnational,
from the border to the center and back. Shen worked in Menglian in
rural Yunnan and catered to Beijing reporters at the heart of party
power, her Simao superiors in more central Yunnan, and the Australian-
Yunnan Red Cross, her international counterpart. Not only do straightforward distinctions between pure civil society and the state become

boundaries blurred, but so do the distinctions between where power resides and where it resists.[15] Borders and centers constantly highlight the processual and multidimensional characteristics of the Chinese state and reveal how identities are remade as the notion of borders shifts in and out of prevention projects. NGOs collaborate with state bureaucracies in order to carry out HIV/AIDS behavioral surveys and prevention in the borderlands, and in turn the state greases the wheels for NGOs to spread international HIV/AIDS discursive practices in a post-socialist state, one that not long ago closed off possibilities for discursive international exchange. State and society are integrated at the level of individual everyday AIDS practices, where modes of action are discursively constructed across time, space, and borders and where risky bodies and risky practices cast shadows on geography and epidemiology. The habitus of state actors inscribes their political subjectivity, and through their everyday AIDS practices these actors in turn inscribe the sovereignty of the state onto minority subjects. As I discuss in chapters 3 and 6, minority subjects themselves then inscribe their own identities in relationship to the state and in particular to the Han majority.

Here political subjectivity means that state government bureaucrats must balance their own emotions, their own personal moral and political convictions, with the goals of the state, and simultaneously, resist the unavoidable. Their political subjectivity is deeply influenced by the historical events that influenced their generation. Dr. Hui was of a revolutionary generation protecting the achievements of the Maoist state, while Lao Yan and Shen were of a Cultural Revolution generation whose lives were disrupted by the great departures in socialist governance and the upheaval of youth sent away from home to help rural peasants. Then there is the generation of Dr. Jing, who grew up in a later era and embraced the campaigns of modernization, including scientifically proven prevention methods such as harm reduction. In the end, late-socialist economies of prevention involve more than just biological power over everyday lives; they involve intimate feelings, political and moral ideals that influence government discourses through individuals working for the late-socialist state.

PART TWO

Narratives of Jinghong, Sipsongpanna

INTRODUCTION

If prostitutes constitute one of the key narratives of how HIV/AIDS is spread across the globe, it is essential to understand just what is happening at the local level in establishments that exchange sex for money. Equally important is an understanding of the construction of the places themselves. In the four chapters in part II, I turn my ethnographic lens inward toward sex tourism in the Chinese border town of Jinghong, Sipsongpanna Tai (Xishuangbanna Dai) Nationality Autonomous Prefecture. I thus move from the dominant political and scientific discourses around HIV/AIDS toward more local conceptions of the everyday practices of sexual modernity in the southwest border region of Sipsongpanna in the late 1990s. How has late-socialist development transformed the rural villages of Sipsongpanna into urban Jinghong, and how do tourism, sex tourism, and now AIDS affect this urbanization?

In these chapters I argue that Jinghong has a particular resonance in China as a place where the fantasies of sex, travel, and minority ethnicity come together. In the city of Jinghong I examine how fantasies of exotic Tai people are experimented with and fulfilled through prostitution with Han women, and how Han women in turn imagine and construct fantasies for Han male tourists through mimicking Tai women. The development project in Sipsongpanna is a story about how a small town on the Lancang (Mekong) River became a tourist destination and then later a place where sex tourism thrives. To understand why the city of Jinghong is now marketed as a sexy tourist destination, one must know its history.

Chapter 3 provides a social history of Sipsongpanna and the city of Jinghong. I introduce two key characters in Jinghong, a madam and one of her customers. Chapter 4 zeros in on a hair salon and the daily activity and lives of the women and men who work there. Chapter 5 looks specifically at prostitution, risk for STIs and HIV, and marketing of condoms in Jinghong. Chapter 6 analyzes China's changing sexual morality and some of the practices that mark sexuality as intrinsic to the urban and modern in Jinghong. It draws on my twenty interviews with men and women of diverse occupations, including prostitutes and their clients in Jinghong. Throughout these chapters, I explore how sexuality, ethnicity, tourism, development, and disease come together as a leitmotifs for modernity in a small border town.

CHAPTER 3

Sex Tourism and Performing Ethnicity in Jinghong

On a sweltering afternoon, so hot you can almost hear the sidewalks sizzle, grandmothers fan sleeping grandsons under the palm trees that line south Nationality Road. As fat black pigs rest on the dusty market tarmac, chain-smoking hooligans *(liumang)* laugh, joke, and watch plumes of blue smoke rise. As night falls, quietude disappears and motorcycles and red taxis filled with finely dressed tourists race to discos and bars blaring Japanese karaoke and American rock and roll. In this liminal time, subtle changes are taking place in terms of who occupies the streets. By day, locals go about their daily affairs; at night some of the two million tourists who flock to Sipsongpanna every year emerge from their air-conditioned hotel rooms, bringing with them a taste for a blend of commerce, capital, and commodity fetishism.

JINGHONG, XISHUANGBANNA

This chapter takes us to China's southwest border region of Xishuang-banna Dai Nationality Autonomous Prefecture (hereafter referred to by its Tai name, Sipsongpanna) in southern Yunnan in the late 1990s. Development in Sipsongpanna is a story about how a small town on the Lancang River became a city of sex tourism, where Han migration and China's state tourism policies transformed a series of large Tai villages into the cosmopolitan city of Jinghong. How has late-socialist development transformed the rural villages of Sipsongpanna into urban Jing-hong? Jinghong resonates in China as a place where the fantasies of sex, travel, and minority ethnicity come together. Examining how travelers, migrants, and locals negotiate imagining Sipsongpanna and visiting and living there enriches our understanding of Chinese sexual modernity and one contemporary Chinese "site of desire." In this exploration of sexuality and sexual practices, I note that while the popular press often marks late-socialist China as making strong breaks from previous regimes, such as the Maoist era, I see a continuum of thinking and prac-tices around sexuality. Recent Chinese literary accounts of the Cultural Revolution have pointed toward the sexualization, as well as the in-crease in birth rates, during that epoch as evidence that even a regime represented as gender neutral and conservative had its sexual peaks and erotic desires (see Zhang Xianliang 1991; Min 1997).

I present my argument about Chinese sexual modernity and desire in three parts. First, a brief social history points toward current construc-tions of Sipsongpanna and the city of Jinghong as sites of desire in con-temporary China. Second, I explore how exoticism in Sipsongpanna is marked by celebrating an ethnic erotic practiced by Han women per-forming and playing on the cultural characteristics of Tai-Lüe ethnicity. I explore how fantasies of the exotic Tai are experimented with and ful-filled through prostitution performed by Han women and how in turn Han women imagine and construct fantasies for Han male tourists through their practices.[1] I discuss this eroticization of ethnicity in my ethnography of two people connected to the New Wind Beauty Salon in Jinghong: the madam who owned the salon and a businessman and cus-tomer. Third, I conclude with an analysis of China's changing sexual morality and some of the practices that mark sexuality as intrinsic to modernity in Jinghong. What emerges is a place that is, by virtue of both geography and ethnicity, on the margins of the Chinese nation. Al-though Jinghong is at the very tip of southern Yunnan Province in an au-tonomous minority prefecture, it is actually not so marginal or so tradi-tional after all.

GLOBAL CONSUMPTION, TOURISM, AND PROSTITUTION

Jinghong is a city of prostitution *(piaocheng)*, according to the local folklore, and in terms of the local economy, it provides Han Chinese male tourists with a lucrative sex tourist destination. Male tourists come to Jinghong to consume Tai women. However, as I have pointed out, the majority of prostitutes are not Tai but Han women from Sichuan and Guizhou who often dress in Tai clothing to attract Han male customers. They, just like the men who solicit them, provide an allure that is marketed in tourist brochures. As a site of desire, Jinghong encompasses what is unique about emerging sex tourism in China and about Chinese ethnic boundaries in Sipsongpanna.[2] Practices of sex tourism are, again, part of these global sites of desire. With the re-emergence of a culture of conspicuous consumption comes the conspicuous consumption of women. In Jinghong, as in the nearby country of Thailand, business culture is often seen as contiguous with the culture of sexuality and sexual consumption. Jiemin Bao (1998) writes that Chinese businessmen in Thailand partake of Thai business cultural norms by seeking out sexual entertainment from bar girls and prostitutes. In Jinghong, a similar phenomenon occurs when businessmen who vacation there seek out sexual entertainment. The venue for this entertainment is the hair salon–cum-brothel. Hair salons that function as brothels are common throughout East Asia, including Japan, Korea, Taiwan, and Hong Kong (Allison 1994).

Thus this market is not unique to China but rather is part of a larger circulation of sex as a global commodity. In many tourist spots around the world, including Sipsongpanna's southern neighbor Thailand, both foreign and local men seek the pleasures of other local women and men (Odzer 1994; Bell and Valentine 1995; Manderson and Jolly 1997; Bishop and Robinson 1998; Law 2000). In the Caribbean and parts of West Africa, it is female tourists from North America and Europe who seek the pleasures of these exotic lands by consuming sun, sand, surf, and the companionship and services of local men.[3] While the relationships between Euro-America, Southeast Asia, and Africa are obviously complicated and intersected by unequal power and political relationships, there are also sex tourism sites in almost all large cities in the United States. The most well known are the several counties in Nevada where prostitution is legal and where men come from all over the world to exchange money for sexual favors.

Constructing this site of desire out of the rural jungle that is southern Yunnan Province involves conceptualizing an urban journey into a place that is idealized as both a tropical paradise and an exotic home to an ethnic erotic. To market Sipsongpanna to greater China and Han Chinese, the notions of a peripheral space—a space outside the norms of urban living in Shanghai, Guangzhou, Nanjing, or even Kunming—must be maintained. Tai women are depicted as sexual exotics in everything from images on clothes, to films about Han youth sent down to rural minority areas during the Cultural Revolution to educate the great masses, to canvases of the Yunnan School of painting that capture their bodies (see Zhang Luanxin 1985). These markets eroticize the ways Tai women represent their sexuality—large uncovered breasts, thin waists, and tightly wrapped sarongs (see Gladney 1994; McKhann 1995; Lufkin 1990). Sipsongpanna is marketed as a rural paradise complete with an urban center that coordinates, manages, and filters such rural pleasures as elephant riding and Tai women bathing in the river. Jinghong, like many global tourist destinations, holds an exotic fantasy world for those embarking on a journey there, while it provides the amenities of urban modernity. This notion of modernity, like that in much of North America, embraces sexual desire and pleasure as legitimate while it simultaneously castigates purveyors of prostitution as dangerous, polluting Others.

A BRIEF HISTORY OF SIPSONGPANNA

Prior to the thirteenth century, Sipsongpanna (literally, "twelve rice fields") was a de facto former kingdom of Thailand, with links to the other three major northern kingdoms of Lan Na, Keng Tung, and Lan Zhang (Hsieh 1995:308, Ai Feng 1995). According to Tai historian Ratanaporn Sethakul (2000), the Tai-Lüe state was unlike other Tai states in that it remained a confederation of a dozen or more allied, ruling classes related to each other by kinship *(chau or panna)*. The Tai-Lüe kingdom was weakened by the interference of its two powerful neighbors, China and Burma, as both wanted to keep Sipsongpanna as a buffer state to ensure peaceful frontiers. According to a popular Tai legend, the region was once part of the sea, which receded to reveal a beautiful oasis; but a demon came to rule and took it back into the darkness. A young Tai man fought this demon for seven days and seven nights, until he finally took a sparkling pearl from the darkness. He hung this pearl on a coconut tree, and it lit the darkness of the city with the light of dawn, and the people shouted "City of dawn!" (Ai Feng 1995; oral accounts from informants). Sipsongpanna became a Chinese tributary state as early as the thirteenth century when the Mongols ruled much of Yunnan, although they did not interfere in the kingdom's internal affairs. With the rise of the Taugoo dynasty (1531–1758) in Burma, Sipsongpanna became a state with two suzerains, and allegiance was paid to both the Chinese emperor and the Burmese King (Sethakul 2000: 69–74). The Sip-

songpanna kingdom became Xishuangbanna Dai Nationality Autonomous Prefecture on January 24, 1953, when the Communists integrated
this suzerainty into mainland China as part of the process of Sinicizing
all regions of China (Hsieh 1995: 315). In northern Tai, Sipsongpanna
also translates as "twelve townships." These regions originated from the
Tai federation of twelve states that ruled the region. Sipsongpanna is
unique in terms of its geography, which is both mountainous and tropical, and its diverse ethnic groups. China has designated several regions
that have a high percentage of China's fifty-five official minorities as "autonomous" and given them a pseudo-autonomous governing structure.

Sipsongpanna has a land base of nineteen thousand square kilometers and is situated on the Yunnan plateau, which is divided by the Lancang River. The river winds down from the northwest to the south of the
prefecture and continues into Southeast Asia, where it is known as the
Mekong. Sipsongpanna is divided into two counties and one main city:
Menghai County to the southwest, Mengla County to the southeast,
and Jinghong city, the regional capital, close to the center.[4]

In the early 1950s the Han population of Sipsongpanna was around
5,700 (less than 10 percent of the total); it increased to just under
230,000 (more than 30 percent) by the early 1970s. By the end of 2003,
the total population grew to 873,694, of which 75 percent were ethnic
minorities, the Tai being the largest at 35 percent of the total population. In 1986 Jinghong city's population was 30,000; by 1996 the population had increased to over 130,000; and by 2002 it was slightly over
371,000, a more than twelve-fold increase in sixteen years (Jinghong
Publicity Department 2005). The population increase in both these
waves of migration consisted of Han Chinese, who currently make up
over 30 percent of the urban population.[5]

Zhang Li (2001), in her work on Beijing migrants, shows that this
large floating population (liudong renkou) has spread out across China
in search of work opportunities that are not available in local townships
and farms. Not only do migrant workers uproot themselves, but with
increasing mobility and disposable income, Han Chinese tourists also
travel to Sipsongpanna to escape their work-a-day lives in the metropo-
lises of Shanghai, Nanjing, and Kunming. Although 90 percent of Sipsongpanna's tourists are mainland Chinese, the immigrants are drawn
from the wider Asian diaspora—the Singaporean who cuts hair in a
salon owned by someone from Macao and the Pakistani who travels
from Burma to sell jade (see Qin 1995). Migrant Chinese workers also
come from Sichuan to drive taxicabs, from Hunan to sell imported Ko-

rean clothing, and from Guizhou to run beauty salons–cum-brothels *(meirong ting* or *meirong yuan).* It is Han tourists from urban China with high incomes who sustain the tourism industry, just as it is Han migrants who provide service work, including "sex work."

Historically, Sipsongpanna was not a Han tourist destination. The Han Chinese came to Sipsongpanna in three distinct waves of migration: in the 1950s to plant rubber; in the late 1960s through the late 1970s, during the Cultural Revolution, as educated youth "sent down" *(xiaxiang)* to serve poor minorities; and in the 1980s to further develop local state resources such as manganese and rubber, the largest cash crop in the region.[6] As Grant Evans (2000) points out, from 1949 until 1978 China had almost no significant foreign trade with Yunnan Province, and it lived up to its name as a "mysterious land south of the clouds."[7] In the late 1980s and early 1990s, several Tai villages south of Jinghong were demolished in the process of building a new economic development zone for joint venture hotels, restaurants, and tourist parks. According to local rumors, little or no compensation was given to village leaders for confiscation of their lands.

Under provincial policies in the late 1980s, Han authorities opened trade routes into the Golden Quadrangle of Laos, northern Thailand, Burma, and southwestern China, clearing pathways for future transnational flows and migrations of people. The central Beijing government viewed Sipsongpanna as a critical gateway into Southeast Asia for trade, goods, and tourists (Zheng Lan 1981). Opening this gateway also meant marketing the region through tourism (see Liu Dajing 2004). Recently numerous tourist websites have sprouted to describe the pleasures and wonders of a place that retains one-sixth of China's incredible plant diversity and thirteen of Yunnan's twenty-two ethnic minority groups (see Tropical Forest Ecosystem Management Project 1999; Margraf 1999; eChina Romance 2001). Sipsongpanna was the launching point for emerging ethnic and ecological tourism into tropical rain forests, Buddhist temples, and Tai villages in the mid-1980s. In 1993, UNESCO designated Sipsongpanna as a world biosphere reserve because of its incredible plant and animal life. Due to its tropical rain forests, biodiversity, and three main nature reserves, in the late 1980s, Sipsongpanna had also become a honeymoon spot for Han couples, a place of rest and relaxation for businessmen, and a prime destination for government-sponsored, all-expenses-paid work unit meetings *(danwei kaocha).* By the early-1990s, a very different kind of tourist arrived in Jinghong, the middle-aged male with money to spend in brothels and on dancing girls and gambling. In Jinghong, sex tourism is practiced under the guise of new occupations in karaoke bars, hair salons, barbershops, massage parlors, saunas, and bars, where services extend beyond the karaoke microphone and the blow dryer. Massage parlors not only provide massages but also have on-site escort services through which young women may entertain men in the privacy of their hotel rooms.

In 1995 more than 1.5 million tourists came to Sipsongpanna, of which more than 90 percent were newly prosperous Han Chinese from greater China (Qin 1995). Almost ten years later, in 2004, the number of tourists increased to 2.71 million Chinese (99 percent) and around 33,000 foreign nationals (1 percent) (www.bndaily.com.cn March 29, 2005). The largest majority of tourists are middle-class Han Chinese who come to Sipsongpanna for rest and relaxation at the end of their Kunming-based business meetings. Jinghong is a forty-five-minute flight or twenty-four-hour bus ride from Kunming. The regional development office now paints what Evans calls a Disneyesque picture of the future, capturing the world beyond China's very real and enforced borders (see Anagnost 1989 & 1997; Ren 1998 & 2005; Evans 2000). Sipsongpanna provides a unique case, for although few Chinese have passports to travel overseas, they can go on excursions to Chinese-controlled border towns in both Burma and Laos.[8] Once there, tourists can spend Chinese yuan in Chinese-run businesses, thus benefiting the Chinese on both sides of the border. The local development office now plans to resurrect the largest Tai temple torn down during the Cultural Revolution and to bring Southeast Asia closer to the relatively closed borders of China in a theme park (Evans 2000; Ai Kham 2002). By 2000, a three-hundred-meter-long bridge was built across the Lancang to connect the industrial district with the commercial center of Jinghong. Sipsongpanna benefited from some of the larger Association of Southeast Asian Nations (ASEAN) development projects, such as building a superhighway between Yunnan and Thailand. Li, a young man of twenty-nine who works for the provincial public security bureau *(sheng gonganjü)*, pointed out that key leaders of the local police went to a conference in Las Vegas in 1995 and returned with visions in their heads of turning Singhong into the Las Vegas of China.

As economic development took root under Deng's dictum "To get rich is glorious," the state appropriated collective farmland and redistributed it for private redevelopment. As four-star international hotels (built by Thai Chinese, Taiwanese Chinese, and Shanghainese developers) rose from these fields, rice cultivation in the two adjacent Tai villages of Manjinglan and Manting were eliminated.[9] Tai were critical of this appropriation, while most local Han understood it in terms of progress and development. Wu, a Han woman of twenty-five, was born and raised in Jinghong and was a teacher by profession and a tour guide and secretary on the side. She told me this story:

> Jinghong was very poor prior to economic reforms; everyone was treated the same and served the same, respected everybody's spirit *(women feng-xian jingshen)*. When I was growing up in Jinghong, the only large buildings were the prefecture's Communist Party headquarters. The site of the Xishuangbanna Hotel was a Tai village called Manyun. Now the Tai villagers are landlords, they have become rich subdividing the bottom dirt floors of their houses into rooms for let. Before, the peasant's trade market was just vegetable fields: the road to the Teacher Training School was just dirt. Everything changed with the airport; with planes came new businesses; with new businesses came the underworld or Chinese mafia *(heishe-hui)*. Prostitution came in 1992 and gambling in 1994. Jinghong is definitely now a town dependent on the tourism industry *(lüyouye)* . . . we have moved from an idealistic to a realistic society.

For Wu, China under socialism was very idealistic, but under Deng Xiaoping's strive for market socialism it had become more realistic, providing jobs outside the work unit *(danwei)* system, as well as encouraging newfound leisure activities. No informant, including Wu, could give me an exact genealogy of prostitution; however, many stated that "it came with the airport," as if flights and sex went together. These new-found pleasures and entertainments are what I term "icons of modern Chinese sexual morality." Since what drives this sexual consumption is the marketization of the ethnic and ethnicity, I now turn to conceptions of race and ethnicity in China.

CONTEMPORARY CHINESE NOTIONS OF RACE AND ETHNICITY

The Communist Party came to power in 1949 and, in the early 1950s, sponsored a program of ethnic identification, sending hundreds of ethnographic researchers to the border areas to distinguish the Han from the non-Han (see Fei 1980; Guldin 1994; Harrell 1995). Applying Engels's reworking of anthropologist Lewis Henry Morgan's stage theory of evolution, the Maoist researchers identified the Han majority as occupying the scientific pinnacle of civilization, and the non-Han, a lower economic stage on the evolutionary scale. Under Mao Zedong, race *(minzu)* was understood as synonymous with class, and racial minorities in China were counted predominantly in relationship to poverty. The definition of a minority was based on Stalin's four criteria for a common nationality: territory, language, economy, and nature. By 1956 the results were to create fifty-one officially recognized minority groups that constituted 8 percent of the population, with the remaining 92 percent of the population being the Han majority. Among the fifty-five ethnic groups China recognizes today, the largest groups are the Mongolian, Hui, Miao, and Uygur. The Tai are the seventeenth largest with just over 1.1 million people (Li Dexi 2003).[10]

In contemporary China this notion of race is still prevalent, but it is intersected by other conceptions of race and ethnicity. Rey Chow (2002) points out the slippage between the concepts of race and ethnicity, race being associated with sociobiology and physical determinism, and ethnicity being perceived as a cultural category. In China this slippage is more apparent than elsewhere. In the Chinese language *minzu* means "nationality," but it is often translated as "ethnicity," as in *shaoshu minzu* or "minority ethnicities." Other ways of interpreting Chinese conceptions of race and ethnicity that are critical to my argument include those articulated in Emily Honig's (1992) work on the Subei of Shanghai. As in Jinghong, "native-place" and rural roots came to define the Subei as having a secondary and often derogatory status among the Han population. Race in the Middle Kingdom was not only a highly contested category but also subject to what Louisa Schein (1997) and Dru Gladney (1994) term a new kind of orientalism—"internal orientalism."[11] Schein (2000: 101) argues that there is fascination with the idea of a more cosmopolitan Chinese culture read against minority exotic cultures, which produces an array of gender divides—most prominently, the minority as represented by rural women, and the Han observer as represented by the urban male.

In Sipsongpanna, ethnic groups are divided not only by economic class and occupation but also by geographic space—where they live. The landscape in Sipsongpanna is subtropical. The Tai minority controls the lowland wet-rice fields, the Bulang minority the middle hillsides, the Akha the mountaintops, and the Han Chinese the townships of Mengla, Menghai, and Jinghong. However, there is more to these differences than their brief description suggests. The poorest villages in Sipsongpanna often consist of the minority groups that represent the smallest proportion of the population: the Jinuo, Yao, and Wa. The question remains: how does an implicit hierarchy of racial typologies operate in daily practice? The trajectory that development takes in contemporary

China leads to the creation of particular racial and sexual subjects, subjects that emerge from the ashes of the prereform era. In her work on colonial Southeast Asia, Ann Stoler (1998) examines the confluences of sexuality, race, and ethnicity, rather than treating them as distinctive categories. The practice of empire building in the nineteenth and early twentieth centuries, and its attendant construction of a racial Other, meant that European sexual discourses read the colonies as a world apart from European sensibility. Europeans often portrayed the natives as wild and sexual, and themselves as staid and proper. If defining oneself as "proper" requires defining oneself against an Other, Han China would perceive non-Han China as a repository of pleasure, a China that is as highly sexed as it is raced. The postreform Chinese state is a key player in these representations of the borderlands *(bianjiang)* and their association with pleasure, sex, and desire, because economic development in the form of tourism uses these representations for marketing purposes (see Manderson and Jolly 1997).

As for the city of Jinghong and the eroticization of local minority women, there is an historical precedent here. The Han-educated youth "sent down" to the Sipsongpanna countryside during the Cultural Revolution relayed, through their literary works and films, popular Han stories of the Tai as an erotic and promiscuous ethnic culture. Deng Xian's (1990) *Dreams of China's Educated Youth (Zhongguo Zhiqing Meng)* and Zhang Luanxin's (1985) film *Sacrificed Youth (Qingchun Ji)* both portray the Tai-Lüe as more sexually enlightened than the Han Chinese.[12] Beginning in the late 1980s, a school of painting, the Yunnan School (Yunnan Huapai), emerged, composed of predominantly Han artists depicting minority people (Lufkin 1990). Much of the work of the Yunnan School itself focused on the eroticization of minority women, Tai women in particular. A catalogue from a Yunnan School collection typically features portrayals that resemble eroticized pinups from the West (see Sun Tairen 1995). Here not just beautiful minority women are being consumed but also a representation of them as the embodiment of Western sexuality read through Tai-ness. The Yunnan School of painting was extremely popular in Europe and North America in the late 1980s and early 1990s, and now many Han Chinese, at least in Yunnan, are also purchasing these works.

In Louisa Schein's work on the dichotomy between Han and non-Han, there is also a third category that is not presented here, the Western white women (Schein 1994). Although she is not illustrated in the Yunnan paintings of Tai women, she is present in depictions of sexual promiscuity and in places of sexual consumption. In the hair salons where I conducted fieldwork, posters representing Western white women lined the walls, and these images carried over to magazines and photo-novella comic books used for HIV/AIDS prevention. In the local context of Jinghong, only a small percentage of tourists were foreigners or whites. Here they include mainly the Lonely Planet backpacker variety en route to Laos, English teachers (four to six at the local college), and a few businesspeople who are experimenting with coffee cultivation. The concept of whiteness is also present in some massage parlor and hair salon owners' alleged refusal to service "white" and "black" foreign customers for fear they had HIV/AIDS. At other times, people such as Madam Liu wanted me to encourage foreign customers, as she saw them as a more lucrative clientele. And finally, whiteness also appears in the form of the ethnographer.

After being denied permission to study Tai village life in Dehong Tai-Jingpo Minority Autonomous Prefecture, a county with high prevalence of HIV/AIDS, I was redirected to Jinghong and Sipsongpanna. My earlier discussions with local authorities about the Tai prompted their speculation that because the Tai in Dehong Tai-Jingpo had high rates of AIDS, so might the Tai in Sipsongpanna. In this process, I came to study less the life of people living with AIDS in villages than the life of a city in transition, a city very much part of ethnic tourism and the rise of urban pleasures—trading sex for money in karaoke bars, beauty salons, and massage parlors. However, reaching out to an illegal industry with the face and body of a Western white women held both challenges and opportunities: the male clients often eagerly accepted me, while the women did not, and it took me two fieldwork trips to be accepted into the underground "sex worker" culture.[13] In a way, I became a player in these narratives and stories that I collected; I was a player in my performance of ethnography (Ebron 2002).

PERFORMING ETHNICITY

As previously stated, several sinologists have argued for a more careful reading of Chinese ethnicity, one that views ethnic categories as fluid and socially constructed through both time and space (Gladney 1991 & 1994; Harrell 1995; Schein 2000; Litzinger 2000a; Mueggler 2001). In exploring the social construction of ethnicity, it is important to recognize the nuances between social representations of the Tai and actual Tai cultural practices. In Jinghong, because Han migrants and tourists both claim to appropriate authentic images of Tai culture, ethnicity is an especially malleable category. However, even the fluidity of ethnic boundaries has its limits. Louisa Schein (1997 & 2000) has noted in her work on tourism and the Miao minority that the Han often construct the non-Han as feminized minority Others. In Sipsongpanna this is evident in the local market economy for sex tourism. Consumers—Han men—drive the market for ethnic women, who are in fact Han women who mimic Tai culture for profit. But money is not the only desired form of profit here: what these Han women can do away from home, away from watchful eyes, is also important. Over and over again, people remarked that Sipsongpanna is the land of freedom, unbounded cultural limits, and promiscuous sex. Also, ethnic boundaries in Sipsongpanna are very much shaped by its recent history of what might be called a colonizing process. In Jinghong, depictions of Tai-Lüe minority girls are eroticized in everything from advertisements for karaoke bars to dance halls— including a sign in the town of Mengla encouraging tourists to watch Tai-Lüe bathing beauties (see Hyde 2001). In an effort to understand local representations of the Tai in Sipsongpanna, I present here a few of the images of minorities.

A contemporary belief among other ethnic groups in Sipsongpanna is that the Tai are the most intelligent, clever, and enterprising of the minority ethnic groups. They have culture *(tamen you wenhua)*, unlike the Bulang or Lahu, in that the Tai possess a written language based on ancient Pali-Hindu texts and are practicing Theravada Buddhists who train young males in the old traditions.[14] These beliefs are mitigated by the influence of Chinese (Han) entrepreneurs who remark that "the locals" (an epithet for the local minority groups) are stupid because they do not have a clue about how to run a business: "Locals don't know how to eat bitterness" (Bendi ren bu hui chi ku). "To eat bitterness" in China has multiple meanings, but here it means that one must work hard and suffer in order to later reap the benefits of one's labor. When outsiders say the locals don't know how to eat bitterness, they mean they don't know how to delay gratification. This further illustrates the instability of stereotypes, but it does not negate their overall power.

The Tai have in fact become economically and socially marginalized in urban Jinghong because of their absence from one of the main businesses, that of selling sex. Local Tais explained this absence as linked to their strength in maintaining cultural values and traditions. Here the local Tai read themselves as superior to the Han, who have forgotten traditional Confucian notions of fidelity. However, although people while in the Tai villages upheld notions of traditional culture that read against images of sexual promiscuity, in the city of Jinghong local Tais often internalized their inferiority. Many local Tai entrepreneurs who were engaged in business similarly mentioned that their friends and family members did not know how to work hard or simply did not like to work. When I asked Ai Yang, the young owner of an appliance store, how he could call his Tai compatriots "lazy, unable to eat bitterness," when he was successful, he shrugged his shoulders and said, "I am different, not like other Tai."

In Jinghong, Tai villagers no longer grow as much sticky rice as they once did, because they have become landlords for the local Han immigrants who live beneath Tai homes in the spaces formerly reserved for farm machinery and pigs. Though Tai locals joked about Han living in spaces formerly reserved for the pigs, the Han migrants' situation was very precarious because the government could crack down on illegally registered tenants at any time (Evans 2000). By 1996 one could no longer purchase a transfer of one's right to permanent residence *(hukou)* and thus to local benefits and state protections and services. Prior to 1996 a wealthy migrant could purchase a local *hukou* for three thousand yuan, but by 2000, one could apply for only a temporary residence permit *(zhanzhu zheng)*. Tenants purchasing residence permits are mainly Han migrant youth, both male and female, who come to Jinghong from China's hinterland in search of employment and the good life. Another consequence of the Hanification of Sipsongpanna is that Han businesses are buying out the Tai. In 1995 on Manting Street, three or four restaurants were run by local Tais, but by 1996 there were no substantial Tai-run businesses. Han businessmen had bought most of the Tai-owned restaurants and then turned them into clubs replete with pseudo-Tai dancing, dinner table massages, and pseudo-Tai food. By 2002 all of the street signs and message boards that were once bilingual, in Mandarin Chinese and Tai, were now in Mandarin only.

One local teacher, Ai Lao, thirty-four years old, complained bitterly that the breakdown in Tai culture has been detrimental not only to Tai farming methods but also to traditional cultural practices. Ai Lao was involved in several projects intended to revive Tai culture: playing in a local all-Tai rock band, teaching at the local temple school, and organizing cross-border exchanges with Tai-Lüe in Burma, Laos, and Thailand. For Ai Yang and Ai Lao, the city of Jinghong embraces both the promotion of Tai culture (it brings in money and capital) and revulsion against and destruction of that culture (by sanitizing Tai practices through refusing to promote the old Tai language, rebuilding old temples only if they agreed to be tourist sites, and paving over village farm plots). The consequences of this production and destruction of Tai culture means Sipsongpanna Tai are looking beyond China to the former borders of the Tai nation for support and capital for such endeavors as training young monks, preserving the Buddhist palm leaf scriptures,[15] and investing in Tai businesses (Hsieh 1995).[16]

Although the Han eroticization of Tai ethnicity has altered Tai subjectivity, it is precisely this Han representation of Tai women as beautiful, sexualized, and at home in their tropical paradise that makes Sipsongpanna a desirable travel location. When the Han Chinese majority in Sipsongpanna configures the Tai in their own imaginations as licentious, free, and lazy, the Tai are conceptualized as weak, eroticized subjects for people in greater China. Here the logic of internal orientalism takes root: the Tai are constructed as an Other and are sexualized in the Han imagination, in the way that desire has been fused in China with both the sexual and the political (see Schein 1996). The eroticism of the Tai body has been written over in what Schein calls "a palimpsest of other meanings," including the political meanings of freedom, individualism, progress, and critiques of morality (1996: 144). In Sipsongpanna, the Han women represent and perform Tai-ness for a Han audience in order to achieve secondary gains in their own economic status, personal freedoms, desires, and amusements. What we see here is precisely what Schein defines as the engendering of ethnic groups—women represent traditional minority culture and men modern Han Chinese culture.

In Jinghong, what is Tai sells, and therefore one merely becomes Tai in order to profit. This applies most readily to the many Han women who dress in Tai clothing to attract Han male customers. Local Han entertainment workers—including those in occupations that do not involve sex such as tour guides, restaurant servers, and singers and dancers—dress in a facsimile of traditional Tai women's clothes: the close-fitting, floor-length *longyi* and a cropped, long-sleeved top with many small snaps in place of buttons. Since Han Chinese women from Sichuan and Guizhou who work in the brothels, nightclubs, and karaoke bars all dress in traditional Tai costumes, they are often at first glance perceived as local Tai by Han tourists. All one has to do is speak with these women to know they are not from Jinghong, for their accents often give them away. However, this impersonation is also perpetuated because, when asked, most of the Jinghong prostitutes would say they are locals.

What concerns me here is how performing ethnicity can be read against Judith Butler's (1990) notion of the performativity of gender. In brief, Butler argues that the body provides a material surface on which various acts and gestures acquire gendered meanings, as opposed to the body being the natural ground of an ontological essence. By focusing on drag, cross-dressing, and the sexual stylization of butch/femme identities within American lesbian culture, Butler suggests that drag performance has the virtue of showing that being feminine or masculine entails performing specific bodily signs rather than being specific bodies.

I do not read ethnicity as authentic or nonauthentic, but as part of China's invention of a modern identity as the country rapidly moves in the direction of the global markets that consume ethnic identity, status, and stigma. As the Chinese government capitalizes on its multicultural and multiethnic quilt in producing touristy visions of the small China in Shenzhen or the ethnic minority parks in Beijing and Kunming (see Ren 1998), so do individual Chinese citizens capitalize on multiculturalism by adopting ethnic dress and styles in the sex trade. Dressing and acting Tai makes prostitutes in Jinghong more valuable. There is also a certain irony here in that, though valued as Tai, the women are chastised as prostitutes. It is precisely this mimesis of Tai-Lüe ethnicity that creates the impression that ethnic Tai women predominate in Jinghong's sex trade. This impression is read against its opposite, that Han women are asexual or less sexual than their ethnic Other. The women working at the salon were also looked at with a combination of distain for engaging in transactional sex and admired for their business acumen—just as Madam Liu was perceived.

FEMALE FANTASIES OF WORK: MADAM LIU'S BEAUTY SALON

Madam Liu begins by shouting at men passing by: "Do you want your hair washed? How about a massage? My girls here give great massages!" Most men ignore her or just stare, others opt for the hair wash, and then she begins negotiating with them over additional services. A massage is a euphemism for a hand job. Most of the on-site services never go beyond a massage and a hand job, but sometimes local men request a particular woman for the evening, often Xiao Wang—her beauty is in high demand.[17] She plays her cards carefully, commenting, "If I don't like the looks of someone, he's a nerd (shudaizi), or I would rather just chat with you, I refuse a potential customer." Overhearing this, Madam Liu yells back at her: "You're so lazy—so beautiful but so lazy."

I spent my summer evenings at Madam Liu's, where she cackled in her Guizhounese accent and joked about the excellent massages provided by her "foreign staff"—referring to me. Madam Liu operated this beauty salon that in many ways was a front for a type of brothel.[18] I use her story as an ethnographic canvas to sketch how sex tourism in this border region actually instantiates the social imaginary that tourism provokes. Prostitution temporarily functions as a quasi-legal business under the gaze of the state. I define it as quasi-legal because prostitution functions under the guise of barbershops and hair salons. Although the salon is legal, the back rooms are illegal. The local policemen warn some of their favorite brothel owners when a nationwide government anti-crime campaign (yanda yundong) is about to begin. There is definitely a complicated but often cohesive and cordial relationship between legitimate businesses; businesses on the periphery, such as hair salons that are also brothels; and the local police, who represent the Chinese state. None of the activities associated with sex tourism are legally sanctioned by the state, but they are allowed to function in certain guises. The sex industry masks itself under certain types of hair salons that are spatially divided by task: the outer storefronts are hair salons; the middle rooms are massage parlors; and the inner sanctums, small rooms with beds, are the brothels.

Liu, a Rubenesque Han woman in her late thirties, says she is divorced from her husband, who remained in Guizhou province. A resident of Jinghong since 1994, Liu and her lover Tan, a tour bus driver, own the New Wind Beauty Salon. In our conversations, Liu said she was extremely glad when she came to Jinghong; it meant an escape from drudgery and her miserable marriage. Madam Liu liked to tease me by asking provocative questions about my sexuality. "How can you know China without tasting Chinese men?" she often asked. "In Sipsongpanna, men taste like sticky rice (nuomifan), in Thailand like pineapple rice (boluofan), and in Guizhou like plain white rice (bai fan)." She asked me what American men taste like.

Liu regularly works from one o'clock in the afternoon to one in the morning, doing haircuts in the afternoon and at night dispatching her staff out on calls. The majority of the sex conducted through the salon consists of sensual massages (anmo), hand jobs (tuiyou or "pushing-out oil," or the local euphemism dafeiji, or "hit the airplane"), and sometimes sex with hair salon customers back in their hotel rooms.[19] Sex acts that were unsafe (exchanging bodily fluids) and required condoms were conducted on these out-calls. Men negotiate these encounters by driving or walking up to the salon and discussing the price and place with Liu. She then yells to a woman to come over and accompany the man to his hotel. When I met Liu, she had four women working in her salon—*all* ethnically Han.

Throughout Jinghong in 1997 there were about one hundred hair salons. Some were genuine beauty salons that only cut hair; others, like Liu's, cut hair and conducted a prostitution business on the side; and still others were complete facades. For Liu's salon workers, Sipsongpanna is the land of opportunity, but an opportunity that has to be masked, for they cannot share their professions with their families in their natal homes. Because the use of hair salons as fronts for prostitution is so widespread, even mentioning that they work in a salon could be dangerous. Just as prostitution has to be hidden behind the facades of beauty parlors, these women had to lie to their families about what they do.

As mentioned earlier, to understand Sipsongpanna, one must look at tourism as creating an experience outside the mundane; tourism and tourist practices build on the fantasies through which people ascribe meaning to urban living (King 1996). To travel to Sipsongpanna is to move from the profane to the sacred, to move outside of everyday lives into fantasies marketed by re-creating authentic Tai-ness. Sipsongpanna is that fantasy, and sex with Han women who look like beautiful Tai women is one of the pleasures it provides. However, prostitution is not a monolithic enterprise; its myriad forms are expressed in different ways at different times and in different geographic locations.

I turn now to one tale among many diverse male fantasies of Sipsongpanna. While women prostitutes capitalize on their beauty and mimic Tai ethnicity, it is men who consume such images by consuming these women. If women come to Sipsongpanna for money, profits, and freedom, the question remains: why are men coming?

MALE FANTASIES OF PLAY: MANAGER ZHOU

Head counts on each of the flights from which I disembarked in Jinghong in the late 1990s revealed that most planes were full of men. On some flights of two hundred passengers, I was one of only two or three females. A few times, all-female work unit tour groups skewed the balance to around 60 percent males, 40 percent females.

As China enters international markets, new products must be invented to ensure the increasing prosperity of its citizenry. Leisure travel, sexual products and the consumption of sex, and the exchange of money for sexual favors all become part of what it means to have a modern urban sexual identity. Chinese male tourists come to Sipsongpanna to chase young Tai women as an expression of their modern consumption practices. These wealthy men perform their roles by consuming not only dinners, fancy hotel rooms, and bottles of XO cognac but also the fantasy women they pay for. Only certain categories of women are consumable—not all women and certainly not all prostitutes.

Sipsongpanna's sexual pleasures carry connotations far beyond intrinsic physical satisfaction to cultural capital. In Sipsongpanna, it is precisely these nouveau riche male tourists who come to consume sex and women. Even though the Yunnan government condones neither prostitution nor gambling, several informants described Jinghong as one of the most popular places in China to seek both (for other locales, see Allison 1994; McClintock 1995; Manderson and Jolly 1997).[20] Sitting in his friend's café, a wealthy Hong Kong businessman asked a local businessman what he should invest in. The local man told him, "Why, prostitution and gambling—that is where the money is." Although Liu's female workers such as Xiao Ling, Xiao Gu, Xiao Yue, and Xiao Wang have varied relationships with the city of Jinghong, the tourists and businessmen are the ones who ultimately drive the eroticization of images. Their relationship with the place provides another picture of Jinghong. To illustrate this drive to eroticize place, I turn to Zhou, a man in his mid-forties and an assistant manager of a trading company in Jiangxi. He was in Sipsongpanna for an extended business meeting and vacation.

After numerous requests from Liu's customers to join them in the nightclubs, one night I acquiesced and went out on a date with Manager Zhou, who frequented the hair salon for massages.[21] I decided it would be an ethnographic exchange: he wanted to discuss American politics as we gambled and danced the night away, and I wanted to find out why he came to Sipsongpanna. The majority of sex worker clients are urban officials and businessmen under the age of thirty-five who are part of China's project to develop its midlevel cities (Settle 2003: 6). After several hours of gambling at the "Elephant Spring Hotel" (a pseudonym), I finally got my nerve up to talk about Liu. I almost fell off my chair when he asked me the rhetorical question: "Of course, you know she is not a hairdresser?" I replied affirmatively that I most certainly did.

When I asked him how he and his colleagues came to engage in massages, he laughed: "I'm on vacation, away from my wife; of course, I want some relaxation accompanied by beautiful women." A friend of a friend of mine articulated his feelings about infidelity this way: "Sex is like eating. If I eat cabbage *(baicai)* every day, I may want some fancy seafood *(haiwei)* once in a while. If you eat seafood every day, you want cabbage. For one cannot live by eating the same thing all the time. It gets boring!"

Manager Zhou did not discuss his trips to Sipsongpanna with his wife but said that going to Sipsongpanna was a frequent treat for him. He did not consider gambling out of the ordinary, and he told me that the slot machines in Sipsongpanna were rigged. The owners of the hotels were not honest gamblers: they cheated him. For Manager Zhou, Sipsongpanna was not only a place of fantasies come true but also a break in his routine, a chance to both work and play in a freer environment. He repeated like a mantra that in Sipsongpanna even the Han women are more open because of the influences of Tai culture and that their openness about sexual promiscuity *(luanjiao)* made this place desirable for him. Promiscuity is then represented as attached to the actual geographic space of Sipsongpanna and to the Tai who influence even local Han women's behaviors.

NOTIONS OF MODERNITY, MORALITY, AND SEX

Many studies of prostitution create an unproblematized binary between the exploited (prostitutes) and the exploiters (customers). Such static binary oppositions cannot fully address a more nuanced reading of ethnicity and sexual entertainment in Sipsongpanna. We have not just two groups, the exploited and exploiters, but in fact several groups. If we only read "Han wives" (living in China's hinterland) as virtuous and "Tai girls" as uncivilized in their rural paradise, we miss the Han single and married women who are prostitutes (the unvirtuous) and Han single and married men who are buying sex (another unvirtuous category). While I do not intend to dismiss the very real matters of the power dynamics underlying exploitation and discrimination in prostitution, I seek to tease out who is exploiting whom, at what time, and in what place, and perhaps even by what ethnicity. As Judith Farquhar (2002) and Virginia Cornue (2003) demonstrate in their work on sexuality in Beijing, new forms of urban life have emerged that touch on personal ambivalences toward sexual behavior and arise from following multiple moral codes as well as from claiming new identities. Many female informants, both Han and Tai, who did not work as prostitutes felt ambivalent toward the practice of exchanging sex for money, as well as toward the role of Han migrant women within cosmopolitan Jinghong.

The increase in prostitution is only one facet of the rise of the multiplication of sites wherein sexuality seeks expression. In Jinghong, I heard many of my informants (both Han and Tai) fervently say that sexually, they, unlike promiscuous Westerners, are very cautious and conservative. Yet I knew that at other times they engaged in all kinds of sexual activities that completely contradicted the way they talked about themselves. Here sex and the sex industry are not about Han repression and Tai promiscuity but about how sex as a commodity is circulated and also stigmatized. Representations of sex are everywhere in China, in a plethora of sex toy advertisements, condom packages, videos and films, anti-HIV/AIDS campaigns, hair salons, sexy clothing, and even stories about sex in the news (see Hyde 2000 & 2004). As a result, the desire, among tourists and locals alike, to consume newfangled leisure amusements includes the consumption of sexual commodities.

What is important for a tourist "site of desire" is to manage the image of the place rather than develop strict moral imperatives regarding sex. Often in Jinghong, what gets repressed is the circulation of, or the will to know and to openly acknowledge, what is being practiced (Foucault 1980). One friend in her thirties in speaking about taboo acts said: "In China we just do: we act. We never speak about what we have done." Thus, in almost every Chinese city, one sees street posters advertising fly-by-night pseudophysicians who claim to cure sexually transmitted diseases, male impotence, and AIDS, yet such cures are not openly discussed (Farquhar 2002). As mentioned in chapter 2, in Jinghong these posters are prominent only in the alleyways where locals venture; they are torn down wherever tourists are apt to view them. The idea that dangerous sex must be concealed in order to promote tourism fits with the notion of competing moral universes: a modern sexual morality promotes sex tourism, while a parochial one hides the consequences of unprotected sex. In fact dangerous sex is concealed in seemingly legal businesses such as hair salons and massage parlors. Underlying all of these practices are conflicting moralities, or rather competing discourses that often simultaneously challenge and embrace Confucian notions of Chinese sexual behavior and Maoist notions of restraint (Farquhar 2002; Dikötter 1995; Zito and Barlow 1994; Ruan 1991). While I discuss these two competing modes of biopower in chapter 4, here I note only that this is not an attempt to declare outright a teleological march through history with an accompanying dismissal of previous regimes; rather I argue that the past is always here through the present. When informants note that contemporary postreform China resembles the Republican Era (1911–48) more than a post-Maoist or post-Dengist nation-state, they are referring to the rise in prostitution, gambling, and drug use.

If the contemporary sex industry signifies a kind of liberation of sexuality (the rise of modern urban pleasures) wherein market forces revolutionize certain social practices, the sex industry, I argue, has commodified sexuality in Sipsongpanna; it has become a commodity fetish in the Marxian sense of the term. Conservative forces favor the return of earlier regimes of moral order, and the police often view the sex industry in Sipsongpanna as symbolic of the rise of urban moral decay and crime. Nonetheless, several female informants alluded to their "sex work" as a sign of modernity—the idea that modern China embraces sexual liberation and affords the freedom to capitalize on one's sexuality. Wu explained the commodification of prostitution this way:

> Prostitutes make quick money . . . they think about the impressions of marriage and the lights of the city . . . most are from the countryside and outside the province, and it [sex] is just a fashion for society . . . there are so many single women in Jinghong, the women who make up the sex industry are in highly paid occupations, and that is why prostitutes are plentiful. There is a saying in Jinghong, *yang xiao bai lian,* which means "to raise a small group of young handsome men." If women can keep a gaggle of handsome men around and just work [exchanging sex for money] . . . cultivate this group . . . just take care of these elegant boys, the boys will take care of their girlfriends in return. To have a nice-looking man to look at and take care of you while you provide the money is pleasing.

For local women such as Wu, prostitution signifies the numerous opportunities women have to make money and become wealthy. It also signifies the possibility of taking care of a small army of young men. This is clearly a usurpation of traditional gender roles. Here the practice of sexuality, the selling of one's body for money, completely transgresses older notions of proper gender hierarchies under Confucianism. Sexuality in 1990s China both shapes and is shaped by the dynamics of human social life that bring the rural into the urban city of Jinghong (via representations of Tai culture) and the urban cosmopolitan into rural Sipsongpanna (via the sex trade). These competing sexual morals pivot around the eroticization of the Tai, for the entire sex tourism industry in Sipsongpanna survives and depends on this eroticization.

BEYOND THE DISNEYESQUE

Sipsongpanna offers the escapist pleasures of an exotic location and the comforts of an urban setting. Han migration and China's state tourism policies have transformed a series of large Tai villages into the cosmopolitan city of Jinghong, a city that caters to Han tourists seeking an escape from Han China. As an escape that remains within China's geographic and linguistic borders, Jinghong is titillating yet not threatening. Sipsongpanna itself provides an instructive example of China's ethnic quilt. The place demonstrates the notion that all minorities are cousins, but the Han are the oldest *(laoda)*; therefore, the older and wiser Han must teach their younger cousins the Tai.[22]

The infelicitous coupling of market reform and sexuality within the context of modernity has transformed China, resulting in the proliferation of people living, working, and traveling in this borderland. Newly blossoming occupations span the legal and the illegal and encompass women who cut hair, own beauty salons, work as prostitutes, and serve as tour guides. All of these people create a modern vision of Sipsongpanna that bolsters its reputation as a fantasyland. Other locals, such as the police, have developed even grander visions of Sipsongpanna, beyond the Disneyesque Tai pleasure ground, based on their own transnational crossings. Sipsongpanna is marked as a key site in the Han imaginary, a place of desire: the desire to work and tour and the desire to consume and produce images of the exotic. It is quintessentially what Schein (1999) dubs an "imagined cosmopolitan" of late-socialist consumption, because people consume not only products but, along with them, practices and new forms of subjectivity. Understanding how travelers, migrants, and locals negotiate the ruptures between imagining Sipsongpanna and living there every day enriches our understanding of Chinese sexual modernity in one site of desire in 1990s China.

Hershatter (1997) calls the Chinese world of prostitution "a conversation about many things." In Jinghong, it is a conversation about Chinese sexual modernity and how prostitutes are perceived simultaneously as receptacles of contamination and victims at risk for contracting AIDS and other STIs. Because sexuality both shapes and is shaped by the dynamics of social life, prostitution in Sipsongpanna reflects the changing political-economic dynamics in a newly emerging regional tourism capital. Han migration and China's state tourism policies transformed a series of large Tai villages into the city of Jinghong. These arrangements, while ethnically unique to Sipsongpanna, are not unique to urban China. The coupling of market reform and sexuality within modernity has meant a rise in numerous occupations and activities on the periphery—prostitutes, karaoke girls, and gambling salons—that are obsessively quasi-sanctioned by the state in urban and semiurban centers. If the contemporary sex industry signifies a kind of liberation of sexuality and the rise of post-Mao urban pleasures, market forces have, in a classic Marxist sense, revolutionized social practices, including sexuality. In contrast to the discourse of liberation, sex and the sex industry are laden with references to the rise of moral decay and crime, especially because they are associated with Tai women and now with AIDS. Several of the women I spoke with see themselves as part and parcel of a larger project that embraces sexual liberation, and seek to maintain the freedom to capitalize on their sexuality. Where lies exploitation? If capitalizing on taking care of "elegant boys" *(yang xiao bailian)* means providing for oneself and one's family, these Chinese women today are not returning to preliberation gender roles (concubines and mistresses), but neither do they embody the tropes of self-actualized strong women from the Maoist era. Although labor migration may be a giant step toward economic liberalization, it has not always been a forward step for all migrant women (see Zhang Li 2001, chapter 5).

CHAPTER 4

Eating Spring Rice

Transactional Sex in a Beauty Salon

The evening sky mirrors the colors of the Lancang River—brown, tan, jeweled, and gold—and in sibilant silence swirls them together, as the gray cobblestones try hopelessly to absorb the evening's heat. With this heavy heat in her body, Madam Liu unlocks the large metal pull-down door and tangos one-by-one with several plastic armchairs. She places them all carefully on the gray pavement stones, adding a large circular white table. She yells at the top of her lungs to Xiao Wang, Xiao Gu, and Xiao Yue. "It's time for work, get ready for customers." I peek around the corner of her parlor's red awning. "*Aiya, Hai Sangdai,* it's you . . . It's work time, but why don't you join us for tea and beef kabobs?" I ask, "What about the customers?" Laughing and waving her hands, "*Aiya,* seeing you here won't chase them away; it only attracts them." Madam Liu sits down at the white plastic table and jokes that I should get a massage by Yuan, her nephew. Yuan sheepishly smiles at me. "Yes, I have hands made of steel that can stroke your tired muscles. See?" He produces his hands. "No," I jokingly protest, "perhaps Xiao Wang would be better since you like her the best." Xiao Wang sniffs the air. "Shit," she screeches, "why would I want such a hooligan like him, such a bastard like him, to even touch me!" All the while she is stroking his hair, running her fingers down his neck, and gently biting his arm. "Him . . . such a brat." We all laugh at her displays of affection.

To conceive of sex in Madam Liu's salon as "transactional" *(xing jiaoyi)* is to foreground both the subjectivity of those negotiating the exchange of sex for something else and the uneven relations of power structuring the possibilities of such an exchange.[1] In chapter 3, I explored how representations of women in Sipsongpanna reveal not only images of virtuous Han wives and unvirtuous Tai girls but also several other categories, most notably the complex performances of ethnicity, including the mimesis of the exotic Tai. In linking both representations and performances back to the main topic of HIV/AIDS, I begin by discussing the figurative and literal links between AIDS and prostitution. Then, I present one view of the world of transactional sex in Jinghong by moving into the space of Liu's salon. Keeping in mind that contemporary sexual identities are caught in the cross fire between the old Maoist state and the Dengist postreform state (Liu 2000; Farquhar 2002), I conclude with a discussion of the commodification of sex and return to the problem of two regimes of power—the police and the health department. Here the productive power of the old Maoist state, which sought to abolish prostitution on the grounds that it exploited women, collides and congeals with the productive powers of the postreform state. How have the images and discourses of sexuality in this tourist area been mediated by the flow of capital and by economic development? At the same time, this productive power creates an interesting paradox. Although the Maoist state sought to liberate prostitutes through Communist government campaigns in the early 1950s to eradicate sexually transmitted infections, the postreform state has inadvertently, through market socialism, reinstantiated the scale and visibility of "sex work." In the Foucauldian sense, the biological control over everyday life, or biopower, operates in these two regimes in their very different attempts to control sexuality and sexual expression.

WHY PROSTITUTION?

My research on the HIV/AIDS epidemic in southwest Yunnan focused in part on prostitutes because they are a stigmatized and often misunderstood risk group for the transmission of HIV/AIDS (see Xia Zhongli 1996). Several epidemiologists and physicians in Kunming shared my research agenda, although our specific goals were antithetical to one another. For them, I was the social scientist, the anthropologist, who was going to provide key cultural clues as to why the Tai were promiscuous by cultural habit and therefore predisposed to AIDS. These physicians are not alone in their assumptions. Around the globe, prostitutes are marked as a high-risk group in the public health literature; however, it is a dual-edged and often sexist sword, because sex workers are as likely to be at risk from their clients, especially those who refuse condoms, as the other way around. In addition, previous studies of prostitution have often relied on the unproblematized binary between the exploited female prostitutes and their exploiting male customers. These neat oppositions cannot fully address the nuances involved in sex work in Jinghong.

There is a vast literature on prostitution in feminist theory, gender studies, anthropology, and most recently, Chinese studies.[2] Before moving into the lives of contemporary women who work exchanging sex for money, I want to examine notable texts that are useful in thinking through some of the issues I present in this chapter. Sexual practices are often contested practices that lend themselves to multiple and divergent interpretations. Prostitution is not a monolithic enterprise. Its myriad forms are expressed in different ways, at different times, and in different geographic locals. In Luise White's (1990) ethnography about prostitutes in colonial Nairobi, she situates the economic and the physical where we find different economic classes of prostitutes, depending on their historical and geographic location. Academic studies of prostitution suggest an arena where a kind of epistemological and theoretical redemption is sought by reclaiming women as self-actualized erotic subjects rather than only objects for male desires. Few Chinese scholars have addressed prostitution from the perspective of the prostitutes themselves, but European scholarly literature has. In many Western European countries, prostitution advocates speak in the language of sociopolitical contracts, occupational protections, and workers' rights (Kempadoo and Doezema 1998). Prostitution in the West exists at least in part due to the subjugation of women and the double standards of sexual behavior for men and women. Much information on prostitution has been misconstrued to perpetuate misnomers and misunderstandings, reflecting little or poor qualitative research. One of the most contentious debates is that among Euro-American feminists over whether prostitution is sexual slavery or a bona fide occupational choice; these two perspectives are often presented as the "agency approach" versus the "violence approach," or in more heated commentary, as those of "sex-positive" versus "liberal-radical" feminists.

Frédérique Delacosta and Priscilla Alexander's (1987) groundbreaking work was the first to publish the voices of sex workers in both the production and writing processes and their work is emblematic of the agency approach. In contrast, Ryan Bishop and Lillian Robinson (1998) actually reinforce the idea that sex workers have no agency and that sex work is an entirely dependent economy, subject to the nefarious whims of global capitalism. Their work reflects the violence approach. Although Kamala Kempadoo and Jo Doezema (1998) build on the arguments presented in Alexander and Delacosta's earlier work, they paint a global canvas; we hear the voices of women organizing for better protection and rights across the globe, from the Netherlands to Japan and Taiwan. In anthropology, several works are notable. Angie Hart's (1998) work in Spain presents a phenomenological view of power in which clients, sex workers, and anthropologists all have key roles to play in the power worlds of prostitution. Hart argues that to examine one of these groups without examining the others creates an oversimplified impression of a very complex sexual economy. The American anthropologist Cleo Odzer (1994) is remarkable for her controversial stories about how she as an American anthropologist conducted fieldwork in the underworld of illegal prostitution in Thailand, at one point taking a Thai pimp as her lover.[3]

DEBATES OVER TERMINOLOGY: SEX AS WORK

Gail Hershatter's (1997) beautifully researched history of prostitution during Republican Era Shanghai focuses on how prostitution was a barometer for the political and social morals of the time. She advocates understanding prostitution as a kind of labor and labeling Chinese prostitution as "sex work." In this vein, political scientist Elizabeth Remick (2003 & 2004) argues that many of the state projects in Canton around the turn of the early twentieth century were funded through a tax on prostitution. In a personal conversation with me, Remick noted that Yunnan Province had some of the highest taxation rates for prostitution at that time.[4] As for the local level, several informants in Jinghong believe that prostitution needs to move out of the hands of the Chinese police and a corrupt mafia and into the hands of the regulated state for the sake of public health, reduction of drug use, and protection against sexually transmitted diseases. This is often expressed in Chinese as a move from the rule of the people to the rule of law *(renzhi fazhi)*.

Among recent studies of prostitution in China, Chinese sexologist Pan Suiming (1999: 23–25) conducted a groundbreaking study of contemporary Chinese prostitution in three towns and devised a scale that

TABLE I. THE SEVEN TIERS OF THE SEX
INDUSTRY IN CHINA

Tier 1	*baoernai*	Second wives or mistresses of wealthy men; defined as prostitutes because the women actively seek out men with rank and money who can provide them with long-term accommodation and a regular allowance
Tier 2	*baopo*	Hired by wealthy men as temporary wives during a business trip or vacation; temporary wives for business purposes
Tier 3	*santing*	Work in karaoke bars, dance halls, and restaurants and receive tips for their services; may go to hotel rooms for sexual services
Tier 4	*dingdong xiaojie*	Solicit customers by telephoning hotel rooms*
Tier 5	*falangmei*	Work in hair salons, beauty parlors, bathhouses, and saunas; this is where the New Wind fits in to the hierarchy
Tier 6	*jienü*	Street workers or streetwalkers
Tier 7	*xiagongpeng*	Work among proletariat or peasant migrant workers at the worksite

SOURCES: Pan 1999; Jeffreys 2004: 168–69.
*The practice is so widespread that men have solicited me on my hotel room telephone.

represents the different types and levels of sex work (see table 1). Pan argues that, given the rise in corruption and exchanges of capital for sex, a more egalitarian approach is needed for regulating and policing prostitution in China than is afforded by simply targeting the lower tiers (4 through 7), often the least well-off economically, and letting the rising entrepreneurial class of prostitutes and their clients remain beyond the law (tiers 1 and 2). He argues that government should either follow through with a 1950s-style campaign of abolition or apply punitive punishments in an egalitarian manner.

Ronald Weitzer (2000) notes that in discussions of prostitution there is often a passive neglect about defining exactly what kind of work prostitutes perform, in what location, and for which forms of compensation. As Weitzer notes, " 'sex work' is a generic term for commercial sex services, performances, or products given in exchange for material compensation" (5). "Sex worker" is also a term that emerged out of the "sex war" battles in the United States and Europe. Liberal feminists in the late 1970s and 1980s denounced all forms of prostitution as gender oppression and sexual slavery. These feminists essentialized all prostitutes as victims, as opposed to viewing sex work as a viable job with fewer hazards than many other occupations. In contrast, Elaine Jeffreys

(2004) argues that China's market-socialist economy and its tiered system of prostitution, ranging from high-class government officials and businessmen's second wives to ordinary street walkers, means that it cannot be reduced to labor or (the more common term) "sex work." Jeffreys argues that the 1990s' incarnation of the sex industry has relatively little to do with work, and thus the sex work approach of many sex-positive feminists merely reflects the liberal sexual-historical subject of Euro-American political thinking.

One of the problems of this critique is that Chinese public health workers and reformers have appropriated the terms "sex work" and "sex worker." By the late 1990s, in some social-work circles in Yunnan—for example, at the Women's and Children's Law Project in Jinghong—the Western term "sex worker" *(xing gongzuozhe or xing fuwuzhe)*[5] was appropriated as a modern term of respect for women who trade (see Hyde 2003 & 2000). However, as Marjolein Van der Veen (2001) points out, the term itself also reifies a particular identity, rather than acknowledging that these women have other multiple identities such as mother, sister, and daughter and are not just workers (35). Furthermore, Steven Gregory (2003: 353) suggests the label "sex worker" also reveals the tendency to view sex work as either simply *work* or as essentially dehumanizing. The problem remains that there is really no easy choice other than using very long-winded expressions, such as "those who sell sex" or "those who buy sex." Therefore, in order to represent these differing subject positions, I switch between "prostitutes" (mimicking my informants literal use of the term *jinü*), "sex workers" (when talking about them as a general category of worker), and "female entertainment workers" (covering a broader category than just women who exchange sex for money), depending on how they are used by my informants and for the sake of precision.[6]

LINKING HIV/AIDS AND THE SEX INDUSTRY

An ethnographic view of the multiple identities and representations of prostitution in Jinghong reveals a more complex picture than just the exploited female prostitute (the vector for AIDS) and her exploiting male customer (the victim of AIDS) and enhances our understanding of contemporary sexuality in China. The global links between an ethnic Other and disease have been repeated in country after country struck by the exponentially growing HIV/AIDS pandemic (Sabatier 1988; Farmer 1992). Although not only prostitutes who were targeted as vectors for AIDS—trucker drivers, migrants, and foreigners were, as well—

prostitutes remain one of the key foci of AIDS discourse in China. The Yunnan Provincial Health and Epidemiology Center reported data from sentinel surveillance sites in Yunnan, showing that by October 2001, 2 percent of prostitutes and 2 percent of STI patients had HIV (Yu Huifen 2001). By 2005 those numbers had increased to 11 percent in some areas, compared to rates of almost 20 to 30 percent in Thailand ten years before (Settle 2003: 6). Furthermore, the conflation of prostitution with ethnicity in Jinghong meant those "Tai" women working as alleged prostitutes were singled out, often as sole vectors for this ubiquitous disease. As sexual transmission is now identified as the next wave for the Chinese AIDS epidemic, female entertainment workers are currently viewed as the bridge population to the general population through their male clients (see also Porter 1995 & 1997; Jeffrey 2002; Gregory 2003). State interpretations of sexual risk have become highly gendered and accompanied by notions of blame.

The plethora of transactional sexual practices *(xing jiaoyi)* is only one facet in the rise of local sites where a modern sexuality seeks expression and embraces global forms of HIV prevention. Properly understood, Chinese gender and sexuality do not mean that sex is about excess in the reform era and repression under the Mao era. The attacks against prostitution in the 1940s and 1950s were, from a strict Foucauldian perspective, about the discourses and obsessions with sexuality, and thus were similar to changes under the reforms: both are productive discourses of sex and sexuality. What has changed are the ways images and discourses of sexuality are linked to particular tourist destinations, and how the flows of tourists and discourses of development mediate this linkage. Sex is circulated and reproduced in a way that links visions of sexual repression to the very same visions of sexual access. As Schein (1999) points out, with the fascination of the market, a kind of imagined cosmopolitanism also emerges that is closely related to her concept of internal orientalism (see chapter 3). Even though the locals in Sipsongpanna often talk about living in a backwater of China, they simultaneously imagine themselves to be part of cosmopolitan China, precisely because they live and work in this urban town in the midst of tropical forests. The local Han immigrant women see themselves as part of an eroticized ethnic culture that caters to visitors from more cosmopolitan places.

Although the borderland here has been identified with HIV/AIDS, what is not known is whether prostitutes are more at risk when they work in the border regions in China or when they work in Thailand;

both are perceived as a "high risk" activities. This is especially true now that Thailand maintains a 100 percent condom use policy in most of its establishments where sex is exchanged. That would suggest a reduced risk for contracting STIs and AIDS and raises the question: where is high risk located? In Jinghong the women who worked in places classified as midlevel brothels by sexologist Pan Suiming (1999), the *falangmei*, performed a variety of services that ranged from safe sensual, nonsexual massages to unsafe intercourse. In addition, Jinghong is a borderlands city where the rates of HIV/AIDS are lower than in other Yunnan border cities (Zhang Xiaobo et al. 2002; Yu Huifen 2001). Because AIDS is a sexually transmitted disease and prostitutes are engaged in exchanges of sex for money, they are marked as high risk for transmitting AIDS to their customers the world over (see Huang et al. 2004).

Picking up Patton's critiques (1996 & 2002) of responses to HIV prevention, we balance indecisively between a focus on bodies or places, infectious pools or infectious locations. This indecision in the 1990s lead to public health measures that often left out large groups of equally vulnerable peoples and areas. In China the early focus on the border regions meant that epidemics in the center were ignored. It was far more advantageous to reduce the epidemic in the borders of the Chinese state, particularly those with a long history of epidemics in tropical climates. This kind of thinking augmented government denial of the central China epidemic among Han Chinese peasants who had contracted AIDS through illegal blood pooling practices. Furthermore, discussions of AIDS in Asia have feminized the epidemic through the belief that prostitutes were predominantly responsible for bringing AIDS into Southeast Asia, specifically Thailand. What this meant is that sexual deviance pivoted around notions of the feminine, including the idea that prostitution fed the epidemic rather than tourists who could have been carrying AIDS into Thailand from the West. In other words, if prevalence rates are so high in a given area, the only means of control is "containment marked within spaces for destruction" (Patton 2002: 116–17).[7]

Little is known about prostitutes' daily interactions with customers or other business owners, or about their relationship to the Chinese nation-state, which defines prostitution as a crime (Farmer, Connors, and Simmons 1996). My research on HIV/AIDS sought in part to fill this information gap by focusing on the daily interactions between the women and men who worked and played in the New Wind Beauty Salon. I began to capture the liveliness of everyday life that existed beyond the organizational hierarchies in the health department, beyond the meanings of collective nouns such as "prostitutes," and beyond the reified epidemiological categories of "persons at risk" and "persons creating risk." In addition, as one internal medicine specialist pointed out, condoms were still not a sanctioned method of birth control in China in the late 1990s, and thus they were not included in work unit birth control subsidies. The most common subsidized forms of birth control remained sterilization (mainly for women) and intrauterine devices (IUDs) (Greenhalgh 1994: 7). If you wanted condoms, you had to buy them in pharmacies or hotel gift shops. Fortunately, a new law was enacted in Yunnan in early 2004 that required public places to provide condoms free of charge, or at the very least at low cost (Zhang Zizhuo 2004). I offer a much fuller explanation of condoms, condom use, and efforts at marketing them in chapter 5. One of the major concerns of nongovernmental organizations (NGOs) conducting AIDS prevention programs in Yunnan and Sipsongpanna is that if no prevention education exists, how can women be expected to even begin to protect themselves and their customers and partners against AIDS?

ENTERING THE NEW WIND BEAUTY SALON

As few epidemiological surveys had been conducted, let alone ethnographic work on prostitutes' everyday practices in Jinghong, there were rampant misconceptions among the public health community about what actually occurred in these so-called brothels. As I began to unravel information about the complex sex industry in Jinghong, my own fears got in the way. I entered Wang's small salon, which was sandwiched in between the only government department store in town, the Baihua Dalou, and the police headquarters. Wang, a fellow outsider from Macao, invited me in for a hair wash and head massage. I thought this might be an opportunity to start this part of my research, as there were several very heavily made-up women, who I assumed were sex workers, sitting on a couch in the salon. Wang, however, had an entirely different agenda. He was looking for a wife and a ticket out of China. I appeared to be the solution to his cross-border transportation problem. After my hair wash, I gave him my card, explained my research to him somewhat vaguely as looking at the history of Jinghong and the rise of certain businesses such as his. I was careful not to mention AIDS in case this would scare him away. The magistrate of the next county had warned me that AIDS "is still a very sensitive and secretive topic in this part of Yunnan." Wang called me several times on the phone, each time mentioning what a perfect pair we made, and this each time meeting with my disapproval and rejection. I became frustrated; perhaps I was not suited to this research. Might it have something to do with my particular personality? If Cleo Odzer could conduct research among prostitutes in Thailand, I wondered, why couldn't I in the "Thailand of China"?[8]

I also visited several other salons. One was Li's old run-down beauty salon (called simply A Beauty Salon, with no proper name), next to a fishpond on the dusty road to several large dance halls and nightclubs.[9] Li's was a salon in name only. A few bottles of shampoo were scattered about, along with a jar of greasy hair gel and a broken mirror. On a couple of torn plastic–covered brown couches, two young women sat. One woman was from Simao, the other from Sichuan. It was eight o'clock and Li, the owner, a young Jinghong Han resident in his early thirties, had just opened his doors for business. Upstairs and around the back were four closet-size rooms, each with a single chair, trash can, vinyl-covered single bed, and either curtain or door. He seemed to have no interest in talking to me, or rather, he just answered my curious questions with a simple yes or no. In addition, the squalor of the place did not make it very inviting.

A couple of more attempts and several months later, in the summer of 1997, I found a more appealing salon. This time the owner was a woman, Madam Liu. I met Liu through her nephew, who I jokingly called Yuan Shikai (an emperor wannabe of China). He ran the bar and café next door to the salon, and seeing me walk by everyday, he struck up a conversation. Eventually, the women working at the salon, who were close friends with Yuan, also came to chat. Madam Liu and her boyfriend, Tan, were planning to marry and set up house in a new apartment complex behind the town's designated tourist development district. Unlike Wang, Madam Liu invited me to come live with her and Tan whenever I returned to Sipsongpanna. I often provided her and her staff with beer, soft drinks, food, the occasional cigarette, and AIDS prevention information. Liu was also quite forward in her requests for me to provide everything from American college scholarships to business connections, pictures, books, and postage stamps. And on occasion, she joked about me working for her. Overall, she appeared genuinely happy that I came into her life, and in return I was happy that she came into mine.

THE SPACE OF A BEAUTY SALON

The dirt and disorder of Li's salon is in sharp contrast to Madam Liu's place, with her whitewashed walls and large red plastic awning, which blows in the warm wind. Her white-painted front room presented the conventional accoutrements of a beauty salon: chairs, bottles of sham-poo and conditioner, brushes, combs, curling irons, blow dryers, and a large electric water boiler. Another room next door had three massage tables, frilly flowered curtains dividing the space between each table, and a larger electric water heater above the sink with a door leading to a bathroom in the back. Liu's two rooms had different decor: one was shadowed with tinted glass, and the other was bright with white tiles. On the walls were posters depicting both white and Asian women with various hairstyles. One of these large posters looked like a facsimile of an old Coppertone advertisement: a white blond woman lies lan-guorously in a skimpy bikini, while a small dog pulls at the strings of her bikini top—her expression is one of seductive surprise.

Madam Liu's place was one of my main fieldwork sites in Jinghong. The hundred or more small salons like Madam Liu's in Jinghong in 2000 reflected both different businesses—beauty salon, hair salon, mas-sage salon—and their attendant levels of status or prestige. The New Wind Beauty Salon (a pseudonym) was a legitimate salon as well as a massage parlor for middle-class tourists who stayed in the nearby three-star hotel. The spatial divisions in the salon circumscribed my daily dealings with the women and men there. I had full access to the hair salon in the front room but not to the massage tables in the back room. This had as much to do with my exercising respect for the women while they were working as it did with my reticence to enter the forbidden space of prostitution. None of the women working would enter the back room unless they had a customer.

Madam Liu commanded the patterns of time for her staff; they slept, ate, worked, and rested when she said. When Liu closed up shop, she sent everyone home, either to her spacious apartment, a short five min-utes away by bicycle, or to their own rented rooms in the old Tai village of Manjinglan. Liu had four women actively working for her when I first met her—Xiao Wang and Xiao Yue from Ruili (a border town in northwestern Yunnan) and Xiao Gu and Xiao Ling from rural villages in Sichuan.

The people working in the salon exhibited a culture of practices through signs of physical affection. Caught off guard and somewhat em-barrassed, I usually playfully joked when she asked me personal ques-tions. Nevertheless, embarrassment is too mild a term to describe how I felt when one afternoon everyone was chatting and giggling about fe-male body parts: breasts, genitalia, and pubic hair. Madam Liu grabbed Xiao Wang's shirt, unbuttoned it, and said, "Look, she has such beautiful nipples." She then pointed to Xiao Gu and said that, because she had a child, hers were dark, large, and ugly. I immediately protested, "How can you say that everyone has the same taste?" She then unceremoniously grabbed my shirt, opened it, and examined my nipples. I laughed nervously, and after everyone at the table approved, she remarked how fortunate foreign women were to have such ample breasts and nipples *(fengman naitou)*. I kept up the playful banter in the conversation that followed this investigation of the roundness of my nipples, the whiteness of my skin, and the thinness of my body. This was the body business, and I had moved beyond common courtesies.

That afternoon when I left, somewhat shocked by this performance, I realized I had leaped over what I understood as clear-cut Confucian, particularly distinct Han, boundaries around bodily space and between strangers. Another evening, Xiao Yuan kept teasing that he lived with two sisters who are both crazy, so he calls Xiao Yue "seductive slut older sister" *(sao jiejie)* and Xiao Wang "crazy younger sister" *(fengzi meimei)*. Then Liu hit Xiao Wang in her chest, yelling at her to cover up her tits, all the while laughing in a playful manner, while Xiao Wang screeched "Ni ma bi!" (Your mother's cunt!). Despite these displays of bodily intimacy, the women rarely touched each other's faces. Even as some parts of the body are intensely focalized, others are ignored. Through these bodily displays, I had entered Liu's shop, her family, and her life.

PORTRAIT OF A MASSEUSE

The women at the salon came to Sipsongpanna from different places and for various reasons. What they all had in common was that they were under thirty, were Han Chinese, and came from outside Sipsongpanna. Xiao Wang, from Ruili, came to Sipsongpanna on vacation and stayed because her cousin was working in a Jinghong gambling salon making lots of money—she boasted over three thousand Yuan per month. Xiao Wang had been working there for only two months when I left at the end of August 1997, and was still working when I returned in 2000. She was not necessarily representative of all prostitutes working in Jinghong. She was the favored worker in the salon and the most sought after by customers. One Lancang transport worker who maneuvered cargo boats between Thailand and China said that Xiao Wang could do ten men in one night and never tire.

When I first met Yue, she was twenty-three years old. She had come to Jinghong from Ruili only a month earlier because work opportunities were better. She said: "In Ruili the hair salons employing prostitutes operate only for local businessmen, not tourists. You cannot make as much money. Local businessmen are not interested in paying local women for their services, but in Xishuangbanna you become something special" and can remain anonymous. Wang, also twenty-three and from Ruili, came to Sipsongpanna to visit her cousin, who worked in one of the gambling salons. Her cousin made really good money. Although Wang wasn't making as much as her cousin, she preferred Jinghong to Ruili. She admitted that, unlike me, she had not excelled in school, finishing only elementary school because she was too busy flirting with the boys. She smiled, the dimples on her cheeks deepening, and said, "I have always loved men." Xiao Wang is very close to Liu's nephew, Yuan (the owner of the bar next door and the person who introduced me to Liu), and another woman in the salon, Xiao Yue, is a *yuanqin* (a distant relative).

Xiao Gu, who at twenty-seven was the oldest of the women working for Liu, had listless, dark, sad eyes. When I asked if she missed her home, she said, "Of course I miss home and especially my son. He is only six years old and I only get to see him a couple of times a year." Xiao Gu said the work is good because there are no jobs for someone as uneducated as she in her hometown, upriver from Chongqing in Sichuan Province. Xiao Gu had a lover, Xiao Wang, who spoke in beautiful clipped Mandarin and had impeccable manners. Later, I discovered he was actually her husband. Xiao Gu told me that her parents are peasants and she has not told them what kind of work she does in Jinghong. Her biggest frustration is that she misses her son, whom she gets to see only at Spring Festival *(chunjie)*.

Yue, Wang, and Gu all said they can make between 200 to 300 yuan a day, 70 percent of which they give to Liu. On good days they take home 100 yuan, meaning that they can clear 1,000 to 2,000 yuan a month, or four to six times what shop assistants or restaurant workers make. If Xiao Wang makes that much, and Madam Liu's cut is 70 percent, she clears at least 2,000 yuan in one month on one masseuse alone. While Yue and her sister spend most of their earnings on themselves, on fancy clothing, perfumes, and jewelry, Gu, the married woman from Sichuan, sends a portion home to her family.

One typical evening, Madam Liu perked up when a well-dressed male tourist arrived. She gestured for Xiao Wang to come forward, but Wang yelled back in Yunnanese, with a note of sarcasm in her voice, "I don't want to go." Another customer appeared and everyone laughed behind his back, calling him a nerd *(shudaizi)*. Later, two men walked in and asked what services Madam Liu was offering. Madam Liu said, pointing to me, "A massage from the foreigner." Then she pointed to Xiao Wang to take one of the men to the back room. Xiao Wang was always loud, often yelling and screaming into the street and then laughing hysterically. Xiao Yuan had a crude tattoo on his upper arm that says, "Wo yiding dengzhe ni" (Of course, I will wait for you). Yuan teased me that he was waiting for Xiao Wang.

Wang and Yue were the most popular women in the salon, perhaps because they often dressed in Tai clothing, beautiful batiks that were closely cropped to fit their figures. Regarding her dress, Yue explained that the men who come to Xishuangbanna really like the Tai look, and to attract customers and keep Liu happy, she often had "Tai" outfits made in one of the small seamstress shops down the block. While she laughed at the idea that anyone could mistake her for a Tai woman, she said that Tai clothes are so beautiful that men come in just to look and that brings more customers into the salon. Even though Xiao Wang was very beautiful, Madam Liu liked to point out she had facial wrinkles *(zhouwen)*, just like me. She said we should both get better face massages to smooth these *zhouwen* out, since men find them unattractive. Xiao Wang also often talked about the gifts that customers gave her in addition to their payment—for instance, the gold rings that a customer from Beijing bought on his trip to the Myanmar border. She often wore expensive, twenty-four-karat gold jewelry and laughed at my fourteen-karat earrings. They were not real gold!

From my point of view, the women working in the salon are important because they are the ones engaged in both risky behaviors, such as having intercourse without condoms, and safer sex practices, such as giving hand jobs—but it was Madam Liu who represented opportunities for women in Jinghong. She was not only the owner of a small business but a successful one, to boot.

MADAM LIU — MONEY, WEALTH, AND SECONDARY GAINS

Liu provided housing for her workers, paid their medical bills, bought them clothes, told them what to wear, and directed when and how they were to receive customers. Madam Liu was in effect a *patronne,* and she and her staff were in a patron-client relationship. This does not mean that the staff had no power to negotiate or maneuver within the confines of the salon or within the larger community in Jinghong. Staff members

often refused a customer based on the way he looked or the car he drove
or just out of boredom.

Though many people in Jinghong speculate about the prostitutes'
high incomes, in reality it is the madams who are accumulating the
money. For Madam Liu, money is the most important acquisition. She
generates and consumes it in large quantities. Madam Liu liked to say
she was really only the secondary boss *(xiao laoban)* and that the real
laoban (her boyfriend) was "making money." She often carried her
wealth on her body. Madam Liu had a beautiful twenty-four-karat gold
necklace with a light green jade pendant of Guanyin, and on other occasions she wore a gold necklace lined with rubies and sapphires.

One Sunday I went over to Madam Liu's house for lunch and a game
of Mahjong. The purpose of this dinner was to meet her boyfriend, the
tour bus driver, who complained that Liu was too fat. Her apartment
was a spacious modern one down the street from her shop. By Jinghong
standards she had all the modern conveniences, including a large new
apartment, a gas stove, a refrigerator, several bicycles, new furniture, internal plumbing, and a telephone. This apartment was only temporary
housing for Liu and Xiao Wang, Xiao Yue, and her nephew, Xiao Yuan.
She and her boyfriend, Tan, had purchased an apartment in a new building in the tourist development district beyond the gold gate. She said
that apartment would be equipped with even more luxurious furniture
and facilities. While Xiao Gu and Xiao Wang cooked, the rest of them
played Mahjong. Liu kept asking me to join in, but because they were
gambling, I declined. In any case, the game went so fast, I could barely
keep up, even though I was just watching the tiles fly around the table.

Lunch was served, with many delicious dishes cooked Sichuan-style
in hot oil with peppers. I spent the afternoon drinking beer and talking
to Liu's staff and friends. Afterwards, Tan arrived and was most curious
about my research. He was one of the first people I met who said that
he felt modernization in Jinghong had made the Tai *less* promiscuous
rather than more. He said they used to bathe naked in the rivers in plain
sight of others, but now, for fear of outsider's wandering eyes, they
bathe fully clothed in the river.[10] Tan had lived in Jinghong for over ten
years, and it was clear that he saw it as the land of opportunity. Tan
helped pay for the clothes Madam Liu had bought in Thailand—her
azure-blue polyester dress and gold jewelry. She usually traveled to
Thailand once a year and was planning on going in the coming September. She wanted to know if I could go to Thailand with her. As Madam
Liu said jokingly, "That way I could buy her another pair of expensive

sandals"—they cost over four hundred Yuan, or four days' work for her employees.

By Jinghong standards, Madam Liu's lifestyle suggests that she makes good money, although she politely refused to tell me how much. But Madam Liu has a penchant for Mahjong and gambling. One day, after the return of Hong Kong to China, Madam Liu drew a long face and said that her finances are not as they should be. That day she lost over one thousand yuan playing Mahjong. She was upset about her loss but continued to eat a large durian fruit, whose juice and peel Xiao Wang claimed you couldn't get off your fingers without applying motorcycle grease.

Madam Liu often commented that these days making a living on Ganlan road was very difficult and that the only people in town making money were the Tai on Mantinglu, the busy street next to one of the remaining Tai villages. She also commented on how tidy and clean the Tai are: "They have houses above the dust and dirt and they sweep and sweep and sweep." Then again, it was the low season *(danji)*, and not the high season *(wangji)* that brings busloads of tourists to Sipsongpanna. Even at the local cafés that cater to foreign backpackers, the owners commented on how few tourists there were in the summer of 1997—people just strolled down the streets *(guang jie)* without even buying a tea. I now turn to the views of local people working in other businesses in Jinghong.

PROSTITUTION IN THE LOCAL IMAGINATION

In Jinghong a popular saying referred to young women and their occupations: *"chi qingchun fan"* (youth rice bowl, or eating spring rice). A play on an earlier, socialist-era metaphor, the saying implies that youth rice bowls do not last forever, and, as young girls fade into older women, they can no longer live off their youthful beauty. Under late socialism, the saying expresses how young women are living off of their youthful appearance and sex appeal, in this case, as female sex workers.

Li San is the Mosuo owner of the Nihao Cafe, a large beautiful bamboo structure with small bamboo tables and chairs, a woven rattan ceiling covered in local batiks, and her husband's artwork on the walls, which are covered in bamboo mats traditionally used for the floor. Li San says she often passes herself off as Tai-Lüe but is actually "Lolozu" (or Lolo) another name for a branch of the Naxi called the Mosuo.[11] Li San explained she is not proud of her heritage and often passes herself off as

Tai-Lüe instead of Lolo because being and looking Tai is more desirable than Lolo. When I asked her about prostitution, Li San reiterated the common notion that prostitutes would not talk to me and that my field-work in the Chinese mafia world was dangerous. She said, as many other legal business owners in Sipsongpanna claimed, "Prostitutes are part of the Chinese mafia *(hei shehui)*." I laughed and said, "I am careful, and conducting AIDS research means understanding even prostitutes."

While locals claim brothels are part of the underground society, these businesses are actually more essential to Jinghong than Li San's café. Xiao Ge, another friend and small shop owner, told me the story of a neighbor of hers, a prostitute from Shanghai, who frequently made purchases in her small shop. One night, the police raided the hotel where her friend worked, and she and her customer ran out the back door with nothing on. She asked Ge to vouch for her, because the police were going to arrest her. The woman claimed to the police that the two of them were married and that she had run out for fear and nothing else. Ge had never seen a marriage certificate and could not have provided proof even if she wanted to. The police arrested her friend. Though fear of police raids plagues the daily life of prostitutes, more important to my argument are the modern plagues of STIs and HIV/AIDS.

Several informants countered the view, espoused by several members of the All-China Women's Federation *(fulian)*, that "women are just being exploited again . . . we are back to preliberation China and what have we gained? One step forward and two steps back." What appears as a marker of difference between the preliberation sex industry and its contemporary appearance is the fact that a number of young women consider prostitution to be a viable occupation rather than a form of ostracized servitude. Other informants remarked that "it is much easier to get a job, a good job, as a female than a male. There are just many more opportunities." Service sector jobs in Jinghong include restaurant workers, shopkeepers and assistants, dancers and singers, and hotel service staff from front desk clerks and managerial staff to maids. When asked about differences between female tour guides and prostitutes (usually young women under the age of thirty) an informant said: "While there is not a big monetary difference, prostitutes don't get to admire their work." Although these young women earn amounts close to tour guides' income, they have to pay for everything—clothing, makeup, and the like—whereas a tour guide's job is all inclusive, the companies even providing uniforms. In addition, education plays a large role in who gets to be a tour guide and who ends up in the sex industry. Those with little more than an elementary-school education do not end up with lucrative tour-guide jobs. Therefore, among the economic migrants, prostitution becomes a choice among a limited range of choices.

I distinguish between occupations that directly involve exchanging sex for money and those that are merely filled by a majority of female workers. Due to Sipsongpanna's recent transition from an agricultural economy to a more service-sector tourist economy, many job opportunities have opened up for young attractive women in the three townships. Many new jobs, from working as a hotel maid to being a local tour guide or running a massage parlor, are only technically open to women. These service-sector employees, much like their prostitute counterparts, are often under the age of thirty and can earn large sums of money from their commissions and tips collected from tourists. Li San said, "A prostitute makes a roughly a minimum of a hundred yuan per job a night, and some women make over six thousand yuan per month, but then they must pay for clothing, makeup, and paying off the police, among other things. Tour guides make around one to three thousand Yuan a month and everything is theirs to keep because the uniforms are provided by the tour company." As tour guides tend to be better educated and have legitimate and respectable jobs in the eyes of the community and their families, there is a marked difference in cultural capital. Most of the tour guides must have command of a second language, such as Japanese or English, while the majority of the prostitutes spoke only dialect-influenced Mandarin. Class status is embodied not only in being "branded on the tongue" but also in level of education (wenhua).

One of the things that separate many prostitutes from the wealthiest tour guides is the prevalence of heroin smoking and injection among the former. A heroin habit in Sipsongpanna costs at least one hundred yuan per day, and much of one's income goes to servicing it. I do not suggest that all prostitutes are heroin addicts, as some Jinghong police officers are wont to say. In fact, to my knowledge, no readily available studies have linked the rates of injection drug use to prostitution in Jinghong. None of the women I mention here used heroin, although some of them smoked cigarettes. Several female escorts I spoke with who said they did not use heroin also said they enjoyed their work because it provided a much better income than they could expect to obtain back in their natal homes, their villages or townships, or in their parents' rice fields. While income was a key factor in their choice of occupation, the problems attendant to prostitution are numerous, especially the constant reminder by the police of the illegal nature of the work.

POLICE HARASSMENT AND THE
COMMODIFICATION OF SEX

The beauty salon itself was also a ludic space open to possibilities for subversion from within the business itself, including subversion against the Chinese state, which classified selling sex for money as a crime.[12] Although it may be illegal to prostitute and operate brothels, there is clearly a quasi-sanctioned relationship between the police and the brothel owners in Jinghong. In fact, several informants explained that the police inform their favorite brothel owners of an impending strike-hard anticrime campaign *(yanda yundong)*, so that the owners can close their brothels or, in the case of hair salons, return to cutting hair for the three weeks the campaign runs. A dusty ramshackle salon on the road facing toward Burma was always closed during the strike-hard campaigns; it was clear that the police had informed the owner when the raids would begin.[13]

The government networks keeping surveillance over prostitution include the government-run clinics, anti-epidemic stations, public security bureau, and the local police stations. Because prostitution is an extralegal activity, it is constantly subject to disciplinary surveillance by agents of the Chinese state. Michel Foucault (1980) argues that with the rise of a medicolegal state apparatus, there is increased control over the individual in the name of greater protection of the state. Liu noted that in Sipsongpanna, there is a common understanding that you must throw water in someone's face to divert their attention—*dianshui*—which is what she had to do to the police in Jinghong. Though the police are the only official figures to actually extract large fines and bribes from the madams *(jimama)*, as well as arresting young female prostitutes, the public health anti-epidemic stations and drug centers are also involved in preventing prostitutes from working. If the police pick up a prostitute, she is often tested for sexually transmitted diseases, and occasionally for HIV. Sometimes her madam pays the police off (often up to ten thousand Yuan per *jinü*), and she may be released. At other times, explained Lao Yan, a policeman from the Jinghong drug prison, prostitutes are sent to re-education centers and then driven to Simao County and let loose. Liu often noted that for business it was imperative to "wo hai yao gei dangguan de qian" (provide monetary bribes to Chinese officials). This approach demonstrates a certain acquiescence by those public security officials who did not adhere to the 1960s Maoist-style campaign for abolition that would remove all sites of prostitution and prostitutes. However, while the arbitrariness of fines and arrests might appear moderate on paper, those involved in the "sex industry," trading sex for money and favors, did not see it that way.

In Jinghong the police are very visible. Every night in the winter of 1996, a paddy wagon—a brand-new Toyota Land Cruiser—accompanied by a motorcade of flashy black Taiwanese motorcycles, cruised the streets and alleys. A friend working in the public security bureau said, "It is like that in your country—the police must go on patrol. In Sipsongpanna we have the additional burden of being too close to the Lao and Burmese borders. There will always be the criminal element that comes here, because this place is too open. We need to capture them."[14] To paraphrase another public security officer, the police may try to get rid of prostitution, but like "poisonous weeds," it keeps growing back because the tiny roots are still there. If policemen round up prostitutes in Jinghong, all they can do is drive them to the rehabilitation center in the county seat in Simao. In two days they are back on the streets working again. Despite these harsh critiques of prostitution, the policemen I knew did not condemn the crimes committed under the business rubric of prostitution as severely as they did the first gambling-related murder in Jinghong, which occurred in the summer of 1996. Whereas gambling was viewed with suspicion, prostitution was almost seen as a way of life, even by members of the public security force.

Although sex workers were regularly rounded up and fined around six hundred yuan or put in drug prisons or rehabilitation centers, that does not mean they did not resist these incursions. Madam Liu's staff disliked the police with a passion and often made crude jokes about them. Xiao Wang and Madam Liu often called them bandits, swearing as they argued that the slogan on the side of the blue and white police vans, "Wei renmin fuwu" (To serve the people), was a fictitious statement. One night after eleven o'clock, when the police had raided a neighbor's salon, extracting over ten thousand yuan in fines, Xiao Wang screamed into the street at a police patrol car, "Nimen wei ni ma bi" (You only serve your own mother's cunts!). Madam Liu complained bitterly to me that the police are the new bandits of China, wearing official uniforms.

The human body on which the practices of prostitution are inscribed provides a site for simultaneously exercising the disciplinary powers of the state and nurturing new kinds of subjectivities, new forms of resistance, and potential transformations of pre-existing power dynamics.

Linda Singer (1993) points out that the disciplinary apparatus that emerges with the ostensible purpose of limiting or abolishing certain forms of sexuality can work only by itself becoming the site of the production of a new set of sexualities. This statement best describes the recent re-emergence of prostitution or sex work in the postreform era. Even though the state aims to control and often eradicate the sex industry, it also contributes both literally and figuratively to its staying power through both censorship and incorporation. In many ways the jobs of the public security forces are a means of extrastate power. With a decline in strict state regulation and surveillance in the form of shutting down the brothels or jailing prostitutes and their customers, the police themselves are benefiting in ways that reflect the current rise in corruption associated with state-appointed officials and employees.

These women's lives were surveyed and criticized not only by the state but also by their partners, lovers, and husbands. Most of the women I met at the New Wind in 1997 were there when I went back in 2000. However, one, Xiao Cui, a bright young woman from Sichuan, who often came into the salon during her off-hours, was painfully absent. Her jealous boyfriend had killed her for taking a new lover and withholding money from him. She was supporting both her boyfriend and her lover, but she complained that every time she gave her jealous boyfriend money, he would use it for his wife. He apparently was incredibly jealous of her and her work, decided to take matters into his own hands with a knife, and then wrote in blood on the floor next to her body, "This person deserves to die." He was imprisoned after her sister found the body and traced the killing to him. I also learned that he disliked me because I was bringing the idea of AIDS to Jinghong and that in his eyes, I would tarnish the town's reputation and the economy would decline. While AIDS is treated epidemiologically as any other STI, it was spoken about much more frequently in the salon than other STIs due to the stigma attached to it. Although several individuals in Jinghong, including health workers, NGO representatives, and tour guides, pointed out how disgusted they were with the exploitation of young women, they blamed equally the prostitutes and their clients for the rise of sex tourism.

TWO REGIMES OF POWER

In terms of HIV/AIDS, the now obvious links between risky behaviors, including unprotected sexual intercourse, and the spread of HIV among sex workers demands critical rethinking about the illegality of the sex industry. While police arrest women and use the condoms they find on them as evidence of their illegal trade in sex, there are also positive notes to consider. The current practice of providing condoms to those both selling and buying sex, and the proliferation of condom sales in Jinghong, shows at least the potential for marketing safer sex practices within a sex tourism site. Finally, the performances of ethnicity, gender, and sex must be weighed equally in understanding the everyday practices of AIDS and public health officials' focus on prevention for a specific subset of sexual practices. The performance of identity and of specific sex acts should also be clearly identified prior to developing prevention strategies for those individuals associated with sex tourism in contemporary China.

If Han men are buying into a mimesis of Han women performing as Tai, ethnic identity and gender are markers for a Chinese modernity in this hinterland paradise where conspicuous consumption includes the practice of buying women for the evening. Sex workers themselves are caught between two regimes of power that emerge and re-emerge at the site of state intervention: the anti-epidemic stations and the public security bureaus. The police in Jinghong have also seesawed between those two regimes of power, which I first mentioned in chapter 2. They are trying to prevent the spread of commercial sex work by rounding up prostitutes and testing some of them for HIV/AIDS, and at the same time are capitalizing on prostitution through the imposition of fines. Although I was unable to research how much local revenue is generated through prostitution, many sectors of the local town economy appear to benefit from the industry. By linking the return of prostitution in postreform China to the rise of new consumption practices that capitalize on the performance of ethnicity, I have opened an ethnographic window onto prostitution in Jinghong, revealing, I hope, a larger, fuller picture than the reduction to either two sides in the sex wars or opposition between "exploited female prostitute" and "exploiting male customer."

CHAPTER 5

A Sexual Hydraulic

Commercial "Sex Workers" and Condoms

In the summer of 1997, I walked into the newly constructed "Elephant Spring Hotel" (a pseudonym) in Jinghong to discover one of the most charming small tourist shops I had ever seen. The glass front display case was divided into two sections, one with toothbrushes, cards, towels, and film, and the other with every kind of condom imaginable. A Guangzhou brand called International *(guoji)* had a picture of a young white couple on the cover, the woman in a sexy pink-flowered sheath dress and the man in a white suit. The two were caressing each other in a languorous pose on a grassy knoll. The caption read, "aixin + fangxin = chengxin" (Love plus feeling at ease equals speaking from the heart). A smaller packet of condoms had a diffused soft-light image of a Chinese woman seen from behind. She was naked, her long black hair reaching to the middle of her back. The yellow lighting focused on her round buttocks, where her hands lay against her body. This Tianjin brand of condoms was called Harmonious and Happy *(hele tao)* and had a caption that read, "Biyun, yufang, jiankang, kuaile" (Prevent pregnancy, prevent disease, and be healthy and happy).

THE STATE, THE MARKET, AND THE CONDOM

When I inquired about how well these condoms sold, the clerk, glancing down at her wares, replied that they had the best display in town and that although the hotel was not yet renting rooms, they were making money on the restaurant, the shop, and these condoms. Here I argue that there is a dialectical relationship between the decline in direct public health intervention and the rise of popular sexual consumption practices in shaping condom use. Moving from a socialist health care system, where health care services were often free of charge, to one where many services are privatized means that medical care has become market oriented for much of China's population. With increasing pressure on even state-run public health hospitals and clinics to generate income, many clinics have attached pharmacies where items such as condoms can be purchased. In addition, local private clinics, department stores, and sex shops also provide condoms and medications for the prevention of pregnancy and disease. While many large Chinese cities also have these conveniences, in Jinghong they are integrally connected to an overt sex industry. All of this leads us to a paradox in which two kinds of power are manifest: the state's power in regulating STIs through clinics that cater to heteronormative couples and the countervailing power of market forces that promote birth control and disease-prevention techniques to anyone with the money to buy condoms. These two kinds of power are evident through the on-the-ground practices described here.

Although condoms were still not openly sanctioned by the Chinese state, in 2000 they were in evidence in fancy display cases like those at the Elephant Spring Hotel and in many other small Jinghong pharmacies and shops. Condoms were plentiful in Jinghong by 2000, in part because of the small salons-cum-brothels that are part of the tourism industry.[1] As condoms became available in private stores, the central government's regulation of birth control devices and medical appliances struggled in many ways to keep up with the market. Although condoms are used globally to reduce population, they are not sanctioned as an official means of birth control in China. Condoms reflect the desire of the market to promote romance and love (see Erwin 2000; Farrer 2002). In contrast to the lively and sensual visual depictions of sexual conduct, there is another side to condom promotion in China. In late November 2003 several television advertisements promoted condom use in time for World AIDS Day on December 1. One advertisement stated, "A woman says she feels safe because they use a condom when she has sex with her boyfriend." This was a remarkable event. In 1998, just five years earlier, a condom advertisement had appeared on buses in Guangzhou, and in 1999 a international public condom advertisement appeared on CCTV (one of the main government-run stations), but both ads were pulled after public criticism that they were in contravention of regulations banning advertisements relating to sexuality or obscenity (*China Daily* November 28, 2003).

When the state and the market compete, a fascinating paradox emerges: when state-financed health care is in decline, the market economy opens the door to new kinds of sexual practices and provides a potent weapon against sexually transmitted infections and AIDS through the sale of condoms. I do not mean to imply that condoms are never available through government-run clinics; however, to illuminate why prostitutes and their clients prefer to buy condoms on the market rather than receive them free of charge from the state I first discuss prostitution and STI prevention.[2] Then, to explicate how the state ethos of birth control changes with regard to the different locations of Chinese citizens, I turn to a public health history of China and the discourse on the representations of prostitutes and their risk for HIV/AIDS. I analyze the changing relationships between the state birth control ethos and the modern condom. I argue that the market in one sense allows individuals to sidestep the state family planning apparatus by purchasing birth control through the market rather than in state-sanctioned hospitals and clinics. The paradox of the modern Chinese state is presented through several different ethnographic examples: individual prostitutes' discussions of STIs at the New Wind Hair Salon; stories about selling and buying condoms and sex toys; and state practices that limit HIV/AIDS prevention, including a condom advertisement ban in Beijing and a Jinghong doctor's effort to prevent sexual liaisons with people with AIDS.[3]

Since AIDS is a sexually transmitted disease and prostitutes are engaged in exchanging sex for money, prostitutes are perceived as an epidemiological threat to their customers the world over. Many countries have noted that the sexually transmitted epidemic has spread along transportation lines and truckers' routes, which are often lined by small brothels. Therefore, the global AIDS pandemic universally stigmatizes female sex workers' bodies. In parts of sub-Saharan Africa, the AIDS virus is traced through truckers' routes in Tanzania, Zambia, Uganda, the Central African Republic, South Africa, and the Congo. However, regarding sex workers in the United States, several studies have pointed to a different narrative in which prostitutes are more vigilant about safer sex practices than women in the general population. For example, in San Francisco, prostitutes have developed unique ways to protect themselves, such as putting on condoms with their mouths so their clients are less aware of the procedure (Stewart 1999).[4] However, although up to

44 percent of the prostitutes in Southeast Asian countries such as Thailand are HIV-positive, the lack of access to public health interventions means that the methods used to protect against sexually transmitted infections are not well understood by public health workers (Beyrer 1998: 23). In China, Pan Suiming and William Parish (2004) suggest that low rates of STIs among local prostitutes in China imply that they are at lower risk than women in other parts of Asia. Others consider the lag time between infection and actual testing and suggest that Pan and Parish's assumptions are rather optimistic. On Hainan Island in 2000 the rate of infection among prostitutes was 2 percent, which was considerably higher than among the general population.

The questions remain in facing a rising AIDS epidemic: What are the consequences for a small border town such as Jinghong? Who is marketing whose sexuality? Jinghong itself did not become an overnight tourist success without the collusion of several factors, including the idea that the Tai-Lüe people are highly prized for their customs and beauty, the role of Sipsongpanna during the Cultural Revolution, and the exploitation of local natural resources by Communist development. In answering these questions, I trace China's unique history with respect to sexually transmitted infections and link this history to the current practices of selling sex and sexual services and to the market role in shaping condom use in Jinghong.

SEXUALLY TRANSMITTED INFECTIONS:
FROM THE TANG DYNASTY TO THE POSTREFORM ERA

STIs are not new to China or to the border regions of Laos, Burma, and northern Thailand.[5] STIs have a long history that is tied to late-eighteenth- and early-nineteenth-century waves of globalization and commercialization. Historian Carol Benedict notes that bubonic plague traveled quickly (1772–1898) through China from the southwest and Yunnan Province to the eastern seaboard, and then northward, along transportation lines and among workers building China's complex transport system (Benedict 1996).

In 1868 Dr. George Thin observed that Chinese doctors and scholars had identified venereal diseases with "some precision" by the late Tang dynasty (A.D. 618–906) (MacPherson 1987: 221). The physician Tou Han Ch'ing noted that Chinese study of syphilography was fully developed by the northern Song dynasty (960–1279) (MacPherson 1987: 221). According to Dr. Tou, syphilis in China was first detected in Canton (contemporary Guangzhou). The Chinese were also the first to use mercury treatments for syphilis. The Infectious Disease Act, established in Britain in 1866, was extended to Britain's concessions in China and the Shanghai settlement. While scant statistical data was collected on the prevalence and incidence rates of STIs, qualitative speculations abounded concerning an increase in STIs in the 1920s (S. Watts 1997). These arguments are mirrored almost 130 years later. STIs were believed to spread in Shanghai because, (1) as a seaport, it attracted a large number of prostitutes within its limits; (2) it had a large floating population that brought in diseases from elsewhere—for instance, the Japanese were often blamed for the increasing incidence; and (3) its local female prostitutes were "the chief source of danger . . . [and] infested the set-tlement" (MacPherson 1987: 219–20). While Chinese xenophobia blamed the Japanese for infestations of STIs, the local Chinese prosti-tutes were blamed for the diseases' spread, though foreign prostitutes, with a more respectable clientele, were thought to be cleaner. Edward Henderson, the police surgeon and municipal health officer for Shang-hai from 1870 to 1898, explored this subject in *A Report on Prostitu-tion in Shanghai,* a study sponsored by the Municipal Council and pub-lished in 1871. It indicated that between 1865 and 1870, roughly 20 percent of the male patients in the General Hospital were treated for venereal diseases (MacPherson 1987: 219).

In the late Qing dynasty (1893–1911), STIs were known as venereal diseases and often referred to simply as "sexual diseases or maladies" (*xingbing*). The most common STI was syphilis, or *meidu,* which trans-lates as "plum poison." Gonorrhea, on the other hand, was referred to as "strangury" *(linzhuo)* during the late Qing dynasty, and currently is known simply as "dripping illness" *(linbing)* (see Dikötter 1995: 127).

Gail Hershatter (1997) notes that warnings about the dangers of STIs appeared in documents written for foreigners in Shanghai as early as the 1870s and were quite common by the 1920s. Based on data from sev-eral Chinese medical journals, Christian Henriot (1992 & 2001) esti-mates that 10 to 15 percent of urban dwellers had syphilis and almost 50 percent had gonorrhea. Other occupational groups targeted as hav-ing high infection rates included soldiers and policemen, at 35 percent, and merchants, at 32 percent. By comparison, the general urban and rural population was estimated to have an infection rate of about 20 percent. Prostitutes were said to have the highest rates of all and to be "the pestilent link in the chain of transmission" (Hershatter 1997: 230;

see also Sommer 2000). According to Frank Dikötter, by the 1920s, venereal diseases had become a standard feature in Chinese reformists' writings about prostitution, which were tinged with social Darwinist overtones which suggested that in fighting prostitution, one was fighting for China's survival. However, Dikötter (1995) argues, when the Nationalists unified China and established the Ministry of Health in 1928, "they lacked the financial resources and the political will to combat STIs effectively" (137).

On the eve of liberation, in October 1949, there were an estimated ten million persons with STIs (Fan 1990). Mao's militaristic strategies to eliminate STIs began in 1950 under the guidance of the Central Research Institute of Dermatology and Venereology (M. Cohen 1996). This campaign comprised four key strategies: training paraprofessional and public health personnel, mass screening and treatment, propaganda (health education Mao-style), and the elimination of prostitution. According to a handbook on the prevention of sexually transmitted infections, after the Maoists took over in 1949, the new Communist government rehabilitated female prostitutes through re-education and re-employment programs centered on a Maoist-feminist analysis that labeled prostitutes' work as a perpetuation of the exploitation of women. Prostitutes did not "hold up half the sky" *(banbian tian)* (Fan 1990).[6]

According to a report on the country's development in the agricultural sector, every county was encouraged to eliminate STIs in the early 1950s. Several articles published in China between 1959 and 1964[7] reported that China's State Council *(guowuyuan)* declared STIs to have been eliminated through the efforts of on-the-ground socialist health care workers and the emergence of small anti-epidemic stations located at the county level (Fan 1990). By 1956 the brothels were closed and prostitutes "liberated." However, the disappearance of all STIs was declared only in 1972. If STIs were in fact eliminated by then, thirty years later they have made an enormous comeback due to changes in sexual consumption patterns, tourism, open borders, and traveling viruses. According to Fan (1990), cases of syphilis, gonorrhea, and nonspecific vaginitis in China have moved from less than one case in ten thousand in 1980 to twelve in ten thousand in 1988, a staggering twelve-fold increase in eight years.[8] By the end of September 2000, there were 800,000 reported cases of STIs in China, representing an annual increase of 30 percent over the previous year (Zhang Konglai 2001). These STIs are surrogate markers for societal risk for HIV (as rates for STIs rise, so does the risk for HIV). They are also cofactors for transmission, as the presence of STIs, genital ulcers in particular, increases the possibility of contracting HIV (Choi et al. 2000).[9]

In 1989 the standing committee of the Chinese National People's Congress passed a law on the surveillance and reporting of communicable diseases. This thirty-first law on the prevention of communicable diseases stated that any medical or health personnel who identified any individual with AIDS *(aizibing)*, syphilis *(meidu)*, gonorrhea *(linbing)*, or venereal warts *(jianruishiyou)* must report that person to the nearest anti-epidemic health station. STIs in the 1990s have now overtaken tuberculosis *(feijiehe)* to become the third most common category of infectious disease in China, after dysentery and hepatitis B *(yixinggan)*. Since the introduction of market reforms in the early 1980s, the Center for Disease Prevention in Beijing has attributed this increase to changes in social mores, the rise in promiscuity, and low levels of risk awareness among ordinary people (*Agence France-Presse* 1999). In 1995, sex education was introduced into the middle-school curriculum under the rubric "adolescent studies."

Between 1984 and 1994, the southern island province of Hainan had a 170 percent increase in STIs, largely due to a rise in the local sex industry (Cowley 1996: 14). According to Dr. Chen Xiangsheng and colleagues (2000), the yearly incidence of STIs has increased on average by about 17 percent a year since 1994, and extramarital infection remains the main source. In fact, at the Health Care East and West Conference in Boston in June 2001, Myron Cohen suggested that the highest-risk group for STIs is wives of high-income businessmen whose husbands engage in extramarital and transactional sex (M. Cohen 2001). The only infectious STI whose rate has decreased since 1989 is gonorrhea. This decline may be due to several factors: changes in sexual behavior; failure to give notification of gonorrhea because the disease is treated by general practitioners rather than gynecological and genitourinary specialists; health-seeking behavior that leads to self-dose therapy; and a lack of screening because, while screening for syphilis in high-risk groups is mandated in China's premarital examinations, screening for gonorrhea is not (Chen Xiangsheng et al. 2000: 141).

According to a Singaporean doctor working in Jinghong in order to diagnose STIs, private clinics use dipsticks to detect protein in the urine. If protein is present, the patient is given medication, usually antibiotics as an injection of penicillin. The clinics do not take cultures to identify specific diseases, and avoid tests, especially on women, involving disrobing or swabbing of the genitals. According to several medical practitioners in Jinghong, examining a man's genitalia is considered appropriate behavior and is fairly easy to do, but female genitalia are another story. Women are reluctant to be examined, and doctors are both shy and scared to examine women. While I was in Kunming, a gynecologist whom I call Dr. Liang reiterated a popular notion that minority women's genitalia were so dirty that it was impossible for doctors to examine them. In addition, four clinics scattered throughout Jinghong display poster boards covered with medical photographs of patients with severe venereal diseases, including one with venereal warts grown as large as grapefruit. These posters serve as both advertising and displays of the public health grotesque to warn those who might contract STIs. But what is most striking about these advertisements is that they were completely absent in the China I knew in the mid-1980s. Sex and sexuality had changed dramatically in the eleven years I had been away. The sheer proliferation of people moving both within and outside postreform China has furthered the spread of STIs and the accompanying HIV/AIDS epidemic (Beyrer et al. 2000).

A VISIBLE SEXUAL REVOLUTION

China is approaching its own visible sexual revolution in terms of the explosion in individual behaviors that is now fueling an exponential increase in sexually transmitted infections. In this context of examining the dual regimes of the market and state, there is a blending of resources whereby new cultural practices represent an adjustment to market conditions but are not simply forms of sexual commodification and consumption. As Judith Farquhar (2002) points out, since the 1980s there has been a rise in post-Mao urban pleasures and an almost voracious consumer drive "that places sex at the center of just about everything" (247). China's postreform sexual cultures all point toward what James Farrer (2002) calls a sexual "opening up" *(xingkaifang)* to more liberal practices that are influenced by several national rhetorics and spaces filled by the West, Japan, and Thailand. These practices in turn influence the Chinese through the media, personal traveler's encounters, and entertainment venues—films, radio, television, karaoke, and pop songs. With new openings come newfound sexual delights and also several casualties: divorce rates of over 20 percent in some urban centers, a high incidence of abortion among unmarried women, and STIs including HIV/AIDS (Wehrfitz 1996, Nie 2005).[10] Divorce rates and the proliferation of unprotected sex are merely two symptoms of a Chinese public that no longer adheres to a Maoist regime of sexual conservatism; they also point toward the rise in new markets for abortions, divorce courts, and services for newly divorced singles.

According to Ma Xiaonian, an expert at the National Institute for Family Planning, about 50 percent of all abortions are now among unmarried women (Wehrfritz 1996). Wehrfritz also attributes the changes in sexual practices to the 1979 one-child policy, which in one sense "liberated sex from procreation" and "demystified the sex act," as modern methods of birth control (the IUD and sterilization) became widely available for the first time since the 1950s. This sexual revolution is not something that just broke out overnight in the wake of Maoist conservatism; in fact, Chinese sexologist Pan Suiming (1999) describes the emergence of these new practices as "the rise of fire out of the glowing embers" *(sihui furan)*. While STIs and prostitution were allegedly eradicated after 1949, smoldering embers, those that were never extinguished, have contributed to their contemporary reappearance (Pan 1999:9). It is with this STI history in mind that I locate my ethnographic examples in the market for condoms in local pharmacies, sex shops, and hair salons. The practices these locations evoke demonstrate that a new politics of sexuality is emerging within sight of the HIV/AIDS epidemic in the city of Jinghong. One way to illustrate this is to focus my lens on actual sexual practices in these newfound establishments, the hair salons and brothels in this small city of prostitution *(piaocheng)*.

In the three towns in Sipsongpanna, both Han and Tai locals talk about prostitutes in terms of their debauched reputations. Jinghong is know as a *piaocheng,* which is a play on the term *piaoke,* or "man who visits a prostitute," combined with *cheng,* "city." As Jinghong has attracted both sex and nonsex tourists, its reputation has been built up through these inside jokes and linguistic turns of phrase. Accompanying the new economy are new spaces, new markets marked by locals using new terms.

TALKING ABOUT *XINGBING*

First, let's talk sex. I use several words to describe what are known as sexually transmitted infections in the West. When I present ethnographic information on HIV/AIDS, I do so with the understanding that STIs are surrogate markers for societal HIV risk; when STIs rise, so does the risk for HIV transmission. Second, I am looking at STIs as cofactors for transmission (e.g., genital ulcer disease increases transmission efficiency for HIV). And finally, addressing the prevention of one STI provides a potential public health model for reducing the spread of all other STIs, including HIV/AIDS.[11] According to Dr. Li Xiaoliang, a specialist in preventive medicine at Yunnan Medical College, the more common STIs in China include Chlamydia trachomatis *(yituanti)*; human papilloma virus *(renlei rutouzhuang liubingdu)*, or warts *(you)*; herpes simplex virus 1 and 2 *(danchunpao bingdu)*, or simply herpes *(paozhen)*; and pubic lice *(changbing)*.[12] While these terms are rarely used in everyday speech, they suggest that China is confronting an STI epidemic similar to that of its neighbors Thailand and Burma (Entz et al. 2001).

In the New Wind Hair Salon, discussed in chapters 3 and 4, Madam Liu kept close watch on her staff and distributed condoms to those working out-calls, visiting men at their hotels. On these out-calls, the women would present themselves at the front desk of the hotel as having come to wash clothes, deliver food, or just visit a patron at the hotel. Before a woman left the salon, owner Madam Liu would open one of the drawers in the front room, take out one condom, and ceremoniously hand it to Xiao Wang or Xiao Gu. She would remind them of their code words. "Say you are there to wash clothes, and don't forget to tell them this when you knock on the door." It was on these out-calls that "unsafe sexual practices" came into play. Although the women often insisted that they used condoms, they also remarked that some Chinese men did not like to use them because they decreased sensation. Liu, having traveled twice to Thailand, said that there, by contrast, condoms are the norm, but Chinese men were not used to them.

Everyone who worked at the New Wind talked about AIDS, syphilis, and gonorrhea *(aizibing, meidu, linbing)* and how to prevent them. Xiao Yue, Xiao Wang, Xiao Ling, and Xiao Gu repeatedly asserted that all you needed to do was to *"baohu ziji or baohu ganjing"* (keep yourself clean). However, this phrase meant no more to them, and to Madam Liu, than bathing after servicing a customer and using condoms with those customers who would agree to use them. When the staff at the salon joked about AIDS, it was to accuse one another of having it. Xiao Yuan said Xiao Gu was so thin that she must have AIDS. Despite Madam Liu's request for me to find her more foreigners, the workers at the salon said they would never have sex with foreign men, particularly any from Thailand. They all had AIDS. While Madam Liu would pass out condoms to women working on out-calls, none of the prostitutes in the salon said they came into contact with public health officials, let alone ones giving out condoms. The women who worked at the New

Wind never saw or knew anyone with AIDS in Jinghong. Xiao Wang's cousin, who was also from Ruili and worked in a gambling salon, spoke about a man she knew in Ruili who had AIDS.

A former AIDS counselor in the United States, I often launched into my diatribe about how difficult AIDS is to transmit through casual physical contact, but how crucial it was for Gu, Yue, Ling, and Wang to use condoms to prevent further sexual transmission. In response, they all vociferously agreed. Nonetheless, they often contradicted themselves when it came to the practice of using condoms: sometimes they used them religiously; at other times they used them over their customer's objections; at still others they used them only when customers did not object. However, it was apparent that condoms were in plentiful supply. As we have seen, Jinghong was full of shops carrying them: they came in small boxes promoting "pregnancy prevention covers" *(biyun tao)*, with glossy photographs of sexy white and Han women seductively posed in lingerie.

SEX TOYS AND CONDOMS: SIDESTEPPING THE STATE

With the rise of the market economy, certain state functions have been replaced. Individuals now have the opportunity to purchase birth control beyond the eyes of the state's appointed birth control and local anti-epidemic station representatives. While even in Jinghong the Chinese state still enforces the one-child policy among the registered Han population, many of my young informants told me they preferred the discretion that purchasing birth control through shops provided. This does not mean that married couples and single men and women could not acquire condoms from the state if they chose to, but rather that many young people found it more convenient and discrete to purchase them elsewhere. One interpretation of this preference is that young people were resisting the former Communist state intrusions into their personal lives, through everyday practices of resistance (Scott 1985).

Xiao Mei works in her parents' small pharmacy, which has a large display of condoms. She sells lots of condoms, she says, ranging from inexpensive local products selling for a couple of yuan to expensive imported ones from Japan and England going for over ten yuan each. While examining the small boxes of condoms, Xiao Mei giggled and said that "men often buy the cheap ones and prostitutes the expensive ones." I perused these condoms, examining the small boxes packaged in groups of three, ten, and twelve; condoms were now definitely part of the market economy in Jinghong. I found condoms in plentiful supply in just about every small pharmacy and hotel convenience shop. Not only were they sold in these small establishments, but the men who frequent the brothels in Jinghong do purchase them. While conducting follow-up fieldwork in the summer of 2000, I discovered Jinghong had an even wider variety of condoms available at the small pharmacies and a much more visible presence of STI clinics that provided treatment for STIs than it had had three years earlier. What had changed in my three-year absence was a growing awareness of sexually transmitted infections.

By the summer of 2000, Jinghong also had its very own sex shop that catered to the town's many sex tourists. Xiao Ling, the owner, a young woman in her early thirties, told me they had opened that May and that she was trying to make available good-quality condoms on the local market. Her shop included condoms made by joint ventures, such as those between Germany and China, and condoms that were manufactured in China that cost anywhere from two to twenty yuan for a packet of three. In Xiao Wang's opinion, the foreign condoms were of a higher quality than the cheaper Chinese varieties. According to a report by the Yunnan Reproductive Health Research Association, in 1995 less than 50 percent of the domestically manufactured condoms met the standard (YRHRA 2001: 15).

The idea of higher quality in foreign condoms reflected the packaging of condoms in general. One package had photographs of beautiful seductive Chinese women in black leather with their hands tied behind their backs. In contrast, other photographs on condom packages depicted sedate married couples walking in the park hand in hand. These two sets of images created a marked contrast between the sweet innocent proper citizen and the audacious, wild Asian sex queen.[13] Another brand was called "strong man" *(nanzihan)*—"mutually sexy and ultra thin" *(xiangxing chaobao)*, with "family taste in mind" *(jiating zhuang)*. The bright rose-pink packaging depicted a light-skinned white couple, she with long, flowing blond hair and he with short brown hair and shirtless. They were rubbing noses; she was almost naked as her pink dress fell off her shoulders. The man was holding her face in both of his hands and looking soulfully into her blue eyes. The "strong man" condom package had both English and Mandarin text that promised these condoms were designated for family planning and AIDS control.[14] "Whiteness" here can be read as a sign of sexual and scientific medical knowledge. There was a general perception that white people knew how to have sex and that whiteness was a sign of the erotic (see Schein 1994).[15] Whiteness here also represents the new ways that desire is marketed. The images on these condom boxes did not suggest chaste, fully dressed Han women wandering through a park, but rather depicted pleasurable, romantic encounters between heterosexual partners.[16] The underlying notion represented by these condom package covers is that the local moral economy represents, challenges, and embraces both parochial and modern notions of Chinese sexuality (Farquhar 2002; Farrer 2002; Dikötter 1995).

The multiple markets that promote individual sexual pleasure were not relegated to the periphery: condoms and sex toys were available in mundane settings such as the electronics sections of department stores. In the summer of 1997, direct condom promotion campaigns were not part of the state public health projects to overtly prevent the spread of HIV/AIDS in Yunnan. By 2000, however, condoms and sex toys were readily available. In the capital city of Kunming in Yunnan Province, I found an advertisement insert next to vibrators that were for sale in the electronics section of Wuhua Baihua Dalou (a department store). It read:

> Recently, our country's biggest problem is sex[, and] at different ages people discover many changes in their sexual organs, which cause them much grief. These include impotence and early ejaculation, and because of these many people are worried. . . . Sex is the foundation of marriage. If sexual desire is not satisfied, the woman will seek out affairs, and it is very likely that a woman will discover that her husband is moving toward a criminal path. All these factors lead to the creation of an unstable society. Therefore, these products will provide people's lives with some happiness and well-being, and sufficiently and satisfactorily fulfill your sexual desires.[17]

Embedded in the text of this advertisement are several assumptions about Chinese sexuality and gender roles that reveal the cultural representations of sexual expression between men and women. First is the notion that satisfying the woman is a key factor in sexual relationships, or perhaps in modern sexual relationships. Second, without sexual satisfaction, men will follow a criminal path, including infidelity and other activities leading to an unstable society. Third, there is an assumption that sexual liaisons and happiness, as well as sexual pleasure, remain within the confines of heterosexual marriage (see Sigley 1998: 3). The model this advertisement suggests is a kind of sexual hydraulic linking the trope of national satisfaction to individual orgasmic satiation, especially for the woman. While the woman has natural instincts that must be satisfied, it is the man who possesses sexual agency; if his sexual desires are not satisfied, he will go on the warpath of infidelity—a crime against the Chinese state. These notions at first appear to reproduce what Sherry Ortner (1974) labeled as the "man is to culture, as woman is to nature" dichotomy. Here the nature of woman must be civilized through the man, but there is more operating here than a simple binary; instead, a kind of sexual hydraulic emerges à la Foucault (1980). It appears that both men and women should satisfy one another to produce a healthy nation.

Underlying all of these notions are local moralizing discourses that represent, challenge, and embrace both parochial and modern notions of Chinese sexuality (Dikötter 1995). Historian Gail Hershatter (1997) notes that during the Republican Era (1911–49), sexuality and sexual satisfaction were often discursively linked to the progress of the nation (see also Juliette Chung 1999). Orgasms indicated that things were going well for the nation and in the monogamous conjugal bed. Uncovering the implications of linking the state and sexuality requires understanding what Foucault argues are the social and cultural ramifications of focusing on sex as a national social issue, in this case, one that permeates all forms of institutional and everyday life, even when it is not clearly visible (Foucault 1980). What remains to be seen is the kinds of modern sexual practices that become manifest in an environment of increasing fear of sexually transmitted infections. Further, what sorts of state public health responses become productive and possible within a declining socialist public health care system?

RECLAIMING SEX AS A COMMODITY AGAINST PUBLIC HEALTH RESTRICTIONS

World AIDS Day is celebrated around the world on the first of December every year. During World AIDS Day in 1999, the first national condom advertisement was banned in Beijing. It was considered inappropriate. When one focused the lens farther afield, at a Jinghong hospital, one saw that state public health officials advocated limited methods for AIDS prevention since these tactics encouraged locals who were known to be HIV-positive to avoid all sexual liaisons and marriage.[18] In China's struggle against the perceived external threat of AIDS, a new politics of sexuality and the global marketplace in AIDS ideas and practices converge to produce and reproduce distinctly local forms of HIV/AIDS intervention. By promoting condoms, sex toys, and the privatization of STI screening, this politics of sexuality encompasses market practices

that challenge former socialist health care policies that directly intervened in men and women's reproductive and sexual lives. In terms of
HIV/AIDS intervention, a fascinating paradox emerges in which most
public health officials refrain from openly promoting the most effective
means of STI and AIDS prevention, the condom.

According to Dr. Li, an internal medicine specialist at Kunming Medical College, because condoms are considered not as reliable as intrauterine devices (IUDs) and sterilization, these methods were chosen
over condoms and became the most widespread. Other friends of mine
reported that condoms were not popular in China prior to liberation
and therefore were not included in the Communist Party's efforts to control the population explosion. Condom use contravenes a state ethos of
birth control whereby the target is to reduce births and instill the political demographic ideal of one child per couple. Condoms were and in
many cases are still seen as both a sexually improper and medically in-
ferior method of birth control (see Tyrene White 1985). However, there
is also a marked gender component to the selection of birth control
methods versus STI prevention. Currently the locus of control remains
with women, as they are expected to regulate their bodies in the name
of demography, whereas condoms, used only by male bodies for safer
sex, are given little importance. In fact several of my informants who
were prostitutes and women in other occupations remarked that sex becomes more pleasurable without worries of pregnancy or disease transmission. The language of prevention gets in the way because condoms
are called by the name *biyun tao* (pregnancy prevention covers), rather
than the term adopted in Taiwan and Hong Kong, *anquan tao* (safety
covers). Condoms in many ways rely on personal agency and practical
consistency, whereas IUDs and sterilization are administered by the
state and are semipermanent and permanent solutions to population
control.

Although one might suspect that the local anti-epidemic station
(fangyizhan) would be the center for STIs and AIDS tests, as well as the
promotion and marketing of free condoms, this was not the case in August 1997. While the market in sex tourism promotes active nonmarital
sex, and even dangerous sexual behavior, it provides mechanisms for the
distribution, sale, and marketing of precisely those birth control devices
that best protect against STIs and pregnancy. These different market
mechanisms support and reinforce one another.

Another phenomenon closely related to the prevention of STIs and
AIDS is the rise in roving small private health clinics. Jinghong, like

many other Chinese cites in the late 1990s, had these illegal clinics that provide inadequate and at best rudimentary STI testing services.[19] Often outside the purview of state public health officials, the clinics instead operate in fly-by-night hotels in the quasi–red light districts of large cities, every so often changing their location to avoid the scrutiny of the state. They rely on their patrons' need for discretion and quick injections of penicillin. They also advertise in many southern Chinese cities in locations where transients are apt to see them, such as near railroad and bus stations. In Jinghong these posters actually eluded me at first; only after living there for several months did I find them located off the beaten track, never on the main streets where tourists would see them.

Dr. Su, an internal medicine specialist interested in HIV/AIDS, said: "Promiscuity and excessive sex are to blame for the proliferation of STIs and AIDS. We need to prevent people from having sex outside of marriage." Dr. Su noted that she spent an afternoon in August 1997 encouraging a man who was HIV-positive to not even think about dating, let alone marrying. She told me her method of prevention was direct intervention into his life; she would periodically meet with him to persuade him that bachelorhood was the only way to prevent AIDS. When I mentioned condoms, she forthrightly pointed out that condoms are not a method of birth control supported by state family planning efforts. IUDs, birth control pills, and sterilization are the current methods sanctioned by the state, and therefore other methods, including condoms, cannot be promoted or condoned. Although it would be simple to condemn Dr. Su's interventions, public health officials are conceptually and practically limited in what they can think and do. They cannot directly promote condom use, but they also do not shut down the private roving clinics in Jinghong, nor confiscate their condoms. At Zhongshan University in Guangzhou, a condom machine was placed on campus as part of the effort to prevent both pregnancy and disease. When the machine was discovered, the university claimed it was only for the faculty's convenience, because it is ostensibly against the law for students to have sex while at university.

Once again, the state was dubious about promoting the outright use of condoms for just anyone. Married couples still have access to condoms that are distributed by such organizations as the anti-epidemic stations, the Women's Federations, and many of the NGOs working on HIV prevention in Yunnan, such as Population Services International, Oxfam, Save the Children Foundation, the Australian Red Cross, and Médicins Sans Frontières. State regulation and licensing is catching up

with the market in the sense that cities such as Tianjin are experimenting with regulating prostitution as a legitimate business rather than just
something to be stamped out. Regulation also applies to changes in policies regarding condoms in order to improve their quality and accessibility. While not widely available through hospitals and clinics, condoms
are available in almost all drug stores in major cities in China. In a study
of fifty-eight randomly selected drug stores in Shanghai in 1998, Tu
Xiaowen and her colleagues discovered that shopkeepers believed that
condoms and contraceptive pills were an essential and important convenience for young unmarried couples (Tu Xiaowen 1998 in YRHRA
2001: 2). Condoms in many ways are a way for youth to avoid the regulation of the state and use the market to fulfill their need for both birth
control and STI prevention.

    On the other hand, the migrant prostitutes are only marginally sub-
ject to the regulatory arm of the local Jinghong government, and certainly do not fall under Dr. Su's scrutiny. Instead, they are subject to
their home localities, and therefore they would have a difficult time getting state-sponsored birth control in Jinghong. Prostitutes' only options
are buying condoms at local stores or paying for medical services at one
of the privately run local clinics. Buying condoms, they told me, was
more discrete than visiting a private clinic. What appears at first as a
kind of antistate pleasure actually is a consumption practice that is encouraged by market socialist reforms. What appears as reclaiming sex
from a conservative state and local patriarchy through the act of buying
condoms may actually be an act of consumptive pleasure that the state
actually encourages through the openness of the market for consumers.

    While some organizations, such as the Women's Federation *(fulian)*,
have begun education efforts, they have adopted a top-down model according to which sex workers sit in a room and listen to education lec-
tures, often early in the morning. The sex workers complain that the
workshops are useless and too early for them because they work all
night. The Women's Federation complains that sex workers are not interested in prevention. However, other projects in cities such as Shanghai have been more successful (Xia Guomei 2003). Shanghai sociologist
Xia Guomei (2003) has been conducting research among female entertainment workers around Shanghai and reports that everyone she spoke
with preferred peer education as the most important and effective way
to deliver HIV/STI prevention information, rather than programs that
were modeled on top-down structures similar to the Women's Federation approach.

SIDESTEPPING THE STATE

In much of contemporary, postreform China, public subsidized care is on the decline and in its place are a myriad of markets including those for sex toys and sexual protection for birth control and disease prevention. Market economies, whether in socialist countries or not, require new markets to the degree that with increasing pressure, even state-run public health hospitals and clinics have to generate income. This has meant that state- and privately run clinics, pharmacies, and hospitals sold items found in many private pharmacies the world over. In Jinghong the proliferation in items associated with sex are integrally connected to its overt sex industry. All of this leads us back to the paradox in which two kinds of power are manifest: the state's power in regulating STIs through clinics that cater to heteronormative couples, and the countervailing power of market forces that promote birth control and disease prevention techniques to anyone with the money to buy condoms. These two kinds of power are evident through the actual on-the-ground practices described here.

If the contemporary sex industry signifies the liberal opening up of sexuality and the rise of post-Mao urban pleasures, we could say that responses to market forces have revolutionized social practices as an act of necessity. As China enters international markets, new products must be invented to ensure the increasing prosperity of its citizenry. Sexual products, the consumption of sex, and the exchange of money for sexual favors become parts of a modern urban sexual culture. Perhaps consuming sexual products is a way of moving toward the market and away from a regulatory state. What is remarkable is that the consumption of condoms in the marketplace is done in Jinghong within the purview of the state public health apparatus. If one wishes to buy condoms, one does not need to consult a neighborhood committee member nor submit to the scrutiny of Women's Federation representatives who carefully survey one's menstrual cycle; however, all business enterprises need permits from the state, even sex shops. Thus condom consumption points toward what I call a sidestepping of strict family planning regulations, rather than consulting the state public health apparatus. If all one has to do is frequent the local pharmacy, department store, or hotel convenience shop, the consumption of condoms marks a potential space for promoting AIDS prevention practices in small tourist towns such as Jinghong. While I have argued it is a simple question of resistance—not deliberate economics, taxation, and surveillance—that has lead to the rise of condom promotion and marketing, there is actually a much more complicated relationship between state economics, public health regulation, and marketing and use of condoms. My term "sidestepping" acknowledges declining state regulatory and surveillance power, while it also points to the expanding markets in market socialism. Chinese citizens' desires for sexual products are attached to notions about what it means to be modern. Condoms in one sense provide both reduced surveillance and increased privacy within market socialism.

If we adopt a strictly public health perspective, it remains to be seen if these marketing strategies for condoms will further prevent the spread of STIs: consumption and actual use are two separate issues. In Thailand, condom use became widespread in brothels only once it was enforced. Men the world over are known for buying their way out of using condoms, as the devices are known to reduce their pleasure. Therefore condoms may not be the panacea with which all public health experts are now so thoroughly enchanted.

CHAPTER 6

Moral Economies
of Sexuality

When Heaven and Earth are in harmony,
I perch my small home on clear clean blue wings.[1]

A stone's throw from the Burma border, the rickety old bus climbs
into the mountains toward a Bulang village. Later, as the bus drives
through the village, I gaze into the eyes of children as they run from
their wooden huts waving and shouting, full of giggles. I cannot
help but notice, beneath this veneer, their torn clothes. They are
wearing no shoes. Their hair is a tangle of black strands. The remoteness of the location means that most of the Bulang in Sipsongpanna do not live or work near the town of Jinghong, and few are
employed in the restaurant and gambling halls where money is
made. The Bulang fit into the stereotypical visions of hill tribes scattered throughout Southeast Asia. [Burma border, August 1996]

Zhang gathers her ebony rayon skirt in one hand and plays busily
with the small gold cross on her chest with the other. She sighs,
"Women are really no longer the property of men. Chinese women
are liberated, we do not have to live under the yoke of one man."
Prostitution, choosing not to marry, and female business acumen
are just symbols of modern life in postreform China that congeal at
the level of desire. [Jinghong, July 1997]

DIFFERENT VIEWS OF AUTHENTICITY

While the above scenarios, revealing the poverty of rural minority hill
tribes and the relative affluence of a young female economic migrant,

present two contrasting and essentializing views of Sipsongpanna, they also provide a glimpse into the divergent worlds that make up modern Sipsongpanna. The two previous chapters set the stage for my investigation of how the cultural politics of the HIV/AIDS epidemic in late-twentieth-century China can be understood as a disease of geography, and of how the border minority prefectures near Laos and Burma became its epicenter. In this chapter, I shift my focus to examine the connections between the formation of a new moral sexual economy and the recent changes in the political and economic landscape that have led to the development and promotion of new leisure sexual activities (see Ruan 1991; Gil 1993; Zito and Barlow 1994). Arthur Kleinman, Veena Das, and Margaret Lock (1997) argue that to understand China, one must understand people's local moral worlds, how they construct and deconstruct their own moral universe. I argue that competing moral economies of sexuality partially explain why AIDS is represented in such a contradictory fashion in these border regions: it is produced by the Tai, it is not produced by the Tai; it is produced by prostitutes, it is not produced by prostitutes; it is due to economic reform; it is a return to the late Qing; it is impacted by tourism, it is not impacted by tourism.

In chapter 3, I introduced three ways of understanding Chinese sexual morality: a *liberal* market morality, a *parochial* Maoist morality, and a Han *nationalist* morality. To these I now add a fourth, the *ethnic revivalist* morality that involves trace actions of counterhegemonic resistance to the Han state. The scope of these local moral ways of thinking covers the following: First, a liberal market morality tells us about what it means to possess a modern sexuality, including prostitution, multiple lovers, and unprotected sex. Second, a parochial morality controls high-risk sexual behavior, especially among commercial sex workers and intravenous drug users. Third, a Han nationalist morality stigmatizes ethnic minority groups, including the Tai. Fourth, a morality of ethnic revivalism challenges both the parochial and the liberal moral codes through counterhegemonic practices. This final set of moral practices highlights a certain Tai voice in Jinghong and illuminates the conflicting responses to my original research question on the Tai and HIV/AIDS. Striking in Yunnan are the internecine battles between these moral practices, as each seeks to legitimize a unique moral universe under the modern Chinese state and under certain kinds of authenticity (see MacCannell 1973). Thus, Han nationalist everyday practices stigmatize the Tai, while liberal moral practices eroticize the Tai. These practices are part of a new moral economy that points toward a modern postreform sexual subject who may have multiple lovers, engage in prostitution, and take second wives (or husbands) as business partners and lovers. However, all four moralities are but conflicting, contested, and partial views of contemporary Chinese sexuality. Anna Tsing (1993) urges allowing local actors to imagine multiple possibilities, so as to permit interpretations of subjects' agency, power, and knowledge of different kinds, and on different levels, such that one interpretation does not supersede the other. Furthermore, I am in no way suggesting a singular theory of socialist modernity or morality; rather, through my informants' acts and words, I weave some key theoretical discussions about cultural transformation in Sipsongpanna.

A MORAL ECONOMY OF SEXUALITY

In the previous chapter, I argued that the Chinese state takes a subsistence approach to sexuality. Sex is considered essential for the rebirth of the Chinese nation, and the state repeatedly demonstrates that if the conjugal couple is happy, so is the nation. This subsistence notion of sexuality insists that sex is never unbounded and free, but rather is proscribed by anti-epidemic station workers, by physicians, and by the police. Sexual economies control morality in modernity, especially, in China's case, through regulations around procreation and the one-child family; the results of unregulated sex are restricted.[2] L. H. M. Ling (1999: 278) points out that with globalization, "modernity means a capital-intensive, upwardly mobile hyper masculinity as opposed to a closed, local, service-based, regressive femininity." However, in Ling's terms this modernity is a hybrid mix of simulacra and local-global relationships. In addition, modern versions of sexuality in China have been shaped by and have responded to earlier understandings of sex and sexuality.

While the meaning of sexuality in China shifted a number of times during the late twentieth century, what Judith Farquhar and Zhang Qicheng (2005) call "footprints" of previous regimes are ever present.[3] Sexuality shifted after collectivization in the 1950s, so that it was no longer considered part of what it meant to be wealthy and prosperous. Under Mao sex became a taboo subject, and erotic attention skirted toward cooperative production for the state, through the family and mothers. Then sex shifted again in the mid-1980s to emerge as part of life separate from reproduction and state demographic obligation (Farquhar 2002: 215–16). Farquhar's discussions of historical memory and bodily practices are a potent contribution to any discussion of contemporary Chinese sexuality; however, her work focuses almost exclusively on the modern city of Beijing.

James Farrer (2002) also addresses contemporary sexuality in China. He focuses on the cosmopolitan city of mid-to-late-1990s Shanghai, with an ethnographic eye toward the confluences of the market economy and unmarried youths' sexual culture. His observations in nightlife spots, university dance halls, and the sexual playgrounds of contemporary youth are stunning in their ethnographic color and depth. Farrer's purpose is to conceptualize the sexual culture of unmarried youth as a broad symbolic field in which actors, scenes, and instrumentalities are as important as acts themselves. In addition, his work, like much scholarship on postreform China, makes a case for conceptualizing sexual cultural change during the transition to the market economy (Farrer 2002: 5–6). However, what Farquhar and Farrer do not provide is a view of sexuality away from the centers of cosmopolitan China. In that regard, I argue that in mid-to-late-1990s borderland China, and in mid-level cities such as Jinghong, the meaning of sex and sexuality has also shifted to reflect a particular kind of local cultural capital strongly influenced by the rise in tourist and economic development.

Another way into the cultural dynamics of contemporary Sipsong-panna is to understand how control over social space contributes to the commodification of age-old practices (prostitution) and ethnic group dynamics (Tai-Han relations). The practice of prostitution marks a unique transition from the Chinese socialist project, which created spaces to entice youth into good, clean fun, away from backward, feudal practices. Since the 1990s, the old socialist spaces have been reconfigured and reclaimed by youth in Jinghong. The cultural palace *(wenhuagong)*, a part of the Maoist project to develop gathering places for youth, is now divided into dark movie theaters where youth go to make out. The former athletic fields are now lined with pool tables and video arcades, which are the new preferred leisure-time amusements. These spaces also provide places where youth can engage in courtship and sexual practices and shoot heroin. Because these spaces are no longer policed in the old Maoist sense, no one is watching what occurs on the edges of these hangouts.

I argue that these spaces, while signifying the changing economic geography of Jinghong, are never really neutral but are highly loaded with latent moral meaning. The Chinese market economic project to create spaces for youthful entertainment has been re-appropriated by local youth who engage in a variety of practices that challenge the state's original vision for these spaces. Spaces that housed Ping-Pong and state-sanctioned films and games have become precisely the spaces where brothels, heroin, and gambling reside, activities that are often referred to as a downside of the socialist market economy. This development also ties in with the competition between the parochial and the liberal local moral economies, just as the earlier condom campaign was first released to the Chinese public and then banned for promoting immorality. Even the 1990s popular television show *Wo Ai Wo Jia* (I Love My Family), scripted by the hooligan writer Wang Shuo, circulated widely and was then banned for portraying an amoral picture of Chinese society.

The bodily behavior of the Jinghong citizen is still regulated in innumerable subtle ways, from signs on street corners that suggest walking in a civil way, to prohibitions on littering, to regulating the sexual behavior of different ethnic groups—all means of internalizing the will of the state at the level of individual bodily behavior (see Brownell 1995; Greenhalgh 2005). In China's border regions, controlling the sexual behavior of different ethnic groups becomes an issue connected to controlling the borders of the Chinese nation. Government policies for developing western China have emerged as means both to quell nationalist sentiments among minority groups and for economic and capital expansion (Rui 2005). In Jinghong, the regulation of behavior is not always as clear-cut as it seems, because competing notions of morality and sexuality operate simultaneously. In terms of my four ways of moral thinking about sexual practices, morality in the borderlands is regulated in part through liberal notions of sexuality, including the idea that a Chinese businessman or -woman can and often does have more than one partner, spouse, or lover, who may also be a business partner. Madam Liu, owner of the New Wind Hair Salon, who had a husband in Guizhou, along with a lover, Tan, in Jinghong, reflects this liberal market morality. As stated above, these notions of morality have shifted since Mao's time.

The new liberal morality furthers the development of the nation by rewarding Han businessmen (and they are mainly men) for their hard work with tourist vacations for sex in Sipsongpanna. Simultaneously, the parochial morality allows sexual liberalism in the form of transactional sex to be punished. Female prostitutes in Jinghong are regularly rounded up and literally driven north into Simao County. This parochial morality, mirrored in much of the colonial thinking in global AIDS discourses, gets inflected with a Han nationalist twist when it is directed toward ethnic minorities. Dr. Qi, a physician in the Jinghong Anti-Epidemic Station, advocates that all women, regardless of their ethnicity, should to be forced to take an HIV test after returning from Thailand—but especially, she adds, the Tai ones. Sexual morality never follows a straightforward path, as it is historically situated and contested every step of the way.

SEX AND DISEASE AS A SOCIAL PROBLEM IN 1990S CHINA

In my own experiences as an outsider in China, I was struck by the startling changes between 1985 and 1995, especially the burgeoning of brash and copious images of sex and sexuality. Long gone are the days when men and women looked and dressed alike in shapeless dark-blue, green, or gray pants with matching loose-fitting buttoned-up Mao jackets. However, accompanying these changes in fashion and behavior are the commercialization of women's bodies and the rampant increase in sexually transmitted diseases, including, now, HIV/AIDS. As Chinese public health officials claim that heterosexual transmission of HIV is on the increase in border towns such as Jinghong, social science researchers need to shift their focus to comprehend local understandings and conceptions of sexuality.

An understanding of HIV/AIDS and new behaviors reflecting new moral economies of sexuality cannot be complete without a discussion of how ordinary people understand these new practices. To address this, I have selected parts of narratives from interviews with Jinghong Han and minority locals who have a particular perspective on the Chinese project of modernity, a viewpoint that includes sexually transmitted diseases and "sex work." Through these interviews, I explore four very different individual perceptions of prostitution and changing notions of sexuality in the city of Jinghong. I selected these particular individuals' stories because their understandings of sexuality, morality, and the links to the political economy of Sipsongpanna reveal the four moral economies I present.

Lian, who is half Tai, suggests that "opening up" has provided some women with better economic opportunities, including the prostitutes who migrate to Jinghong to work in bars, hair salons, and brothels. She also suggests that while the economy has moved forward, prosperity has marked downsides, among them sickness among women and rampant STIs. Tian, who is a member of the Aini minority,[4] enunciates a Han nationalist view of minorities such as herself when she says, "The Tai are lazy and do not work hard." At the same time, she recounts her own memories of being persecuted as a minority student in an elementary school run by a sent-down Han youth from Shanghai. Zhang, a Han businesswoman in Jinghong, provides another view of Chinese women. She chose not to marry because, in her words, marriage only makes women into chattel and slaves. Her point of view is important in that she herself is part of the ongoing civilizing project of the Chinese state: she trains young hotel workers to be more courteous and polite and to serve their customers in what she calls an "old-fashioned style," one more conducive to the market economy than the brusque Maoist egalitarian work ethic.

My final narrative is about a young Tai Buddhist, Ai Lao, who is part of the revival of Tai culture in Sipsongpanna that is occurring through pop music, Tai language fluency, and a Buddhist school. His views reflect an emerging consciousness among a small segment of educated Tai that Sipsongpanna should exist as a region for the minorities who have lived there for centuries, rather than only as a tourist playground for the Han. He too is full of contradictions. Like many Tai, he participates in Han tourism because his family's livelihood depends on Han floaters, the large population of migrants in Jinghong who are the backbone of the tourist industry and to whom he rents small rooms on the ground floor of his home. The majority of his income comes from these illegal renters. He was one of the many Tai I spoke to who was openly distressed about how the Tai are represented as sexually promiscuous and as carriers of AIDS to the Han majority. However, most Tai villagers whom I interviewed found it rather paradoxical that the Han would peg them as promiscuous, as the Tai believe that all of the prostitutes and customers in Jinghong are Han. These four individuals—Lian, Zhang, Tian, and Ai Lao—offer stories about contemporary Jinghong that are partial, unstable, and contradictory as they reveal competing narratives of authenticity, narratives that move back and forth between ideas and practices that both embrace and repel a market morality, a parochial morality, a Han nationalist morality, and a morality of ethnic revival (see Malkki 1995).[5]

LIAN: A YOUTHFUL ENTREPRENEURIAL SPIRIT

I first met Lian, a boisterous nineteen-year-old with dark amber skin and warm brown eyes, when she was the owner of a small shop near one of the elementary schools in Jinghong. Lian graduated from middle school at age fifteen and came to Jinghong, she said, "because one cannot live all one's life at home." She was unemployed and looking for work. Lian often spoke in loud tones and raised her voice in vociferous arguments. I regarded her as a live wire. I later learned that she had led an adventurous life for one so young. By the age of nineteen, she had held several jobs as a teacher, tour guide, café worker, and now shopkeeper. She was born in the town of Menghai, the second largest city in Sipsongpanna, where her parents worked at the local tea research institute picking tea. Her father was fifty-one, her stepmother forty-one, her younger stepsister fourteen, and her stepbrother ten. She laughed in a most delicate and awkward way when I asked about the last. Apparently he had been removed from the family home because he was difficult for her stepmother, a schizophrenic, to handle. Her stepmother now lives in an institution, and Lian hasn't seen her biological mother since she was fourteen. Her biological mother is Tai, so Lian considered herself one of the Han-Tai minorities in Sipsongpanna. Her stepmother and fourteen-year-old stepsister are Ainizu. This stepsister had had a fever as a child and had not spoken since, although Lian insisted she is very smart. That year, 1996, a new school for the disabled (canjiren) was opening in Menghai that would accommodate her sister. Because the girl was very expressive, a local dance troop (gewutuan) had agreed to take her in, provided she could follow directions. Unfortunately, her hearing loss precluded this opportunity.

Lian described own her life in these terms:

> In 1994, I went to Damenlong to work at a jade shop with my aunt's daughter. Then, in 1995, I worked in a gambling salon in the leisure room as a clerk. I then worked as a tour guide because I can speak some Tai and made about four hundred yuan per month in salary, but I could make as much as ten thousand yuan per month with my commissions (huikou). In the early days of tourism in Sipsongpanna [the early 1990s], you could make really good money—before more women came and before each establishment gave tour guides a cut only if their customers bought something. Early on, they made money even when customers didn't buy, just for the service of bringing people by. A prominent Shanghai paper even commented that the tour guides were making great salaries. In contrast, now almost everyone I know has either quit, is out of work, or is looking for better jobs. There is a difference between the low season (danji) and high season (wanji), and now I want to open a small shop with my savings. My parents now have the ability to buy a home for fifty thousand yuan and I want to help them realize their dream.

When I asked Lian about the recent economic changes and the rise in sex tourism, she repeated a popular refrain:

As for economic changes in Jinghong and the rise of tourism, I got to know several prostitutes *(jinü)*, since they lived in a small housing complex down the street from my store. They told me lots of stories. . . . One time, I was asked to verify to the police that a woman was not a prostitute. As she looked at me, I could not honestly tell the police this was her boyfriend. As for why women like her become prostitutes, it is easy money that doesn't require skills. To become a tour guide, one must be local and at least have some education and usually speak some minority language or be familiar with local customs.

Almost all the prostitutes are from outside the area, most from Sichuan and Guizhou. Many women leave home after marrying and after giving birth because they cannot find enough work in their hometowns. They come to Sipsongpanna to become prostitutes. But their lives are really difficult because they get sick regularly because their customers do not use condoms and then they are afraid to go to the local government hospital. Instead, the madam charges one hundred yuan per injection of antibiotics.

Otherwise, the work is easy and they can make around three to four thousand yuan per month. . . . During the day you can play and then only have to work at night. Most go home at spring festival, but those who don't go home are usually the ones where someone in their hometown found out about their work, and they lost face. Work involves performing sex at one hundred to three hundred yuan per customer. But when they get sick, they cannot work. On average they see three to four customers a night. Also because few tests are done, and they don't know what disease they have, they just get an injection of penicillin. The hospital often has to report it, and they don't want to be identified as someone who has too many STIs. There are definitely more prostitutes *(jipo)* working in the hair salons and at the cosmetic salons *(huazhuang benbao)* than when I first came here.

When I asked Lian about who she thought were most likely to get STIs and AIDS, she said:

As for getting STIs, it is prostitutes and their customers, and then their wives and children. There is also a local legend that says there was a guy who had given AIDS to his wife and then his wife gave it to their seven-year-old daughter. The man was one of the male government officials who allegedly come here on trips to promote business, and then engaged with prostitutes during his official business. I also believe that objects in your house can give you AIDS, like food products and utensils.

When I asked Lian about the police presence in Jinghong, she said:

As for the police, and the recent surveillance of customers down in Man-jinglan and on Mantinglu,[6] the people just stay inside until a crackdown *(yanda yundong)* ends—no walking, no business at night, and so on. We have to be wary because one woman hung out with some men who poisoned her food and then raped her. I think our society is becoming crazier. This is certainly true here in Jinghong compared to the town of Menghai where I grew up. The crackdown does find particular people to fine, and other businesses in return must provide bribes *(dianshui)* to avoid these fines.[7] However, the criminals are many and the police are few, and Jinghong is a tourist town and those without anything will always desire to steal other people's belongings.

Lian is clear as to the dual nature of morality that operates in places like Jinghong. On one hand, women are gaining very lucrative employment, especially peasant women who cannot find work in their hometowns in Sichuan and Guizhou provinces. On the other hand, these women entertainers who live off their beauty are the same women subject to China's rising epidemics of STIs and HIV/AIDS, because customers are reluctant to use condoms. In Lian's narrative exists the liberal market morality that encourages and condones women's sexual freedom to capitalize on their beauty. There is also the parochial Maoist morality—or perhaps one may say Confucian values—that shuns women who work in the sex industry. Lian's narrative reflects the idea that these moral economies exist side by side, often waxing and waning, depending on the economic tides that swing through Jinghong. Lian does not link the cycle of disease transmission morally. She understands that customers can give AIDS to their wives, but she does not see that customers also can give it to the female prostitutes. Her discussion about AIDS suggested a particularly gendered narrative. Female prostitutes get blamed for infecting innocent wives, while men get left out of this narrative of blame, as if they have no role to play as customers. Women in one sense are the ones who cannot entirely protect themselves from men—their partners, husbands, and customers—who do not often use condoms. As it has the world over, AIDS in China becomes a gendered epidemic. Several male customers remarked that while they would consider using condoms with prostitutes, they would not with their wives and girlfriends.

TIAN: MINORITY WOMEN AND MODERNITY

In the following narrative, I focus on a beautiful young Aini woman who worked at one of the most expensive hotels in Jinghong. When I first moved to Jinghong in February 1996, I lived across the street from one of the city's oldest and nicest hotels. As guest numbers were low, I was allowed to swim in the hotel's pool, at a premium price. While at the pool, I met several young people working in the hotel, as the hotel workers' guesthouse was directly behind the swimming pool. It was there that I met Tian, a twenty-three-year-old former elementary English teacher from the town of Puer. She was born in 1974 near Puer and at the time of our interviews was an unemployed tour guide. Tian explained her family's history, that she came from a very poor area and had five siblings. Her two older brothers worked in Jinghong, the elder as a policeman and the younger at a local travel agency.

Tian described her life this way:

> My three sisters all live near our home, ninety-eight kilometers from Puer. My parents are peasants, and since peasants never retire, they are still planting wet rice in Meizi. I graduated from a teacher training college in Simao, the same place where I went to middle school, and then spent three years teaching English. I went to an elementary school that was a two-kilometer walk from my natal home, and I couldn't speak Mandarin when I first went to school. When I was a child, we didn't have very much to eat and we often ate corn versus the wet rice that my father planted. My father and mother are now fifty and forty-nine years old, respectively. My first teacher didn't like minority students and I was definitely discriminated against because of my dark skin. My second teacher was one of the Han-educated youth sent down here during the Cultural Revolution, and he liked to beat children. It was also the mining industry that brought more Han like him into the area. When my second Han teacher hit me, I didn't want to return to school, but my father encouraged me because I was too young to work in the fields. My Han teacher discriminated against all minority children as these middle-school kids came from all over Banna [the local moniker for Xishuangbanna]—from Menglian, Simao and also Lancang. Although my grandfather was Han, everyone else down the line is Aini. Almost all of my classmates went on to attend middle school, but only 50 percent went on to high school, and then only 10 percent of the students at the teacher training college are minorities, although we make up over 60 percent of the population.
>
> When I graduated, I went to teach for three to four years and had almost fifty students per class. I was also praised for writing pinyin very well and always got good grades, but didn't get a red scarf *(hong lingjin)* until my second year, because the teacher didn't think I was valiant enough.[8]

When I asked Tian why she came to Jinghong, she said:

> I came to Jinghong during the Tai New Year Water Splashing Festival *(poshuijie)* in 1992 on a school trip. I then returned in 1994 to travel and stayed with relatives. My first job was at the Tai Garden Hotel soon after it opened. I was paid nothing at first in my training classes, which included learning some English, and then 320 yuan per month, and later 800 per month at the front desk, where I was supposed to speak English to foreign guests. However, my English was still limited. I was given two free meals a day and a dorm room that I shared with eight other hotel workers, includ-

ing a communal toilet and shower. I left this job because there was very little freedom, long hours, and almost nothing to do, as we had few guests at
the hotel.

My second job was at the Jade Spring Travel Agency as a tour guide,
where I worked for one year. Later, as a travel agent, I made two hundred
yuan per month in salary and between three thousand and four thousand
yuan in commissions per month. In 1996, I quit when a relative suggested I
work for them in Kunming at a joint venture company, with American in-
vestors who were affiliated with the local tobacco company. The Tai Garden Hotel is also one of their affiliated businesses. Even if the work unit
(danwei) system doesn't work anymore, businesses still take care of those
they see as their own.[9] But you see, I couldn't get a residence permit for
Kunming, and they decided if I had no local residence permit *(hukou)*, I
couldn't possibly work for them. In Jinghong having a local *hukou* doesn't
matter, but in Kunming it does. Also, working as a travel agent, you are on
your feet every day and I worried about being in the sun. My younger
brother said I was beginning to look like a peasant after being in the sun so
much, guiding tourists here and there.

When I asked Tian about the impact of economic changes in Jinghong, she said:

Freedoms have increased a little bit. The old system of the iron rice bowl
(tie fanwan) no longer exists, where everything and everyone was carefree.[10] But now that you are no longer assigned jobs, generating connections is extremely important; to follow your own path is the new way. In
Jinghong there is a talent market *(rencai shichang)* for the tourist industry,
but few people go because the salaries there are not as high as if you find a
job on your own.

When I asked Tian about the sex industry and tourism in Jinghong,
she laughed and said:

Often hotel customers will ask me about finding them a woman to accompany them for the evening. People rarely say they are looking for a prostitute *(jipo)*. They usually charge at least three hundred yuan just to accompany them, but I don't know other prices. Customers always turned to the
male guide to ask him to find someone, and they often use a more discreet
term of "zhao yi ge nü de tanxin" (finding a woman to "flirt" with). At
Peacock Park at night all the women waiting there are prostitutes and these
prostitutes are from outside the town, not locals at all. Also, since regulations *(hukou)* are so relaxed here, they can rent apartments, not just single
rooms like on Mantinglu. However, being a prostitute has its risks, and getting a sexually transmitted disease is just one risk. Also, everyone knows
that foreigners carry AIDS, but if so few foreigners come here, we cannot
blame foreigners but the Chinese men who pursue these prostitutes. In
terms of the prostitution trade, it is like the wind, it blows away and then

blows back again. Because the strike-hard anticrime campaign *(yanda yundong)* in Banna is not explicit, even if they catch prostitutes and fine them or send them out of the county, of course they come back. It would be better if we had a a red-light district *(hong dengqu)*, according to approved rules and administered regulations. Otherwise, there is no way to keep order, and currently the lack of administration over prostitution means it is completely out of control.

When I asked Tian about whether she thought there is discrimination of minorities in Sipsongpanna, she said:

In terms of education, people's levels are not the same, and in people's hearts they are not really the same either. What we need more than anything else is to increase people's level of education. There are just too many people in Banna that are illiterate, and because school fees are getting too expensive for everyone to participate, it is not fair to discriminate against certain children. As for the discrimination against minorities, it depends on your position. The Tai also wear the clothes of the Han, so we cannot distinguish them. All of the dancers on Mantinglu are 90 percent Tai women. The Tai have become rich from selling their land and also renting out their homes. They have the freedom to do with their land what they choose. The Tai are very open *(kaifang)* but have little formal education, while the Han are the hard workers in Banna. And while they [the Tai] also may have little education, they have good hearts, a little like foreign men who are playful and nice. I want to find a husband who is carefree and playful, especially a foreign one!

Tian reveals a sort of hybridity in her views of the local moral economy: her ideas reflect a mélange of the Han nationalist and the liberal market morality. While she criticizes the Han youth from Shanghai for discriminating against her for being non-Han and a minority, she also embraces the local lore that the Han are the hard workers in Jinghong, that they came to develop the mining industry and stayed to develop greater Sipsongpanna. In terms of a liberal market morality, she believes that the Tai have not been left out of tourist development, that they have become rich from buying into Han notions of modernity, and that developing the land and the tourism industry will bring prosperity to the region. Nevertheless, she internalizes local Han ideas about the Tai as she sees them as lazy and carefree, not industrious like the Han. She does point out that in terms of obvious bodily ethnic markers, the Han and Tai often dress alike so that it is difficult to distinguish them. At the end of her narrative, she says that she too would like to escape Sipsongpanna and China and go to another country and into a foreigner's (read: Westerner's) arms.

ZHANG: CHANGING NOTIONS OF FEMALE SEXUALITY

In the third narrative, I continue with the story of the unusual woman I
introduced at the beginning of this chapter, who embarked on a life that
rests on a combination of feminist ideals and her own brand of Catholicism. Zhang was the former owner of a café and a karaoke bar near the
north end of town. I first met her at her café in 1996, when it was located around the corner from an elementary school where I got clothes
washed; it was close to a friend's café. Zhang and I chatted many times.
She often offered to take me to her brother's karaoke bar. She was an
unmarried woman in her mid-thirties, and unlike other women I met in
China, she was not unhappy being single, not being legally attached to
a man. Zhang had a striking appearance and often wore fashionable
black clothes, even in the one-hundred-degree heat. She wore a small
gold chain necklace with a gold cross around her neck, black sandals,
and no makeup on her round freckled face. When she smiled, her
straight white teeth showed. As we talked the nights away, our conversations were gently punctuated by her lilting voice. One evening, I found
Zhang at a popular hangout for the few foreign backpackers who pass
through Jinghong en route to Laos. She was sitting and talking with an
older hippie-looking male from Colorado and a friend of his from Germany, who was accompanied by his Chinese girlfriend (Zhang said she
was an aspiring anthropologist). Zhang was sitting close to the man
from Colorado. He explained to me, as he stroked Zhang's hands, that
he had returned to Yunnan to find Zhang. The two of them seemed quite
physically close; however, Zhang said nothing about their relationship
to me other than that she had guided him to Mengla, where they went
to visit a cousin of hers who was convalescing after losing a kidney in a
motorbike accident.

Zhang presented her life story as follows:

> For a Chinese woman I am rare because I am thirty-five years old and hap-
> pily unmarried. Most Chinese woman want to be married long before
> thirty-five, but then I see my brother, who has a seven-year-old daughter,
> and he is already divorced. I attended the Teacher's Training School (Shifan
> Xuexiao) in Jinghong and then went to Yunnan University (Yunda) to
> study English and education from 1988 to 1991. Then I got a job teaching
> at the Minorities Technical Training Institute (Minzu Zhiye Xuexiao), and
> then later I was working at the tourism bureau. The Minzhi Xuexiao is
> now a training school for the police. As the school was suffering from lack
> of local government funding, the police bought the school last year. Now
> all the minority students have been sent back to their villages. My older
> brother, who started our karaoke bar, has moved on to build an interior

decorating business. He has helped me with the café. It was easy money—
the money came in and then the money went out; breaking even was easy. I
started the café with another friend, but he soon found the hours too long,
and left to start his own business. I had no hard feelings. My own philosophy is that work is work, and friendships are friendships; you cannot place
them together. I then took off five months to play in the central city of
Wuhan, only to return to start another business delivering gas for people's
stoves. With the help of my current boyfriend, I purchased a truck from the
proceeds of the café. I am also working to train hotel service workers in the
art of service. There are too many people here in Banna who have attitudes
left over from the Cultural Revolution, when service was a bourgeois concept. We said we wanted to serve the people, but we never bothered to
serve customers. It was all seen as a bother. My current goal is to raise the
quality and standards of these service workers, to raise their human quality
(suzhi). I really enjoy teaching this class as it is only twice a week for a couple of hours at the Post Office Hotel.

That night, I asked Zhang why she wore a gold cross around her
neck.

When I was at Yunnan University, I met a teacher who was a Christian. It
sounded like a good religion, so I became one at least in spirit. I sometimes
attend the church in town, but no one else in my family is a Christian. My
father worked for the police and my mother was a cashier for a local small
business. They are both from Puer, where the famous tea is grown. My
mother now works in the Sipsongpanna Department Store. She is still alive
at fifty-eight but she has health problems! My older brother, who is thirty-
eight, works as an investigator for the courts because now in Banna there
are too many legal cases for the public security bureau to handle on their
own. My older brother married a local Han woman from Jinghong, and
they have an eleven-year-old daughter. My younger brother, who is thirty-
two, is also a successful independent businessman.

When I asked Zhang about the recent economic changes in Jinghong,
she said:

After the economic changes in the 1980s, the economy of money changed,
people went from a peasant mentality about money—where money was not
so important, most things could be provided by the land—to a completely
new system. The problem with money is that it is a burden: trying to make
money, trying to keep the money you have, and making more money, all
are tiring and cumbersome activities. In terms of more recent changes, finding a job is difficult now, because before, the government work unit or
school would find you a job. Now young people must find their own jobs.
In this town, if one is pretty, young, and a woman, it is pretty easy to find
work. Then again, it is more difficult for men, as they don't have the option
of working as tour guides, because these jobs are almost always reserved
for women. But working as a tour guide is difficult—you work long hours

and deal with difficult people. You must hustle for a percentage of the proceeds from purchases that your customers buy, so you can make up to ten
thousand yuan a month if you are well known and work hard. Then again,
tour guiding happens out in bright sun every day and this turns one's skin
brown, an unattractive trait.

I also asked Zhang about drugs, gambling, and prostitution in Jinghong.

In terms of other changes, I see just as many men as women using drugs;
especially if one member of a couple uses drugs, then the other is just as
likely to use them. Also, young girls working in Jinghong who are not from
here use drugs. In 1995–97, heroin use became popular among the locals;
until then, there were only a select few minorities who used drugs, especially a kind of marijuana, a plant that gets you high, but only a few old
men used this. Gambling is also a problem. I have seen people even gamble
away their homes; gambling is like a drug in that you will sell everything
for it. As for stories, a son of a friend of my mother's who was about thirty
years old used drugs and was sent to the drug rehabilitation center in Jiangbei. After he served his time there, about six months, he hooked up with
the same friends and of course went back to using heroin. Most people use
clean needles and not dirty ones, but what kind of standards do we have
when even the doctors do not use clean needles![11] If people are not consci-
entious, then, of course, this becomes a way of life. It's what's in one's
heart. If you like this kind of life, you become part of it, and it becomes
part of you.
    In terms of regulating crime in Banna, the crackdown is merely a tool of
our bureaucratic leaders to get citizens to behave, to move away from the
rule of man (renzhi) to the rule of law (fazhi), to both officiate and to become the officiated. It is necessary to rely on the rule of law if we want to
change our society, if we want to become modern. This is a slow process,
and maybe twenty years from now things will change. The police also want
to ensure better driving habits among the people, and therefore they are en-
forcing local regulations about having a driver's license for your motorcycle. Otherwise the roads will be a mess; we need the money collected from
tickets to protect traffic safety.

When I questioned Zhang about the rise in STIs, she said:

As for STIs, it is the wives of men who fool around who get them from
their partners. I think women rarely have outside partners, but they can
pass an illness on to their children if their husband or lover infects them.
Now, in Banna, importance is placed on making money, and prostitution is
just another way to make money. At my old business, many prostitutes
lived across the street and would come to chat; most of them were girls
from Sichuan, with a few from Guizhou. It all comes down to economics—
what kind of job are you going to get that permits you to make enough
money to support yourself and to send some money home to your husband

and child? Few prostitutes think only of themselves, most are working for their families to support them. In Sichuan there are not enough jobs, so Sichuanese people can be found all over China. Of course, that means in places like Banna. The local Ainizu and Tai make money because of their culture. In some Aini villages they have children first and then marry, so their educational foundation is not the same as for us Han. As for the Tai, they are rather carefree and not very hard working compared to us Han. For minority women, becoming a prostitute is not that different from their regular customs. However, if one gets sick as a prostitute, shots are expensive, a hundred yuan per injection, and several must be given in one week.

One time, when I was explaining the English expression "sex worker," Zhang laughed at the notion of sex as work, as an occupation, and the idea espoused by some feminists in the West that prostitutes get paid for what many women give away for free. On the subject of marriage, Zhang said:

> In terms of marriage, it is really not the same as prostitution. The goal there is to exchange sex for money, but with marriage the exchange is mutual feelings of love; marital love is not something for you to make money with. Then again, if your connection or relationship *(guanxi)* with your husband is so bad, maybe a bad marriage is like being a prostitute. Women in China now must eat bitterness *(chiku)*, and the moral is not to be a woman. So I decided not to get married and live my life the way I like to, by my own rules. I don't have children to look after, so I have a lot of freedom. Most of all, I like my freedom, and I am afraid of being tied down by marriage. If you are alone, you can do everything; if you are married, your husband scolds you, and your mother-in-law hits you. Then you become responsible for doing everything in the home. After a few years, you never see your husband anymore, because he has taken up with his new girlfriend. Your husband couldn't care less about your home, other than bringing in the money. My boyfriend is a driver but has a terrible temper and often gets into accidents. Do I want to marry into that? As for marriage in general, men often find a lover on the side. I think that now in China, everyone's ideas are wild; in their hearts they are wild. Twenty years after China opened up to the outside world, many customs are coming back from previous eras, such as prostitution and gambling. Twenty years later, the main problems are with the family. Men are not responsible. For men who are over thirty, they want one wife, one child, and one lover *(xiao laopo)*. They want to be able to come home late at night because they know their wives are always at home, always responsible for their children. Of course, men and women are equal in certain respects, and in others, the more things change, the more men and women are unequal.

Zhang's narrative points to the fluidity of moral economies in Jinghong. Though women are free to pursue various jobs and occupations, class differences and native place restrict who can move up the economic ladder. Family background and values make a difference. Zhang's thoughts reflect the Han nationalist morality when discussing her views on policing Sipsongpanna. Yet her ideas about sexuality balance the liberal market and parochial moral economies. She considers herself a Chinese Catholic, but does not believe in the sanctity of heterosexual marriage that Catholicism enjoins, as she was interested in having multiple lovers. Zhang is similar to Tian in that she describes the current political, economic, and cultural changes as evidence that society is "now wild, with wild hearts and wild ideas." Zhang also concurs with Tian in her assessment of AIDS as being a gendered epidemic, where wives are invoked as the unwilling victims of their husbands' sexual escapades. My final tale examines someone who embraces three moral economies—liberal, market, and parochial—and reveals my fourth moral economy of ethnic revivalism.

AI LAO: A TALE OF RESISTANCE?

Ai Lao was one of the few people I met in Jinghong who was seriously, though quietly, organizing to revive Tai culture. In this final narrative, Ai Lao reveals that there is never an easy relationship between Han nationalism and the incipient rule of ethnic power that he saw in everyday acts of policing the Sipsongpanna Tai.[12] These acts encompass discursive practices that turn Han prostitutes into Tai women in everything from films to television to public health journals. He viewed such acts as a kind of colonization of Tai women, making them unjust and unworthy representations of the Tai people. At the same time, Lao Ai was a member of the local Chinese Communist Party in Jinghong.

Lao Ai provided the following narrative of his life:

> I came from Damenlong and married in Jinghong in 1991 a really beautiful Tai woman [his wife, who was present, merely smiled at me]. Originally we lived in Manjinglan, which was actually the only village here. Only much later did the village of Manting move to Jinghong from Lincang in Menglian County. Manjinglan used to have over eight hundred mu of land, and in the last few years we sold eight hundred mu (sixty-four hectares) to Han developers for only thirty thousand yuan. I could not sell my house for that little, let alone an entire plot of land. Also, these days I make almost twelve thousand yuan per year in rents. Now [in 1997], only 10 percent of the businesses on the street are Tai businesses, where the Tai ran almost 90 percent in 1991 when I first moved here. For now, I feel my most important task is the Buddhist school, a place to revive Tai culture and history, a means to promote local Tai culture. But there are problems with recruit-

ment. Currently students are recruited based on their personal connections *(guanxi)* because there is no examination system. However, beginning next year, we will institute new policies and only allow the best students to attend. Now the youngest student is eight years old and the oldest is thirty-six. The problem with the school is that we are not allowed to proselytize, and how can you build a religious base without proselytizing?

In the 1890s, Sipsongpanna was an independent kingdom, and it was only eighty years ago that the Han came here to settle. There was a feudal administrator and a fort *(yamen)* across from land that the Sipsongpanna hotel is currently located on. This is only a vestige of the Han; the administrator didn't really have any impact on how we Tai ran Sipsongpanna. In the 1950s, the the Nationalist Army (Guomindang) fled to Sipsongpanna, and later they fled over the border into the Shan state [rumors abound that they are the ones now running the drug trade between Burma and Yunnan]. Then in 1953, with the liberation of Sipsongpanna, the Communists came in and destroyed the old history books and religion, and with these acts, our history was lost.[13] The only things left were our people's customs and houses. Then, in the late 1960s, came the sent-down educated youth *(laozhiqing)*, and they are reputed to have left many children behind. Han men had children with Tai women, and while a few stayed behind because they were from Hunan and Sichuan, places much worse off economically than Sipsongpanna in terms of living standards, most returned home to Beijing, Shanghai, and Kunming. Then, more recently, miners came in the 1970s, and now the floating populations of migrant Han come to find jobs in Jinghong in the 1990s. However, in the 1930s, Protestants from Thailand came here, but they converted only two villages because only those outcast by the Tai would listen to them: the sick, the infirm, the crippled, those with leprosy *(mafengbing)*, or those thought to have the possession by ghost spirits *(pipaguai)* converted to Christianity.[14] It was the village that everyone labeled as the *pipaguai* that had to move from Ganlanba to its present site. The village near the Sipsongpanna hotel became the present site of the only Christian church, and that building still stands.[15]

One day I ran into Ai Lao at the Buddhist temple in the park called *wanbasi fojiao jinian,*[16] where the Buddhist school is located. I was there inquiring about the local Buddhist school and gathering more information about the temple. That afternoon I came across Ai Lao, who was, much to the delight of the young monks, picking up an enormous snake with a large stick and putting it into a cloth bag. That evening we rendezvoused at Ai Lao's family compound, a large Tai house made of wood and bamboo that had five small rooms downstairs rented to Han migrants working in town. Ai Lao explained that unlike other Tai, "I demand courtesy from my Han tenants—quiet, no karaoke, cleanliness—and if they don't obey, they are asked to leave. My wife and I share two rooms and one guest room on the top floor of the house, plus our courtyard, where we cook and tend our small garden, where the water spigot is." Ai Lao had no television (although his tenants did), no refrigerator, and no indoor kitchen. His lifestyle was very similar to that of Tai villagers whom I visited in the countryside surrounding Jinghong, with the exception of the high brick wall around his compound and the fact his house was made of wood, concrete, and bamboo, not just bamboo. While the electricity was infrequent, there was one weak light bulb in each room, and Ai Lao kept it on during the day.

When I asked about the precarious status of migrants, he said:

> The Han police don't mind us renting out our dirt floors as long as everyone registers with the police. It is the individuals who are fined, and not the landlords, if they don't register. As for money from the government, other villagers receive money from the village head, and contrary to what people say, the Tai receive nothing from the Han government. Even the annual 450 yuan that we receive from village profits on our rubber and rice cultivation, that is not Han compensation.

I later asked Ai Lao about the kinship and linguistic terms for defining the Tai. He replied that there were many misconceptions about the local Tai held by Han scholars of Tai culture.

> As for the common distinctions made between *Huayao-Tai* [the floral-belt Tai], *Shui-Tai* [the water Tai], or the *Han-Tai* [those with one Tai and one Han parent], these are merely words used by the Han to make distinctions and have nothing to do with historical ethnic differences. We Tai do not distinguish which parent is Tai or not, we believe that all Tais are Tai. Last year when I accompanied Grant Evans, an anthropologist from Hong Kong University, to the Tai Studies Conference in Chiang Mai, there was this old Han Chinese Tai scholar who had this theory that the Tai came from Northeast China from the province of Shandong. This scholar's point of comparison was that there were certain symbols such as the peacocks on weather vanes and temple steeples present in both locations. I just couldn't believe what he was saying and told him so. Instead of a scholarly exchange, what ensued was an angry fight. This scholar didn't take criticism lightly. Of course, this was his contribution to Tai scholarship, and I was attacking the heart of his work. If the Han say water is important for the Tai and fire is important for the Yi, for which peoples are water and fire not necessary? It is such a simplistic way of understanding the complexities of culture.

When I asked Ai Lao what counselors or professors in Kunming knew about the Tai, he mentioned Dao Shi Shun. Dao Shi Shun was destined to become the last reigning monarch (*zhaotianling*) of Sipsongpanna. He refused. According to Ai Lao, Dao feared that if he returned to Sipsongpanna, there would be an uprising. Others have noted that he was being courted by Nationalist forces, the Guomintang, and therefore for Communist security reasons had to remain in Kunming.[17] Dao has remained as a professor at Yunnan Nationalities Institute since the early 1950s. Ai Lao's comments on this were as follows:

> Dao never returned to Sipsongpanna after liberation because he feared a war would break out among his people. He held documents that stated the land base was still theirs [the Tais'] and that it was only the government that would change; the Communists would come in but leave the Tai to themselves. Of course, the rest is history that never happened. We are all under Communist rule now.

Ai Lao was very vocal about my research topic on the connections between the Tai and HIV/AIDS. He surmised:

> The Han now have a built-in set of prejudices that induce them to get Han women to dress in Tai clothing and bathe promiscuously by the water's edge. This is actually an infamous Mengla tourist attraction. As for the Hui-Tai, they are merely people who married Hui [Muslims] from villages near Dali [there are two villages near Dali where many Sipsongpanna Hui originate]. You must be cautious about claims made about the Tai, especially these claims about Tai women and culture. If many people in Kunming say that Sipsongpanna is so open, that the people are promiscuous, what they are relying on is their own Han prejudices; they do not really know what goes on. Most Han know only what the tour guides tell them, and most of them [the tour guides] are not Tai either, even if they are local Han girls. This happens all the time: you see Han women dressed in Tai clothes, performing Tai dances, and serving what you think of as Tai food, and of course it is not! It is similar to nostalgic *lao zhiqing* Tai food restaurants in Kunming; the food served there is very bland by our Tai standards [*lao zhiqing* are the youth of the 1960s and 1970s who were "sent down" to Sipsongpanna]. The accusations that the Tai are more prone to transmitting sexual diseases are just as ludicrous as the claims that the tour guides are authentic Tai girls.

Ai Lao's narrative reveals several tropes and tales of what happens when a dominant culture takes control of another less powerful one. What is enlightening about his narrative is that it presents his own counterhegemonic beliefs in this "peaceful former kingdom." The narrative also points to contradictions in a local moral economy where Ai Lao both criticizes the prevailing Han parochial morality and, at the same time, benefits economically from the infiltration of Han migrants into this tourist economic region. More important to my argument about sexuality, modernity, and the Tai is that there are multiple representations of authenticity. Even the local Han suggest there are multiple representations of the Tai. Madam Liu's boyfriend said that when he first came to Sipsongpanna in the 1980s, the Tai were never embarrassed by people watching them bathe, but that now the Han think it is uncivilized, the Tai never bathe within public view. These notions of authenticity are fraught with questions about just what constitutes authentic Tai practice, what has been adulterated by the Han, and also to what degree there is or has been resistance to the Chinese state.

Thomas Borchert (2005) has suggested that resistance and acquiescence are not necessarily incompatible. Not only is the Chinese government facing increasing unrest among Uighur and Tibetan separatists, but in 2004 in Henan and Sichuan tens of thousands of peasant and workers rioted, including those left out of market socialism and those who cannot find sustainable work (Human Rights Watch 2005). This active political resistance continues to be met with harsh punishment, as were the Tiananmen youth in 1989. However, more subtle forms of resistance are much more nuanced and often accepted. If Ai Lao seeks to increase Tai linguistic ability and Buddhist practices among Tai youth, is that resistance or a means of bringing modernity to the Tai minority? If the Tai benefit from the tourist development, are they just acquiescing, or are they merely finding a means of survival in an otherwise untenable situation? To reiterate, while some Tai scholars have suggested that the closer the Tai get to Thailand and Buddhism, the more troublesome they will be viewed by the Chinese state, others, including myself, see the revival of Buddhism as something that goes hand in hand with the Chinese government's goals for developing western China. Tourism, Buddhist religious revivalism, and development all go hand in hand—there are no overt contradictions. Yet this does not mean that developing Sipsongpanna with ever more high-rise hotels does not challenge local Buddhist practitioners who wish for less development and more attention to religious practice through cultural revivals—creating more stringent norms for sending young males into the Buddhist monasteries and developing widespread access to learning the Tai language.

Ai Lao counters the first three moralities with his particular view of resistance. Although Tai resistance is more circumscribed than in parts of China's northwest—where Uighurs, a Turkic speaking Muslim population, are routinely rounded up, imprisoned, and often executed (Human Rights Watch 2005)—it is still part of what James Scott (1985) would label as "weapons of the weak." Ai Lao's resistance against the Chinese state suggests that members of the Sipsongpanna Tai continue to challenge the parochial, nationalist, and liberal moralities. Ai Lao's thoughts and practices reveal the complications inherent in counterhegemonic morality. This is especially evident when he challenges the notion that Tai women are the local prostitutes. His anger and frustration at the representations of his people in the name of development and tourism are apparent. At the same time, he capitalizes on Han economic development by renting his house to Han immigrant youth. While this may appear as a contradiction, he rents his house in a particular way, demanding Tai standards of respect from his Han tenants. In addition, the landlord-tenant relationship is one of unequal power relations, as the landlord has the upper hand over his tenants—and Ai Lao retains the upper hand.

MARKET-SOCIALIST MORAL ECONOMIES?

The market-socialist moral economies in China do not lend themselves to a story that moves in linear progression from the ancient Confucian notion of the proper conjugal bed, through a Maoist code of containment, to emerge into sexual freedom and modernity. It is a story of ongoing and persistent conflicts among alternative regimes of power. Tai resistance to Han nationalist repositioning of sexual containment produces one of the many alternative moral economies. In discussing counterhegemonic practices through my narrative of Ai Lao, I am not merely adding ethnicity to a list of differences but trying to understand how ethnicity and sexuality work together to both stigmatize and eroticize the ethnic Other. Through the Han state's intervention in the sexual practices of local prostitutes' bodies and through its depiction of local minorities as the diseased Other in its discourse on AIDS, China creates a barbarian border people who must be regulated and controlled in the name of building modernity.

Returning to my ethnographic portraits—a Han woman working in a Tai autonomous region, a Han-Tai entrepreneur, an Aini woman tour guide, and a male Tai activist—one may place these narratives together in order to reveal competing new moral economies in practice in post-reform China. Rather than each person fitting neatly into a singular heuristic moral code, the interweaving of the liberal, parochial, nationalist, and ethnic revivalist moralities leads to the amalgamation of several moral economies that represent new social formations and the cross-fertilization of people, place, and disease. While many individuals in Sipsongpanna view the Tai as unenterprising and lazy, others would compare their industriousness to a lazier Other, the Bulang and Wa minority groups. Others attribute the spread of AIDS to the rise in sex tourism and to Tai cultural values and locate the problem as part of the decay in moral values throughout the Chinese nation.

Although Zhang considers herself a liberated woman, she still maintains the notion that sexual minorities' marital practices are similar to prostitution. In other words, because they do not adhere to the exact practices of the Han Chinese, they must be exploiting women in a way similar to prostitution. A lack of understanding about the nuances of cultural difference plays out in Zhang's discussion of how the Tai may have children before marriage, but not multiple partners. While Zhang labels this behavior as suggestive of sexual promiscuity, she fails to recognize the fact that these practices retain their own cultural logic. Another example of this idea is the deeply held belief among Han Chinese about the Mosuo minority in northern Yunnan, which organizes around a matriarchy. Men are the fathers of their children, but these children move through the mother's lineage rather than their fathers (Cai Hua 2001). The Mosuo are often referred to as promiscuous because of this practice (see Walsh 2001). Among the Tai, Sara Davis (2005) points out that after marriage, Tai women actually do have more sexual freedom than do Han women. Sex, gender, and ethnicity all converge here in Zhang's narrative account of being a liberated woman and having liberal notions of sexuality. However, this liberal moral economy is transected by a Han nationalist morality that both stigmatizes and eroticizes ethnic minorities, in particular ethnic minority women as less educated and less modern than herself. Tian noted that even when she was a child, the Han-educated youth from Shanghai would pick on her because of her ethnic status. She also bemoans the fact that local prostitutes do not maintain a sense of pride in their work the way tour guides do.

As in every other chapter, the informants I present here strove to legitimize a unique moral universe that revealed the contradictory and confounding relationships that we find when discussing the endless historical traffic in bodies and diseases in China. AIDS does not discriminate according to lines on a map or persons' origins or their ethnicity or gender; what it does do is cross and recross the maps we draw of sexual morality. AIDS as an epidemic is always more than a disease of signification or moral panic; it is a disease that has made its mark as a major player of the end of the twentieth century and the beginning of the twenty-first.

What Is to Be Done?

In the last year and a half, I have often gone to the hair salons to get styling done, mainly for business reasons. Some attendants at the salon wanted to make extra money, so while they offer a massage, they would also often have sex with their clients. Sometimes I would ask them whether, if a client asked to have sex with them, they would ask him to wear a condom. Some of them would say "yes." They are the ones who knew how to protect themselves. However, some wanted to earn extra money. For an additional fifty yuan, they would allow a man not to wear a condom. For these girls I often leave them with my phone number and try to convince them to quit their job and make a living in other fashions. I remember four women between the ages of eighteen and twenty-three, Misses Du, Zheng, Luo, and Xiao, whom I convinced to quit this kind of job. After educating them, some went back to their hometowns and got married, others went to work in factories, and only one stayed at her previous job, but quit completely from doing that kind of "business" in order to earn more money.

I can feel my time is near, if I don't tell my story soon, after two or three months, I might not be well enough to say anything. . . . [Even] though I know my mind is clear, I know my body is abandoning me. I am also sounding the alarm to the entire country, this disease is in fact not easy to be infected by, but one's carelessness can allow the virus into the body. . . . [We] are already very unfortunate, and I wish people would not look at us with discrimination—people like me would like to have some sympathy and understanding. [Excerpts from stories about Xiao Lu in Tu Qiao 2000 (translated from Chinese)].

Reporter Tu Qiao's journalistic account of her character Xiao Lu, a Chinese man infected with AIDS, takes us full circle: AIDS does infect and infest people's lives with much sorrow, pain, and suffering.[1] Because much has changed in the past eight years, in this epilogue I bring readers up to date, particularly for the period from 2002 to early 2006, when my field was libraries in the United States and Canada. As a public health practitioner and an anthropologist, I conclude with discussions culled from my field notes on informants' suggestions on how to prevent the further spread of HIV in China. But first, I offer this update on AIDS in Asia and in China.

BRINGING HIV/AIDS FORWARD (2002–2006)

Predictions that AIDS in China and India will surpass Africa's epidemics in severity are fraught with discrepancies in terms of the wide range of the predictions; the rise of infections in Asian countries such as Burma and Cambodia, with smaller populations; and the incomplete and unreliable surveillance methods. Currently no country in Asia has experienced a generalized epidemic; however, Cambodia, Indonesia, Myanmar, Nepal, Thailand, and Vietnam have reached the concentrated stage, as have China's Yunnan Province and certain states in India. In concentrated epidemics, prevalence is more than 5 percent in one group (e.g., injection drug users and plasma blood donors) but below 1 percent among women in antenatal clinics (Bloom et al. 2004: 10–11). At the end of 2003, sub-Saharan Africa and South and Southeast Asia still had the highest numbers of people infected with HIV/AIDS (see figure 6).[2]

As my research focused on Yunnan and areas of low infection rate among both the Han and Chinese minorities, I contrast these areas with places where higher infection rates have emerged such as central Henan among rural Han peasants (Gao 2004). As Joan Kaufman, Anthony Saich, and Arthur Kleinman (2004) point out, China's AIDS situation has been unfolding now for over a decade and is accelerating. In an interesting turn of statistics, the Chinese government reduced its figures from 840,000 persons infected with HIV in 2003 to 650,000 at the beginning of 2006.[3] The majority of infections still remain among former plasma donors from central China and injection drug users from Yunnan. Although China's infection rate is less than 1 percent of the population, those infected are concentrated in several provinces and subregions within those provinces. Among injection drug users, who account for 44 percent of all estimated HIV cases, seven provinces—Yunnan,

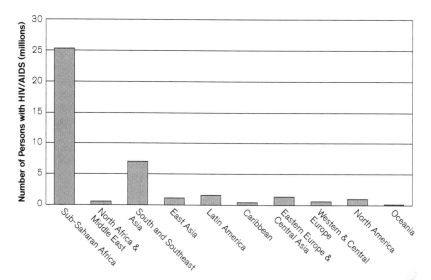

Figure 6. Persons with HIV/AIDS by World Region, End of 2003.

Xinjiang, Guangxi, Guangdong, Guizhou, Sichuan, and Hunan— account for 90 percent of infections (MOH 2006: 1). Henan Province is still the epicenter of high infection rates among commercial blood and plasma donors infected in the 1990s, and in the wake of this epidemic, central China has produced upwards of 200,000 AIDS orphans (Wang Lan 2005). Five provinces account for 80 percent of infections in this population: Henan, Hubei, Anhui, Hebei, and Shanxi.[4] Kaufman notes that even if China were able to keep rates of new infection closer to 2 to 3 percent, as Thailand has, given the sheer size of the population, tens of thousands of people will still require treatment and care (see Kaufman, Saich, and Kleinman 2004; Kaufman 2003; Kaufman and Jing 2002). Currently 20,453 people with AIDS are receiving antiretroviral therapies in 605 counties and twenty-eight provinces (MOH 2006: ii).

In Yunnan itself prevalence rates have changed significantly since I first began conducting research in 1995. According to estimates from the end of 2005, 37,040 people are infected with HIV, with blood transmission accounting for 65 percent of all infections and sexual contact 13 percent (Wang Lin Ganna 2005). Since 1989, the first year in which monitoring of injection drug users in the border areas uncovered cases of HIV/AIDS, infection among injection drug users (IDUs) in Yunnan has spread. By the beginning of 2002, HIV infections moved away from

TABLE 2. OFFICIAL HIV/AIDS
STATISTICS REPORTED BY THE MINISTRY OF
HEALTH, 2006

HIV/AIDS cases (estimate)	760,000
HIV+	650,000
AIDS cases	75,000
AIDS orphans (estimate)	44,000
AIDS-related deaths (estimate)	90,000
Annual increase in HIV cases	30%
National prevalence rate, persons 15 to 49 years old	0.04–0.06%

SOURCE: MOH 2006; UNAIDS 2005.

the border areas to include sixteen districts in 116 counties (including 93.5 percent of all cities in the province) (Zhang Xiaobo 2002: 330) (see table 2). The Yunnan Centers for Disease Control and Prevention report that after testing 95,755 individuals from what are defined as high-risk groups—injection drug users, those engaging in promiscuous sex, and migrants—the incidence rate was 1.5 percent. Seven prefectures are defined as having the highest rates, especially Ruili County of Dehong Tai-Jingpo Minority Autonomous Prefecture, the location of the Dehong-Tai minority. The rates are as follows: The HIV prevalence among male STI patients is 2.7 percent and as high as 13.4 in Ruili County. Among pregnant women it is 0.2 percent but as high as 2.2 percent in Long-chuang County in Dehong. The majority of HIV-positive persons are twenty-to-thirty-year-old males who are injection drug users, Han Chinese, and unemployed peasants. The lowest rate among injection drug users was in Jinghong, at 1.1 percent, while the provincial average is 2.7 percent, mirroring rates in the previous year. Among STI patients at sentinel surveillance sites in 2001, the highest rate among females was in Baoshan County, while no infected people were found in Jinghong, with a provincial average of 0.2 percent. The largest single site of HIV infection in Yunnan still remains Dehong, which accounts for only 22 percent of all cases (Zhang Xiaobo et al. 2002: 330). Some experts estimate that the rates of infection from dirty needles and sexual contact are increasing exponentially and predict an upsurge in the next ten years to almost ten times the number of infected persons by the end of 2010 (Yuan et al. 2002: 78).

Other groups have presented rates of infection that were not even examined when I left the field in 1997. As homosexuality is not openly discussed in much of rural China, data available on men who have sex with

TABLE 3. PROPORTION OF FEMALES HIV+ IN
CHINA, 2000–2004

	2000	2001	2002	2003	2004
Females HIV+ as percentage of all cases	19.4	22.7	25.4	35.6	39.0

SOURCE: UNAIDS 2004.

other men (MSM) is still very limited, and even in urban settings this remains an area requiring further in-depth study. Whereas in 2003 in Beijing, Harbin, Guangzhou, and Shenyang the estimated prevalence rates were around 1.1 percent, in 2006 men who have sex with men accounted for 7.3 percent of all HIV infections (Settle 2003; MOH 2006: 2).

Sexually transmitted infections (*xingbing*), which are surrogate markers for increased HIV, have overtaken tuberculosis to become the third most common category of infectious disease after dysentery and hepatitis (Parish et al 2002; M. Cohen et al. 2000; M. Cohen 2001). Since women are more vulnerable because of the biology of genital tissues and women's personal difficulties in negotiating consistent condom use, they too are increasingly becoming infected at rates that will soon reach or, as some predict, surpass gender parity.

Despite the continuing rates of HIV in Yunnan Province, which made it ground zero of the Chinese epidemic, there have been significant strides made in combating HIV since 1995. Despite many of the problems associated with surveys of the general public, a recent survey by researchers in Dali found that among a sample of two thousand individuals ages sixteen to forty-five, 73 percent answered correctly when questioned about their epidemiological knowledge of HIV transmission. This is certainly a much higher average than when I began fieldwork in 1995 (He et al. 2000: 513). Also, with the combined efforts of the Centers for Disease Control and Prevention in Beijing and the Ministries of Civil Affairs, Education, and Health, many new organizations and joint venture projects have been launched.

When I left Yunnan in 1997, there were very few NGOs working on HIV. The first organizations in the province in 1995 were Save the Children–Hong Kong (SCF) and the Australian Red Cross (ARC); shortly afterward came Oxfam–Hong Kong and Médicins Sans Frontiéres–Belgium. These four groups continue to work in Yunnan and have since branched out into other areas of the country. SCF has a large health care project in Ruili where it sponsors a clinic run by the local health department and the Women's Federation. ARC started the largest youth peer training program and now also runs a project that provides support groups and vocational training for people living with HIV/AIDS (PLHIV). The ARC moved its China office from Yunnan in 2004 to Xinjiang, which is facing its own epidemic among injection drug users. Other organizations in Yunnan working on HIV/AIDS prevention include the International Planned Parenthood Federation, the Hong Kong Red Ribbon Center, UK-China AIDS, Aizhi, the Ford Foundation, the Amity Foundation, World Vision, the Salvation Army, Daytop, Family Health International, Futures Group, DKT International (a condom social marketing agency), the AIDS Alliance, Population Services International, Care International, ActionAID, and Health Unlimited.[5]

In addition to more traditional NGOs, government-affiliated NGOs (GONGOs) that are present in Yunnan include the Buddhist Associations in Dehong and Sipsongpanna, the HIV/AIDS Association, Family Planning Association, and the Yunnan Red Cross (Couzin 2004). Other government agencies that have initiated GONGOs include the China AIDS Network, All-China Women's Federation, Ministry of Health, Railway Ministry, the Army, Ministry of Education, All-China Federation of Trade Unions, and Chinese Communist Youth League (MOH 2006: 8), some of which are discussed in earlier chapters. In Yunnan, Guangxi, and Sichuan provinces, the Centers for Disease Control and Prevention play a key role in surveillance and intervention (Couzin 2004). As new NGOs appear to be heading into China at an ever-growing pace, the above list is by no means exhaustive nor representative of the very latest state of affairs as this book goes to press. However, this list demonstrates the increased national alarm and response to rising rates of HIV in China. There are also the bilateral organizations involved in HIV/AIDS health projects: the Asian Development Bank, the World Health Organization, the U.S. Agency for International Development, the British government's Department for International Development (DFID), and the Canadian International Development Agency. Numerous United Nations organizations include UNAIDS, UNICEF, UNFPA, UNDP, and UNESCO. In many ways, AIDS has become a virtual health care industry in China, especially for NGOs working in health care and STI/AIDS prevention.

In December 2003 Premier Wen Jiabao and Vice-Premier Wu Yi announced a new policy for comprehensive HIV/AIDS prevention and treatment. "The 'Four Frees and One Care Policy' had the following aims: free anti-HIV drugs to AIDS patients who are rural residents or people with financial difficulties living in urban areas; free voluntary counseling and testing; free drugs to HIV-infected pregnant women to prevent mother-to-child transmission, and HIV testing of newborn babies; free schooling for children orphaned by AIDS; and free care and economic assistance to the households of people living with HIV/AIDS" (UNAIDS 2004; Li Hong et al. 2001). Most recently in 2004 and 2005 the Chinese government has begun to implement these policies, with some interesting results. In light of my work among sex workers in Yunnan, there appears to be an increase in the number of female sex workers who have their clients use condoms when they have intercourse. Sentinel surveillance data in 2005 showed that only 9 percent of commercial sex workers (CSWs) mentioned their clients never used condoms. Also, according to sentinel site surveillance, in Beijing the prevalence rates among CSWs have decreased from 0.8 percent in 2004 to 0.5 percent in 2005. Efforts to curb prostitution often contradict efforts to curb disease. One policeman in Liuzhou said, "Dispatching condoms at hospitality facilities is somewhat contradictory to our crackdown on prostitution. But disease prevention is a life and death issue and therefore more important than a crackdown" (Zhou Yan 2005). While Gejiu city has been recognized as a model in dealing with its HIV/AIDS epidemic and, like this policemen, has chosen to prioritize disease prevention above law enforcement, not all cities or all policemen have this attitude. In Jinghong a recent crackdown on prostitution and businesses offering prostitution has moved the practice underground, which makes it even more difficult to regulate or provide protections for workers and clients alike.

According to Peter Piot of UNAIDS in Geneva, China is far ahead of India and Russia in addressing large-scale AIDS epidemics. For Dr. Piot it was the rise of the SARS (severe acute respiratory syndrome) epidemic in 2003 that put an implicit panic and fear into Chinese officials about the destabilizing effects of a widespread epidemic (Yardley 2005; see also Kleinman and Watson 2006). Prevention, however, is not the only arena where strides have been made. The new policies to be implemented in 2006 will institute mandatory condom distribution campaigns like the one in Yunnan, making condoms available in all public places, especially the entertainment industry venues; enhance access to antiretroviral therapies; and expand legal protection for PLHIV. These policies, however, do not come without clear costs. Human rights activists have claimed that in many cases PLHIV are still being discriminated against by the insistence they no longer marry; however, this time the law has been rewritten as "postponing marriage." Furthermore, there are still no legal protections to ensure that PLHIV have access to medical care. Instead, according to the Aizhixing Research Institute, there is a strong emphasis on the "duties" required of PLHIV, including submission to mandatory surveillance and testing even though people whose status is disclosed will have no legal protections nor definitive access to treatment and care. In some cases people who are infected will be fined or jailed for infecting others, which leads to disincentives for getting people to know their HIV status (Aizhixing Research Group 2006).

China has just doubled the amount of money targeted to combat AIDS and has received a Global Fund award of 29 million U.S. dollars (which will be combined with a 20 million U.S. dollars equivalent from the Chinese government) to combat the spread of new infections (see China AIDS Info 2006). However, all is not clear-cut and straightforward in these new prevention measures or in the implementation of new laws and regulations. Policies are still implemented unevenly across China, especially when contrasting rural and urban populations and areas. Antiretroviral therapies are currently available to only 20,453 people living with AIDS, which is but a fraction of current infections (MOH 2006: 9; Office of the State Council Working Committee on AIDS, China 2005). Access to the drugs is still expensive by Chinese standards and unevenly distributed and managed. Furthermore, certain state sectors have not welcomed all the civil society activities on behalf of those with HIV. Wan Yanhai, one of the first activists to bring the plight of Henan's HIV-positive blood donors to the attention of the Chinese government, was arrested in 2002, then later released. Chinese AIDS activists continue to be arrested when they overstep the boundaries of what the government considers acceptable public protest. Following an organized hunger strike to protest detention and human rights violations, several AIDS activists associated with the Beijing Aizhixing Institute, the Chinese Democratic Party, and the Empowerment and Rights Institute in Beijing disappeared after being harassed, tailed, and in some cases beaten by the police.[6] All across China, complaints have been voiced about corruption among local officials, the diversion of funds marked for PLHIV, and milder forms of expropriation of funding. Overall, compared to ten years ago, progress is being made, even though implementing policies set in Beijing takes time and is far from widespread. The question remains: is this progress too late?

WHAT SHOULD BE DONE?

At the end of the day, in tackling any epidemic, it is neither epidemiology nor history and personal narratives that count. What any epidemic evokes is Vladimir Ilych Lenin's famous dictum, *What should be done?* Although few prevention projects are mentioned in this book, there are currently hundreds of efforts under way in China, and many began on the remote borders of Yunnan. Some follow the line of reasoning in the 2002 outbreak of SARS and maintain simple quarantines; others move to provide support groups for people living with HIV (Watts 2003; Piper and Yeoh 2005). However, a note of caution is necessary as the problems with data are widespread. As health economist and African AIDS expert Tony Barnett points out, data collection is done for three purposes—advocacy, prevention, and prediction. Nonetheless, data used for any of these three purposes are but a partial picture, as models by definition are only a representation of reality and cannot capture the full complexity of any given situation (Barnett and Whiteside 2002: 60–61). In the realm of prevention, there have never been easy solutions, especially in particular contexts when local governments prefer to hide and deny rather than openly acknowledge. This was more than apparent in the early days of China's 2003 SARS epidemic, when top government officials were dismissed for burying important epidemiological information and denying an epidemic that struck over three thousand people (Altman 2003: D1). This reinforces a more salient point, one repeated by former UNAIDS head Émile Fox, that while the Chinese face many obstacles in addressing their HIV/AIDS epidemic, the current decentralization of provincial and county power means that in those counties where public health officials are eager to prevent HIV/AIDS, programs exist. In contrast, in those counties where public health officials are reticent, programs for HIV/AIDS prevention take a back seat to other priorities.[7] Others such as William Stewart, formerly with UK-China AIDS, have stated that "all over China we've seen little good projects, but little good projects don't stop an epidemic. What you need to do is to take these projects to scale, and that takes top-level leadership" (Settle 2003).

In many geographic locales in China very little is understood about the relationship between transactional sex and the spread of HIV, apart from the speculation that women and men with many sexual partners are prone to infecting themselves, their clients, their boyfriends and girlfriends, and their husbands and wives (Choi et al. 2000). In addition, the recent decline in national funding and support for the nationwide public health system means that citizens have unequal access to health care. In a recent study, the World Health Organization claimed that the equitable distribution of health care in China has declined dramatically in the past ten years. China moved from a ranking among nations of 144 to 188 due to the increasing privatization of health care and the uneven levels of access to care among China's poor. Zhang Xiaobo and Ravi Kanbur (2005) note that inequality in economic earnings and less government-sponsored health care have meant that the majority of the population does not have full access to health care.

Despite embracing joint foreign NGO projects to build HIV/AIDS education programs for students in middle school through college, too few resources are directed at prevention for this age group, for the general population, and especially for those currently infected—injection drug users and blood donors. Instead the old Maoist regimes of surveillance and quarantine prevail (Hyde 2002 & 1999). In terms of new approaches to HIV prevention, there are quite a few innovative programs in Yunnan. I argue in chapter 5 that when the power of the market and of the state compete, a fascinating paradox emerges. The market economy opens the door to a potentially potent weapon against the further spread of STIs and HIV—condoms. The market in conjunction with the state allows individuals to sidestep the state family planning apparatus by purchasing condoms through private vendors (department stores, pharmacies, small private sundry shops), rather than through state-sanctioned hospitals and clinics.

Not only does the market economy open up space for couples to access birth control methods outside state-run clinics, but also prostitution has brought a source of local tax revenue. As Elizabeth Remick (2004) argues, during the Republican Era, provinces such as Yunnan gained almost 50 percent of their revenues from a tax on prostitution *(jinü juan)*. Pan Suiming (1999) notes that by the summer of 1998, over forty-three cities in China had begun to levy individual income taxes on sex workers and their places of business. Furthermore, Pan argues that since municipalities were now responsible for generating their own income, who could blame policemen for jumping on the bandwagon by fining establishments engaged in prostitution, including everything from karaoke bars to hotels, restaurants, escort services, and massage and beauty parlors? Pan (1999: 324) notes that in one town he studied, the locals had a saying about the police: "Some officials whore when their trousers are off, and clean up prostitution when their trousers are on."

During the evenings and nights I spent with sex workers in Jinghong, I came to recognize just when and where they would take precautions against STIs and HIV. Johanna Hood (2005) has remarked that China in many ways has created a sort of imagined immunity, because having AIDS or being HIV-positive is related to one's status as being uneducated, untrained, and unclean. Similar to the Chinese government, my informants too often placed HIV/AIDS on the bodies of foreigners— including men they would never service, the Burmese or Pakistani jade dealers in town—as certain foreign bodies they regarded as more prone to AIDS than others. Condoms are plentiful in the shops in Jinghong— but women often do not use them, because their customers don't like them. When I asked sex workers about this pattern, they said that they had more faith in the expensive brands and that Japanese and British brands were the best. However, underlying the problem in all of these encounters is that local men do not like to use condoms. In San Francisco, Cianna Stewart, formerly of the Asian AIDS Project (now the Wellness Project), said that in conducting outreach with Asian sex workers, she discovered that they had learned to put condoms on with their mouths without their customers knowing that the condoms were there.[8]

Two San Francisco–based sex educators, Robert Lawrence and Carol Queen, were invited by Mary Ann Burris of the Ford Foundation in 1996 to train educators and staff at the Beijing Women's Health Center, a center modeled after Boston's Women's Health Collective. Queen and Lawrence demonstrated the ways women can use their mouths to put condoms on their partners. Xia Guomei (2003) states that in Shanghai prostitutes are employed in a frontline campaign to promote safer sex among their peers, as has been done in Thailand (see Lyttleton and Amarapibal 2000; Entz et al. 2001). Thailand has seen a dramatic decrease in rates of infection since the early 1990s due to widespread prevention campaigns, the increase in NGO involvement, and most important, government cooperation and investment in stemming the tide of what was seen as a threat to development. The goal was and is to shift normative unsafe sex toward safer practices in brothels and other establishments selling sex. The insistence on a culture of condom use for all sex acts is standard practice in all thirty-six legal sex establishments in Nevada (Schwartz 2000) and in Thailand as well, where 100 percent condom use policies are enforced.[9] Despite the slow pace of research on microbicides, they provide one of the only woman-centered methods, as they can be used without a partner's knowledge.[10]

SEXUAL CITIZENSHIP

Preventing the spread of AIDS and other STIs is rife not simply with scientific facts but with moral judgments about what sexual acts are morally dangerous. The notion that all female sex workers are at high risk for STIs may be erroneous, as the women I have described who worked at the New Wind Hair Salon were often in the business of nonpenetrative sex (Pan 1999; Hyde 1999). This does not mean that sex work is risk free; rather, blanket assumptions cannot be made about all establishments. Dr. Shen Jie, the director of China's National Center for AIDS Prevention and Control, noted in February 2004 that heterosexual transmission would become the major route of infection in China over the next decade. It is necessary within this context to interrogate local practices for what they mean in terms of prevention. For example, what is imbued with moral overtones? Who is representing whose sexuality? And how do older Maoist notions of the sexual in service of the nation now compete with postreform notions of the sexual in service of the market? Differing opinions create both stigma and praise for those exchanging sexual services for money. In many ways, celebrating and promoting nonpenetrative sex could ease the burden on both clients and their customers, providing safer sex outlets in an industry that is unlikely to return to the Maoist closet.

What is encouraging in China is that local sex workers in conjunction with the Women's Federation and certain international NGOs—namely the International Red Cross, Save the Children, and Population Services International—have begun to target prevention campaigns to disenfranchised groups of women. I reiterate that sex acts that require condoms often occur outside the space of the salon; thus China faces different challenges than, say, parts of Africa where unlubricated dry sex is highly desired. Although dry sex may be no barrier for female sex workers in Jinghong, they still complain that condoms hurt, and lubricants are not readily available. Therefore there are no simple answers. Instead the arguments about the solutions must be reframed to reflect not just the increase in the availability of condoms (advocated by condom social marketers such as Futures Group and Population Services International) but also the actual sexual practices being targeted in the first place.

If one were to adopt a prevention model that embraces an array of options that link the scientifically sexually risky (unprotected penetrative sex) to the less risky practices (hand jobs) that the hair salons promote, it would allow a range of sexual practices rather than holding on to a strict utilitarian notion that all sex is unprotected and dangerous. Finally, the hierarchy of risk needs to be reframed as a hierarchy of pleasure. Rather than emphasizing a culture of "risky sex as dangerous sex," a culture is needed that promotes condoms and nonpenetrative sex as pleasurable (see Moore 1998). Perhaps one may take the lead from women's organizations in Senegal that are now promoting the Femidom, a female condom sold with bine bine beads, an erotic accessory that women wear around their hips to enhance the crinkling sounds made by polyurethane during sex.[11] In contrast to the objections to the sounds made by the female condom in the West, African women's organizations have eroticized the sound through local marketing campaigns that promote both safer and sexier sex (Burt 2005: 14).

HIV/AIDS is spreading rapidly in China, but with a prevalence rate of less than 1 percent, it is still considered an emerging epidemic compared to those in India and Burma. China is facing what epidemiologist Kyung-Hee Choi (2000) calls "high prevalent multiple sexual partnerships," low condom use, and STIs as cofactors for infection (118). Yunnan's 2003 seroprevalence survey suggests that injection drug users still have high rates of infection, while the rates for STIs among sex workers, their clients, and pregnant women vary widely (from less than 0.2 percent to 3 percent in Baoshan). In nonborder cities in Yunnan, the rates among people with no known risk factors vary from very high—in Baoshan, Dehong Tai-Jingpo Prefecture, and in Kunming, where there has been 75 percent increase in infections since 1995—to places such as Sipsongpanna, with low rates (Cheng Hehe, Zhang, Pan, Jia, et al. 2000: 74; Yu Huifen 2001). Considering the disproportionate amount of aid money being directed at Ruili, the capital city of Dehong Tai-Jingpo Prefecture, as compared to aid to poor farmers dying of AIDS in central China, the AIDS imagination is very much alive and well.

In developing prevention projects, behavioral change models will not succeed if not accompanied by the political will for socioeconomic change. The reason Thailand is a success story is that AIDS was placed under the Office of the Prime Minister within a multisectoral National AIDS Prevention and Control Office with its own minister, which signaled a high level of political commitment. A massive public information campaign was launched under the cabinet minister Mechai Viravaidya, combined with a policy of 100 percent compliance in condom use among commercial sex establishments (Barnett and Whiteside 2002: 334–35). To link the discursive to the material means creating prevention projects that prevent future suffering. With that in mind I wish to conclude with a few selected prevention ideas suggested by my informants and my own experience.

Madam Liu wanted the police not to presume that just because a young woman was carrying condoms, she was a prostitute and not entitled to protect herself. Dr. Hui suggested that all hotels in major cities should provide condoms for free, like putting mints on the bedcovers. Dr. Li suggested that to change the practice of reusing dirty needles, China would need to return to old-fashioned Maoist health care campaigns to get everyone, including medical practitioners, to refuse to reuse dirty needles and to teach others about safer needle practices. Dr. Hui suggested that drug users must be enculturated not to share needles, syringes, spoons, and other intravenous paraphernalia, and in those places where drug culture discourages needle sharing, to find out why. Furthermore, Dr. Hui suggested that all blood products and all blood supplies should be screened for HIV and that illegal practices in the collection of this scarce resource should be banned for good.

EVERYDAY AIDS PRACTICES:
RETHINKING THE ETHNOGRAPHY OF EPIDEMICS

In this book I focus on two minority prefectures in southern Yunnan, Sipsongpanna and Menglian, in order to examine how certain individuals and groups were represented and treated in the emergent AIDS epidemic in Southwest China. I analyzed how representatives of the state and NGOs, health workers, and ordinary citizens evoke, describe, and stigmatize certain groups of people in the epidemic through their own everyday AIDS practices. However, these cases of stigmatized individuals as traveling vectors for HIV actually fit rather neatly into the larger global narratives of disease contamination. The narratives often follow pattern thinking based on epidemiological risk group models and on colonial tropical disease prevention models emphasizing infection in distinct locations.

In the preceding pages I have drawn together a story about the cultural politics of AIDS and the state in postreform China. Writing on the cultural politics of AIDS, which fills particular spaces created by the onslaught of global consumption, means that the story of AIDS is about more than an infectious disease. At a systemic level, the Chinese government has carved a regime of control around surveying AIDS, controlling prevention, and intervention. China has been praised by international health organizations for its ability and skill at surveillance (Watts 2004). However, surveillance and control are but one part of an epidemic. Through the notion of everyday AIDS practices, I examine the cultural politics behind the Chinese epidemic that brings the epidemic to the forefront from several vantage points: representatives of the state, medical practitioners, NGO representatives, sex workers, and the multi-ethnic inhabitants of Jinghong city. This ethnography differs from previous ethnographies on AIDS, culture, and politics by focusing on how AIDS in China became a part of global discourses and how key scientific rationalities that played out in epidemiological research, behavioral surveys, and public health interventions actually influenced the practices on the ground and vice versa. It is precisely by looking at everyday practices that one realizes that practices transform when actualized.

In popular culture, AIDS is often regarded in one of two ways: as a biological fact or a call to activism. Here I present multiple actors' narratives as if they were marbles colliding on an even tabletop, where their everyday practices reveal the intimate intertextures of an epidemic in the making. The neat dichotomies of social science analysis are meant to be disturbed; compliance and resistance are not contradictory modes of action but function in multiple ways. Taking the narratives of my informants, and combining these with the process or performance of conducting my ethnography and ethnographic interviews, I show that understanding difficult and often taboo subjects lend themselves to ethnographic methods. Much of the work on HIV around the world relies on qualitative public health survey research that leaves the intricacies and complexities of people's lives, particularly their sexual lives, out in the cold. Before I even finished my dissertation research, a major figure in AIDS research in the United States asked me to assist in designing a prevention program that would cover simple, easy-to-use messages for all of southern China. He emphasized that he did not want to hear about local knowledge or languages: "large scale" and "sweeping" were operative words. There is a need for prevention, but in order for it to be effective, it must be heard. In working through much of the material I have presented here, I hope I have convinced readers of the value of local and individual narratives as part of our armamentarium for understanding emerging epidemics.

All these efforts to reduce or curb the spread of HIV inside China require that medical practitioners and public health and security officials see HIV as something that defies borders, ethnic groups, and identity politics within late socialism. HIV does not respect lines on a map or strict global epidemiological markers. In my narrative accounts of this emerging epidemic, I present but a partial view of Chinese AIDS from the late 1990s through 2002. My portrait provides a small looking glass into the cultural politics of epidemics in a postreform socialist country. If the integral role that the market and cultural politics play in how people function is taken into account, HIV prevention can indeed deliver. To build on everyday AIDS practices means to return to a fighter's response and to understand that epidemics are not grounded in one group, one place, or one type of behavior occurring in only one type of person.

The current levels of concern expressed and acted upon by those in power in the Chinese Ministry of Health mean that there is still hope that a massive epidemic can be prevented. In writing this book, I did not set out to criticize any particular institution or person, but rather to critically engage with what I saw, read, and recorded.[12] In understanding our fetishes of postmodernity that circulate with exploding development under late socialism, we must lay bare the stories that people tell about themselves, as well as the stories that epidemics tell us about ourselves. As Paul Farmer (1992: 262) drives home, ethnography has much to offer those who seek rich and textured understandings of AIDS. Coming from the field of public health, I have been converted. Ethnographic accounts based on long-term fieldwork, spread out across time and space and focused closely on situations and people's stories are our strength. Ethnography of epidemics is essential to understanding the complexities of emerging infectious diseases that cross and recross the borders of our twenty-first century. All of this is of no small consequence to those of us who wish for a world without AIDS. As Chinese writer Wang Anyi (1994) so eloquently writes: "From looking at a map, China is only a floating island, and its people a floating body, fluttering toward their eternal destiny."

Notes

1. For a general overview of the American and African epidemics, see Krieger and Appleman 1986 and Fee and Fox 1988 & 1992.

2. In general, an epidemic is a widespread disease that affects many people within a population. It becomes a pandemic only when the disease is global.

3. Because the term "sex worker" is one of contestation, I have chosen to put it in quotation marks. It is an acceptable Western term for women and men who work in the sex trade; at the same time, it links sex to occupation and has been interpreted by some as providing a false sense of agency—thus, occupational choice—to those whose occupational choices are limited.

4. Both Thailand and Cambodia have been tireless in acting to curb the spread of HIV/AIDS, with a resulting drop in prevalence rates for both countries, to 1.8 percent for Thailand and 2.7 percent for Cambodia (UNAIDS September 2002 in Bloom et al. 2004: 13).

5. Cindy Patton has been a tireless AIDS activist, writer, and scholar of the AIDS epidemic since the early 1990s. Two of her earlier works are *Inventing AIDS* (1990), on the emergence of how a disease comes to take over our collective imagination and material practices, and *Fatal Advice* (1996), a critique of current safe-sex education messages. For further discussion linking the genealogy of AIDS and scientific discovery to activism in the United States, see Steven Epstein's (1996) *Impure Science*.

6. According to the *People's Daily* online (http://www.english.people.com.cn) for July 27, 2005, the floating population of China has increased from 70 million in 1993 to 140 million in 2003. While this represents 10 percent of the total population, it is actually 30 percent of the rural labor force. Sixty-five percent moves within provinces, and the other 35 percent moves to different provinces. China's unemployment rate—14 percent in 2004—has also fueled

these processes of migration across and within provinces and between urban and rural areas (Giles, Park and Zhang 2005: 149–170). Social inequality in China has increased substantially since economic reform began in 1979 (Zhang Xiaobo and Kanbur 2005: 189–204). For the argument that temporary migration and HIV/AIDS are connected, see Smith and Yang (2005) and Smith (2005).

7. For excellent discussions of the particular vagaries of Chinese transnationalism, see Ong and Nononi's (1997) *Ungrounded Empires*.

8. On January 24, 2006, China issued a new estimate of the number of people living with HIV and AIDS: 650,000 by the end of 2005, a 23 percent reduction from the official figure of 840,000. The 2006 figure was based on studies done by the World Health Organization and the United Nations AIDS Program and on what Ray Yip, the Beijing representative of the United States Centers for Disease Control and Prevention, called a more complete and robust sampling method (MOH 2006: i; Yardley 2006).

9. India at the end of 2003 had an estimated 4.58 million infections (UNAIDS 2003). Since India and China together account for nearly half the world's population, the concern is that, if the disease is not kept under control, the two countries may eventually have infection rates closer to those in sub-Saharan Africa. In 2002 Thailand had 755,000 people living with HIV and a growing infection rate of 2.15 percent per year (Barnett and Whiteside 2002: 14).

10. The term "nascent" is as much a qualifier as a technical term. Nascent epidemics are those in which HIV prevalence is less than 5 percent in the overall population. In concentrated epidemics, at least one subgroup shows prevalence above 5 percent and among women in antenatal clinics rates are below 1 percent. In a generalized epidemic, the prevalence rate becomes more than 1 percent among women in antenatal clinics (Bloom et al. 2004: 10). Again, this is the nomenclature of international public health and epidemiology. Furthermore, I should explain in lay terms that the incidence rate measures a disease's occurrence in a given population and refers to the annual number of people who get AIDS. "Prevalence," on the other hand, means the number of people who already have AIDS, the grand picture.

11. The term "Tai" refers of all speakers of Tai languages in Southeast Asia and in present-day China; it differs from the term "Thai," which refers to the citizens of Thailand. Gehan Wijeyewardene (1990: 48) points out, "Dai is the pinyin spelling of the word and is used by Chinese speakers of the southwestern branch of languages living in China."

12. Critics of the KABP survey approach—among whom the most vociferous are often anthropologists—warn that there are limitations in reducing sexual and drug-use behavior to a series of isolated and quantifiable events, as if people can just check off their sexual behaviors on a list (Do you use condoms: always, sometimes, occasionally, never?). Catherine Campbell (2003) warns that sexual behaviors involve an array of complex interactions and relationships, as well as emotional sentiments, that are too complex to reduce to mere numbers and quantitative surveys. Other approaches include that of sociologist Yang Xiushi (2003), who has devised a qualitative research method whereby

men crossing the Shenzhen border are asked intimate questions about their sexual behavior by an anonymous researcher via cell phone. He maintains that his research team's results are quite accurate and capture the social intimacies of the ways that Hong Kong men relate to wives, lovers, and girlfriends in mainland China.

13. With a nascent epidemic, I felt that it was imperative not only to position myself in multiple sites—Hong Kong, Beijing, Kunming, Menglian, and Jinghong—but also to embed myself within various identities.

14. There is a vast literature in sociology, anthropology, and public health on the political economy of health; I have merely given the names of some of the key writers who have influenced my own work. For a more in-depth discussion of some of the early work in the political economy of AIDS, see Merrill Singer (1998). The literature on the cultural representations of AIDS is even more vast; I touch only on a few works here. One excellent source is Richard Parker's (2001) *Annual Review of Anthropology* article surveying research on sexuality, politics, and HIV/AIDS.

15. The term "practice theory" is linked with the work of Pierre Bourdieu. However, in analyzing the Chinese state, there is a certain slippage between practice theory and Foucault's notion of discursive practices. Foucault relies heavily on the notion of genealogies in analyzing the rise of certain state practices; Bourdieu, on the other hand, moves away from time-based chronologies. The notion of focusing on the practices of individuals is antithetical to Foucault's radically antihumanist notion of power; however, I have taken the liberty of borrowing from both Bourdieu and Foucault. Ralph Litzinger (2000b) in chapter 1 of *Other Chinas* also makes a strong case for working with Foucault through fieldwork methodologies that focus on the actions and reflections of individuals and their experiences. For an excellent statement on the concept of genealogy, see Jean Cohen and Andrew Arato's (1992) *Civil Society and Political Theory*, chapter 6.

16. While one may argue that I am building on Michel de Certeau's (1984: 29–30) notion of the "practice of everyday life," I am not. De Certeau had a particular take on how practices are mediated through tactics and strategies that are distinguishable in how they are executed. As de Certeau notes, strategies are technical, are "able to produce, tabulate and impose," and operate in situations where one has control and power; whereas tactics are what he called "manipulations," quick decisions made when one does not have power or time on one's side.

17. In late 2003, the Chinese government replaced the former anti-epidemic stations with "Jibing yufang kongzhi zhongxin" (Centers for Disease Control and Prevention) at the prefecture, city, provincial, and national levels. In a personal conversation in November 2005, Dr. Li Jianhua, the deputy director of the Yunnan Institute for Drug Abuse and a psychiatrist working on the prevention of injection drug use and HIV/AIDS, said: "In the United States you have one CDC, in China we have hundreds."

18. As Catherine Campbell (2003: 104–5) points out in her work in South Africa, prevention projects are up against tremendous challenges because fighting HIV must take place on three levels simultaneously: as direct biomedical

control (administration of health care and drug therapies for those already infected); as community-level peer education and condom distribution; and as efforts over the long haul to reduce poverty and empower people to be part of what I call sexual citizenship. However, what currently happens is that projects focus on the easy parts first. In Yunnan that meant developing peer education projects, with or without condom distribution. It is only recently that efforts have been set up to alleviate those who are already infected. As for poverty alleviation projects that directly provide means of alternative employment for drug users and prostitutes, they are few and far between.

19. While there has been considerable discussion of the differences between black and white bodies in terms of acquiring HIV in both the United States and Africa, few have written on the differences among ethnic groups in China. For a discussion of the issues surrounding race in the United States, see Harlon Dalton (1989) and Evelyn Hammonds (1987); for China, see Johanna Hood (2005).

20. Some social scientists both in China and in the broader international community maintain that HIV disproportionately affects minorities. The statistic that 36 percent of all infections are registered to minorities is biased, I maintain, because the early surveillance data were taken only in minority prefectures, and only among minorities. As the blood crisis in central China heats up, with upwards of 10 million infections, the proportion of minority groups with HIV will pale in comparison. I acknowledge that in many small minority communities, such as Liangshan County in Sichuan, AIDS rages among injection drug users who happen to be part of the Yi ethnic group. However, the connection here has less to do with one's ethnic status than with one's poverty and proximity to the drug trade.

21. For an analysis of the eroticization of minority women in the Yunnan School of Art, see Felicity Lufkin (1990).

22. In a follow-up trip in the summer of 2002, I found that the tourist industry in Jinghong appeared to be in decline, as was the status of sex workers. The well-placed beauty salon where I once did extensive fieldwork is now a dingy, run-down salon owned by two rather seedy men from Beijing. The young women working there were still from outlying provinces but now were wearing *modern* clothing.

23. More recent work in minority studies includes scholars such as Jacqueline Armijo-Hussein (1997), who worked among the Hui of Yunnan to reconstruct the history of a Hui explorer who is credited with bringing civilization to Yunnan's hinterland. Louisa Schein (2000) has conducted research on minorities by examining the transnational relationships formed between the Miao (Hmong) in the United States (in the area of Fresno, California) and the Miao of Guizhou province in China. Ralph Litzinger (1998, 2000a, & 2000b) has conducted research on the Yao in Guangxi Province, looking specifically at the relationship between memory work, history, and cultural capital. As far as the question of vector, the problem with focusing exclusively on prostitutes means that their clients, the ones who would be using condoms, are left out of the prevention equation. Also, the clinical and epidemiological gaze turns toward women, often sexually disenfranchised women, rather than men, because the latter are perceived as a difficult population to study and also such studies are

thought to be an invasion of their privacy. Currently, graduate student Elanah Uretsky (2003) at Columbia University is conducting research on male clients in the city of Ruili, in northwestern Yunnan.

24. There is a large literature on the anthropology of suffering. In China the pioneer in stigma studies is Arthur Kleinman, who was the first foreign anthropologist-physician to study the effects of stigma and the embodiment of the terrors of the Cultural Revolution (1966–67). See Kleinman 1986 & 1994; Kleinman, Das, and Lock 1997).

25. The Dai of China are an officially recognized ethnic group living in Xishuangbanna Dai Minority Autonomous Prefecture and the Dehong Tai-Jingpo Minority Autonomous Prefecture (both in southern Yunnan), and also in Laos, Vietnam, Thailand, and Burma. Although they are officially recognized as a single ethnic group by the Han Chinese state, the Dai people form several distinct cultural and linguistic groups. The two main languages of the Dai are Tai Lüe (Xishuangbanna Dai) and Tai Nüa (Dehong Dai); two other written languages used by the Dai in China are Tai Bong and Tai Dam (Black Tai). These four languages are closely related to Thai, Lao, and Zhuang and are part of the Tai-Kadai language family. (*Wikipedia,* s.v. "Dai people," www.en.wikipedia .org/wiki/Dai_people [accessed March 10, 2006].)

26. Aizhi Action Project (Beijing) is a nonprofit organization concerned with AIDS/HIV/STD/sexuality-related information, education, morality, law, policy, and research. The project has a website, www.aizhi.net, and a weekly report on related issues. As of early 2006, the website had been suspended in a government crackdown.

27. This is by no means an exhaustive bibliographic list; rather I am using these few references to point out that anthropology does not have exclusive rights to studies of the state and population that have become popular since Foucault's work on sexuality.

28. Susan Greenhalgh (1994 & 2005), in her fascinating engagement with Chinese demography and the projects surrounding the 1980s campaigns for the one-child family, also builds on Foucault's insights.

29. I do not disregard sociologist Pan Suiming's tireless work (1992, 1999, & 2000) on contemporary prostitution; rather, I am thinking more in terms of works in English.

Since 2002, anthropologist Jing Jun founded the Tsinghua-Bayer Public Health and Media Studies Program in Beijing, and sociologist Xia Guomei founded the Research Center for HIV/AIDS Public Policy at the Shanghai Academy of Social Sciences. Both are actively training Chinese social scientists in AIDS research.

30. Other works in Chinese on prostitution include Huang Yingying et al (2004) on brothel-based female sex workers; for general overviews, see Shan Guangnai (1995) and Wang Shunu (1988).

31. Eastern European studies of the transition from socialism to capitalism preceded much of the work on China. For some interesting discussions of work in Hungary, see Michael Burawoy and Janos Lukacs (1992); for Russia, see Nancy Ries (1997); and for Romania, see Katherine Verdery (1996).

32. In describing the role of the local party-state cadre in the reform era, Ann Anagnost (1985) identifies its members as subjects who through their reor-

ganization of social subjectivity imagine themselves as formidable forces in Chinese society. The local cadre participates in circulating carefully chosen political symbols and practices throughout society, and in that process the party-state is made visible in its displays of government functions. Zhang Li (2001) demonstrates how the political and spatial landscapes of cosmopolitan cities such as Beijing have been radically changed by migrant laborers and their networks, especially through their ties to party-state leaders, and how, therefore, the Chinese state is never totalizing in its control and surveillance of these cityscapes. Another crucial work on peasant migration and postreform market pressures is Dorothy Solinger's (1998) *Contesting Citizenship in Urban China*.

33. David Goodman (1983) was the first to use the term "internal colonialism" in reference to the party-state's efforts during the early years of the People's Republic to unify the country and condense the boundaries of its far border regions. Other scholars building on Marxist interpretations to describe economic and political inequalities between regions and ethnic groups did so long before Sinologists picked up the term. Several Sinologists have developed Goodman's use of the term, in particular Dru Gladney (2002), in reference to internal political struggle in Xinjiang among the Uighur minority of Central Asia (see also Sautman 2000); and Tim Oakes (1995), in reference to minority struggles in Guizhou. Here I refer to Louisa Schein (1996), who uses the term "internal orientalism" when she addresses Edward Said's work on the intricacies of the phenomena of orientalism.

34. In anthropology, early work on ethnicity and ethnic group boundaries can be found in Frederick Barth's (1969) *Ethnic Groups and Boundaries*.

35. More recently, anthropologists Elizabeth Miller (2002) and João Biehl (2001) write about the AIDS imaginary. In her work in Japan on nationalism and sexuality, Miller discusses the idea of AIDS as imagined by the Japanese state. Biehl's work on Brazilian AIDS centers suggests there is a kind of statistical imaginary in terms of low-risk individuals seeking repeated HIV/AIDS testing.

36. In a recent journalistic account, Tu Qiao (2000) writes a memoir of a man who got HIV/AIDS in Thailand and shared his story with her.

37. The People's Republic of China officially describes itself as a multi-ethnic state that officially recognizes fifty-six nationalities or *minzu*. The Han Chinese are the majority at around 92 percent of the population; the remaining 8 percent constitute fifty-five national minorities. As the classification project in the 1950s (*minzu shibie*) designated only fifty-five groups, there are additional groups in China that are still seeking minority status or that classify themselves as minority groups.

38. See also Malkki 1995: 19–52.

39. I would like to thank Mayfair Yang for pointing this out in her commentary at the Ethnographies of the Urban in Contemporary China Workshop in September 1997 at the University of California, Santa Cruz. For a longer and more in-depth discussion of the expression *qingchunfan* see Zhang Zhen's " Mediating Time: The 'Rice Bowl of Youth' in Fin de Siècle Urban China," in Arjun Apppardurai's (2003) *Globalization*.

CHAPTER I

1. I used a literal translation of "Huangyan, taoyan de huangyan, haishi tongji."

2. Because Matthew Kohrman's (2005) wonderful study on the experiences of disability in postreform China was published as this book was going to press, I was unable to integrate all of his insights or do his work justice. His work is important for scholars of China, medical anthropology, and science studies for understanding how a certain kind of biosociality around disability arose in China in the early 1990s.

3. Mary-Jo DelVecchio Good (1995) first used the term to describe how positive statistical outcomes are presented to anxious cancer patients; presenting the best-possible scenario meant statistics retained an aesthetic quality (see also Gould 1996).

4. Judith Farquhar (2002), in talking about China's 1992 nationwide sex survey, observes that behavioral surveys insist that all preferences have existed and will exist beyond the confines of the survey, and thus "sexual behavior enjoys an existence independent of the instrument's written questions and the carefully crafted sociological categories from which they are constructed" (220).

5. There has been very little research in English on hospitals in the reform era. One source that carefully analyzes the hospital as a socialist work unit is Gail Henderson and Myron Cohen's (1984) *The Chinese Hospital*.

6. In her master's thesis, Johanna Hood (2005: 23) analyzes media representations of HIV/AIDS in China with a particular focus on the links between race and place. In chapter 1 she suggests that those with AIDS in China are similar to minorities, and she classifies them as *aizu*, or simply translated, the AIDS minority.

7. Personal communication with Dr. Chen. In addition, as of 2001, two-thirds of the Chinese population is infected with hepatitis B, according to an Associated Press wire report on August 22, 2001.

8. I have not been able to confirm a date for the relocation of the village, nor for when the entire village converted from Buddhism to Christianity. Records of some of the Protestant missionaries remain at MacGilvery Theological Union in Chiang Mai, Thailand.

9. Places such as Sipsongpanna were not integrated into mainland China until January 24, 1953.

10. All key informants names are pseudonyms.

11. Randy Shilts (1987: 157), in his journalistic account of the rise of the HIV/AIDS epidemic in the United States in the early 1980s, points out that while epidemics like Spanish flu and polio were once spread in large viral mixing bowls during the great movements of people across the globe at the turn of the century, with air travel and displacement, viruses like HIV now spread at lightening speeds.

In this Golden Quadrangle, heroin trafficking now follows the old Burma-China road as a major access route through China and on to Hong Kong ports, and finally out of Asia to the United States and Europe.

12. Sara Davis's book *Song and Silence* (2005), on the Tai-Lüe and Buddhist temple singers in Jinghong is a useful source for understanding issues facing contemporary Tai-Lüe in Sipsongpanna. Others who are currently writing on Sipsongpanna include Metta Hansen (1999) on minority education, Susan McCarthy on political power (2001), Janet Sturgeon (2005) on forestry practices among the Akha in Thailand and China, and Sara Davis (2005) on tourism, Buddhism, and the Zanghap singers among the Tai.

13. I use the term "counting bodily behaviors" because all surveys, including those that document knowledge and behaviors, treat each individual as one body count, and thus, due to confidentiality, bodies are not counted as individual histories but as numbers.

14. In China, people who are HIV-positive tend to have two to three symptoms of AIDS before receiving an AIDS diagnosis. In much of Europe and North America, an AIDS diagnosis is determined by lab tests that confirm a helper T-cell count of less than 200 per cubic millimeter. In epidemiological information derived from popular health journals and the popular press, HIV is often referred to as AIDS and there is a certain slippage in the statistics; therefore the definition of a diagnosis of full-blown AIDS continues to change. The "confirmation" test used at the time was the Western blot test, which costs three to four times as much as the original (Elisa) test in almost all countries; therefore, most developing countries settled for either a repeat Elisa or did not perform confirmation tests. This practice, then, slightly raised the probability of false positives.

15. By the time I finished my first round of fieldwork in 1997, the official counts of HIV in Sipsongpanna were still not released to the press, to foreign researchers, or to NGOs working on HIV/AIDS. As for the number of HIV persons reaching ten million, this appears to be a slight exaggeration. China's own admission is an increase of 26 to 30 percent a year, which brings the estimate closer to six million. Again, these numbers must be understood in terms of the problems associated with government reports that may both inflate and deflate statistics, depending on who is reviewing them. Because HIV is also referred to as HIV/AIDS, statistics used for epidemiological information in popular health journals and the press can be imprecise. I try to be sensitive to these slippages and identify them when they are present. A note about statistics collected on HIV: in all countries statistics are problematic, and that includes China. Here I discuss the notion of what Mary-Jo Good (1995) calls the "aesthetics of statistics" and how statistics are embedded with meanings beyond their face value. In other instances, the Chinese government has faced many obstacles in gaining accurate statistics, including the factors noted here—unreliable collection methods, untrained personnel, random or uneven testing pools, and the bias selection, testing some populations rather than others.

16. Kyung-Hee Choi and associates (2003) at the Center for AIDS Prevention Studies at the University of California at San Francisco conducted one of the first cohort studies of men who have sex with men in China, and found that while only 3 percent were infected with HIV-1, over 49 percent reported having unprotected anal intercourse over the previous six months.

17. There are two types of HIV—HIV-1 and HIV-2—and both are transmitted by the same routes of infection—blood, semen and vaginal fluids, and

mother to child. They are clinically indistinguishable. The difference is that HIV-2 is less easily transmitted, has a longer time period before people become symptomatic, and is usually only found in West Africa.

18. Specifically, seroprevalence surveys and blood sampling from six hundred people with HIV from thirty provinces in 2000 revealed that 47.5 percent of the samples were of subtype B, or the same type as that in Thailand. Over 34 percent of the blood samples were subtype C, which is found among drug users in India, and 9.6 percent were subtype E, which is common in Southeast Asia. Subtype B was prevalent in all areas, while subtype C was concentrated in Xinjiang, Yunnan, and Sichuan provinces. Subtype E, commonly transmitted by sexual contact, was concentrated in southeastern coastal areas and southwestern border regions. These data are from Liu Baoying 2000; Cheng Hehe et al. 1996; Beyrer 1998; and Jia Manhong et al. 2003.

19. Although the first case of AIDS in Yunnan appeared in 1987 in an American tourist, Dr. Cheng Hehe noted that most of the foreigners with AIDS in Yunnan were from Myanmar (Cheng Hehe et al. 1994: 5).

20. Current official estimates suggest that in Henan Province alone there were 287 official blood collection centers and many more illegal ones (Brookes 2001).

21. According to Zhang Feng (*China Daily* [Shanghai], July 30, 2004), once the cat was out of the bag about high rates of infection from illegal blood and plasma centers, central China's Henan Province closed all blood stations, both illegal and legal, in an effort to investigate suppliers of blood and to weed out the harmful practices from the healthy ones.

22. To complicate matters, YRC can also be considered an NGO; however, it is a government-sponsored NGO, or what is known as a GONGO.

23. See Zheng Xiwan (1991) for one of the earliest studies on injection drug–using communities in Ruili County, Dehong Tai-Jingpo Prefecture, Yunnan Province.

24. The remaining figures included fourteen persons in Lingchang, ten in Baoshan, two in Jinghong, one in Dali, and one in Lijiang (Cheng Hehe et al. 1996).

25. Personal statements were made during the survey and then taken from my transcribed notes and translated into English.

26. The literal translation of *jiedusuo* is "drug admonish center." For simplicity's sake, I have translated it as "drug prison" because the only rehabilitation that occurs there occurs when prisoners work as unpaid laborers. This can be read two ways: as slave labor, according to international human rights activists; or as labor re-education (*laodong jiaoyu*), following the old Maoist dictum. See chapter 2 for a fuller explanation of this Chinese concept.

The full survey also included another five hundred people in and around Kunming, the provincial capital.

27. The Hani are another minority group, called the Akha in Thailand.

28. The concept of the exposure tour is attributed to one of Lenin's tactics: to get individuals to really understand a situation, they had to be allowed to experience it for themselves. Because Madam Wu was exposed to the Thai HIV/ AIDS epidemic and the government's efforts to alleviate and prevent further

transmission, she was ready to prevent what she called a Thailand-like epidemic. This exposure tour was initiated and executed by the first health adviser to Save the Children Foundation in Kunming, Dr. Nagib Hussein.

29. Actual figures on how many women are crossing the border vary widely. According to the Committee for the Protection of Children's Rights and the International Organization for Migration, both based in Bangkok, less than one hundred women cross the borders to work in Thai brothels in 1997. No one in Jinghong knew of friends and family members who chose to work in Thailand rather than Jinghong. However, in Menglian, Shen reported that she knew of several women who had worked in Thailand, and she tried to contact all of them on their return to China. Historically, according to the National People's Congress in 1989 and 1990, a total of 65,236 people were arrested for trafficking in women and children, of whom only 10,000 had been "rescued by the authorities" (Kristof and Wudunn 1994). Another, more recent report is Feingold 1998.

30. Such sessions have been used among health educators in the United States since the mid-1980s to conduct basic training on information about HIV/AIDS prevention for a variety of interest groups.

31. External Propaganda Office of Simao Prefecture Party Committee and Press Office of the Simao Prefecture Administration 2003 (www.chacheng.cn).

32. Menglian County is part of Simao Prefecture, which is directly north of Sipsongpanna. Simao Prefecture governs eleven counties, four of which are on the border with Laos People's Democratic Republic (PDR), Burma, and Vietnam. Simao Prefecture has a population of approximately 2.5 million, of which approximately 1.54 million belong to ethnic minority groups including the Yi, Hani, Lahu, Wa, and Tai. The area's socioeconomic level is quite low; the average annual income of the people in the urban areas is 4,740 renminbi (RMB), compared to RMB 1,069 in rural areas. The illiteracy rate is 10.2 percent; the dropout rates are 1.2 percent (of which 55 percent are girls) in primary schools and 2.01 percent (60 percent are girls) in middle schools. (All data from Simao Prefecture Party Committee, 2004)

33. One evening, while walking to dinner, I saw an older teenager whaling on a young kid and was so angry that I intervened. I told the teenager to think about what he was doing and asked how he could beat up a small kid—who was bleeding at this point and crying. The guy just looked at me with a blank stare and walked away. The kid kept crying, and I asked if he could get home OK and he nodded. Then I let the people around them have it. Why were they ignoring this child and letting him get the shit kicked out of him? Again, it is difficult to draw the line between where one intervenes and doesn't. But I just couldn't watch while an adult beat up a ten-year-old.

34. Common myths included the ideas that only homosexuals and prostitutes get HIV/AIDS and that the disease can be transmitted via toothbrushes and razor blades and by kissing someone on the lips. In 1994, two farmers in Shandong province destroyed a family heirloom painting because they thought it was spreading HIV/AIDS.

35. The texts of the three speeches were taken from my notes and those of another survey worker. They were not tape-recorded due to the sensitive nature of this research and people's general fear of having their voices recorded. These are therefore not exact translations.

36. Jonathan Mann (1992) uses the term "avidity of statistics" to suggest that there has been an over-reliance on statistics in determining HIV/AIDS outcomes and in the design of prevention projects.

37. All of the names given for places are selected pseudonyms and have no resemblance to any actual place names in this part of southwest Yunnan.

38. Altogether, interviews were conducted in five languages: English, Mandarin, Tai, Lahu, and Wa.

39. On the fourth day, a Saturday, the team went to interview women in the Tai village on the edge of Sanya. There I would interview women who spoke Mandarin, because at that stage I was unable to say much beyond "hello" and "goodbye" in Tai. Then, Sunday, some of us would go to a Wa community, and others to a Lahu community. The survey would culminate in a trip to Tai villages on the Burmese border. I had to return to my field site and did not accompany the group to the border. A sociologist from the Women's Cadre Training School in Kunming was to take my place.

40. This situation reminds me that I have become an honorary male of sorts through conducting fieldwork—or perhaps not so much an honorary male as a city sophisticate who, of course, drinks.

41. Chinese condoms are generally thought to be less reliable or less desirable than European or Japanese brands. At this time in China, especially in a small hamlet like Menglian, nothing was available but Chinese condoms. I also want to clarify that not all Chinese condoms are equal; there are some Shanghai brands that have been tested for endurance, comfort, and reliability.

42. In Mandarin the translation is "Tiaojian cha keshi huanying hao."

43. Much of the information here on the actual statistics in the HIV/AIDS Menglian survey was taken from the final report, Armijo-Hussein and Beesey 1998.

44. See "Yunnan Expands Disease Control along Borders," *China Daily*, April 16, 1996 (originally printed in *Yunnan Ribao*). For an update, see "Yunnan Strengthens AIDS Surveillance amongst Foreign Visitors at Immigration Control Ports," *Yunnan Ribao*, June 13, 2005 (originally printed in *Chunqing Wenbao* [Spring City Evening News] as "Yunnan jiaqiang rujing waijirenyuan aizibing jianguan").

CHAPTER 2

1. As discussed in my introduction, I use the term "everyday AIDS practices" for two reasons: first, to bring practice theory into an analysis of an epidemic, because the term "epidemic" captures a whole array of practices, thoughts, policies, words, and actions engaged in the process of HIV prevention; and second, to bridge the variety and range of human endeavors that are involved in the social practices and discourses associated with documenting and disciplining a new epidemic. The Foucauldian notion of discursive practice allows me to move away from temporal and spatial analyses of a neat chronology of HIV/AIDS. I am more interested in what Liu Xin (2000: 24) calls the uncertainty in practice and in how practices transform themselves in the very moment when they are actualized.

2. This sense of hybridity is not a new concept in terms of understanding power relations in postreform China. Victor Nee (1992) discusses how the market in transition created all kinds of hybrid forms of property relations and mixed different kinds of economies.

3. The literature on civil society and the state in China is so large as to permit mentioning only the works most relevant to this study. China scholars in recent years have debated the power of the socialist state to embrace the emergence of civil society and the degree to which this has succeeded since the post-1979 reforms (Siu 1989; Wasserstrom and Perry 1992; M. Yang 1994; Jing 1996; Anagnost 1997; Madsen 1998; C. Lee 1998; Zhang Li 2001; Tsai 2002; Remick 2004). Following other scholars of late-socialist society (from the post-1979 reforms to the late 1990s), I present here some of the complexities of the changing Communist state.

4. For an alternative to the Foucauldian, networks and webs approach to conceptualizing power, see Laura Nader's (1997) *Controlling Processes.*

5. For an in-depth discussion of the Chinese concept of *guanxi* and how it functions within contemporary Chinese society, see Andrew Kipnis's (1997) *Producing Guanxi*; Mayfair Yang's (1994) *Gifts, Favors, and Banquets;* and Yan Yunxiang's (1996) *The Flow of Gifts.*

6. A couple of informants mentioned that the recent increases in syphilis in Kunming prompted the anti-epidemic station to hold people with secondary and tertiary syphilis against their will until they completed treatment.

7. The written scripts for the Tai language in Xishuangbanna and Dehong Tai-Jingpo are mutually unintelligible, as the two groups of Tai, while often linked by Han Chinese, are ethnolinguistically distinct.

8. Much has been made of the graphic distinctions between Han and non-Han by the Yunnan School of painting. The school is known for often depicting minority women as sexualized nudes, and reprints of the paintings are used in tourism brochures that market minority border areas. These brochures build on the marked distinctions between Han women, who are depicted as conservative, and minority non-Han women, who are free and open with their sexuality. See Lufkin 1990; Gladney 1994; Schein 1997; and chapter 3.

9. Prior to the 1950s, the term for the Tai-Lüe was "Baiyi"—*bai* (white) + *yi* (cloth or clothing). However, a homonym for *yi* means "barbarian." When the Tai were integrated into China in 1953, an effort was made to eradicate the earlier term and replace it with "Tai" or rather the Mandarin "Dai" (see Hsieh 1995 for further discussion.)

10. I thank Jay Dautcher for pointing out that *gui* (ghost) is a long-standing metaphor for addiction and a term of dehumanization. Europeans in Chinese history were often referred to as ghosts due to their white skin. Ghosts were people who had died but were not successfully transformed into rightful ancestors by funeral rites, and they plagued the living.

11. I realize this discussion of men and women at the drug center begs for a gendered analysis of incarceration and treatment. Due to my focus on everyday AIDS practices and the state, I shift my thinking away from gender in this piece.

For an earlier work that discusses women and the state in China, see Christina Gilmartin's (1994) *Engendering China*.

12. Outside of the large urban centers, clean needles are not always used in health care facilities, despite the Ministry of Health's directives for clean syringes.

13. See Lisa Rofel (1999) for her discussion of factory workers and their generational differences in terms of ideas about postreform policies.

14. Historians note that the southwest and the border regions in particular were described in this way. Current infectious disease specialists in Yunnan are concerned that some of these diseases, such as cerebral malaria, are making a comeback with the continued lack of medical care in rural areas.

15. Judith Farquhar and Zhang Qicheng (2005), in a piece published as this book was going to press, points out that "power is generated, sustained and challenged through everyday practices" (303). In her study of the arts of life cultivation (including everything from diet to Taiji to anger management) that exist in many parks and public spaces in Beijing, one discovers that these collective practices are both part of and a challenge to the projects of the Chinese state. In other words, personal actions are not part of what Western political scientists would call the rise of civil society but actually an extension of state power, or what Foucault labels generative or productive power in institutions of everyday life.

CHAPTER 3

1. To reiterate a point made earlier, Han Chinese constitute 92 percent of the population of China; fifty-five minority groups fill out the other 8 percent (Li Dexi 2003).

2. For further explanation of the term "site of desire," see Manderson and Jolly 1997: 1.

3. For other materials on sex tourism around the globe, see Adams and Pigg 2005, Gregory 2003, Ebron 2002, Kempadoo and Doezema 1998.

4. Overall there are forty townships, 198 administrative villages, and 2,095 village committees.

5. According to the Jinghong Publicity Department (2005), by 2002 (the latest figures I could find) ethnic minorities made up 67 percent of the population of Sipsongpanna and Han Chinese 33 percent, while the Tai minority remains the largest of the minority groups with 35 percent of the population.

6. Rubber first came to China in the 1950s, first somewhat informally via Chinese returning from Thailand, then in the form of official state research on rubber. The state began to lower the price of rubber during the 1990s, as it became clearer that China would be accepted into the World Trade Organization. Rubber remains the premier cash crop in the region and farmers plant trees with the assumption that the price will increase again. According to Janet Sturgeon, who is working on a history of rubber in Sipsongpanna, due to global environmental concerns about synthetic and petrochemical alternatives, market demand for natural rubber is on the upswing (personal communication with Janet Sturgeon, June 30, 2004).

7. Currently several scholars are working on the impact of tourism on ethnic groups in China. See, for example, the work of Eileen Walsh (Walsh 2001; Walsh and Swain 2004). Two of the pioneers in this area of scholarship are Margaret Byrne Swain (1990; Swain and Momsen 2002) and Tim Oakes (1998). For recent ethnographic studies of contemporary Tai life in Sipsongpanna, see Sara Davis (2005), McCarthy (2001), and Ratanaporn Sethakul (2000). In addition, Gail Hershatter's (2005) review article in *The Journal of Asian Studies* provides a wealth of information on the geography and timing of the state's research on women in China.

8. As of August 1997, twelve officially designated travel tours were available around Sipsongpanna, including excursions into the border regions in Burma and Laos and further south into northern Thailand (Qin 1995).

9. Sara Davis (1999) notes that the contemporary Mandarin term *man* is an inaccurate translation of the Tai term *ban*, so actually these names in Tai would be "Banjinglan" and "Banting," the old township names.

10. According to Greg Guldin (1994: 108), these nationality policies were at the heart of democratic reforms from 1955 to 1957, and continuing work over the years would add additional minority groups: the Tuijia, Monba, and Luoba by the early 1960s and the Jinuo in 1979. The process continues into the twenty-first century.

11. While both Schein and Gladney use the term "internal orientalism," they do so in very different ways and with different outcomes. Schein (2000) questions the utility of a strict Han-ethnic binary, as ethnicity is a category that is constantly changing, often in relation to the utility of claiming Han or non-Han identities, depending on the circumstances. For example, non-Han minorities were often exempt from the strict one-child policies of the 1980s; thus having a non-Han identity meant that one could have more than one child. Ralph Litzinger (2000) also addresses this question by challenging the neat binary of the Han versus non-Han minority Other. He demonstrates that Yao intellectuals and government officials, often marked as the minority Other, are potent agents through redefining their own positions in the Chinese nation at the same time that they have definite control over their more peasant and poor brethren (230–59). Dru Gladney (2002) argues that Chinese nationalism in the post-1989 era means that subaltern groups within China are the target of increasing colonial and expansionist endeavors to the degree that they are regarded as peripheral and less authentic; but at the same time they help feed a sense of Chinese nationalism. This kind of nationalism takes on a religious fervor that detracts from the growing unrest and social problems of market socialism.

12. It is not only the question of minority status that evokes a sense of sexual openness but also the distinction between rurality and urbanity. In more recent films such as Dai Sijie's (2002) *Balzac and the Little Chinese Seamstress,* we see the sexual awakening of two youth sent to the countryside for re-education during the Cultural Revolution (1966–76); the beautiful daughter of the young tailor tempts the two youths. In these depictions of rural China lies a sense that being rural, or being a peasant, allowed for a closer relationship to the flesh and its pleasures than those working in industry in large cities are capable of.

13. Both a Western foreigner and a white woman, I had easier access to the higher-class, visible salons than to the lower-class, low-income brothels. In these brothels, my first impression was that the owners were interested only in pimping me, not in having me study them.

14. The Tai language has undergone changes similar to those affecting Kazak in Xinjiang. There, as in Sipsongpanna, three generations often cannot communicate with one another through one writing system because of policies that aimed to simplify China's minority languages in the name of literacy. In Sipsongpanna, what is called *lao Tai wen,* or old Tai, is now the official language. However, from 1961 to 1986 a script called *xin Tai wen,* or new Tai, was used in the schools, the media, and official documents. This renaissance in Tai culture can be attributed to links with Southeast Asia, where several other countries' minority groups use old script. China is unique in having raised only a generation or two on new Tai. However, unlike the result of the efforts to romanize ancient Arabic script in Xinjiang, old and new Tai are mutually intelligible. (Personal communication with Tai linguist Gao Lishi, *Yunnan Minzu Xueyuan,* January 1996).

15. Preserving the remaining 83,000 palm leaf scriptures proceeds with a sense of urgency, as palm leaves are not a stable material and are subject to insect infestations and environmental deterioration over time.

16. Simultaneously, many Tai have resigned themselves to what they deem the final stage in the complete destruction of the Tai-Lüe that liberation and the Cultural Revolution began. Other scholars such as Shih-chung Hsieh believe that the closer the Tai are to northern Thailand, the more dangerous the reaction of the central Chinese government may be (Hsieh 1995: 328). I should also note that while Tai women were noticeably absent from the sex industry in Sipsongpanna, I did meet one Tai woman who owned a brothel.

17. In creating these pseudonyms, I have used a term of respect, taking their fictitious family name and putting old (lao) or young (xiao) in front of it.

18. Prostitution is often a symbolically gendered category as the majority of "sex workers" are females; however, not all are women. This ethnography privileges female sex workers because those are the ones to whom I had access. Gigolos (*mianshou*) were rumored to be present in Jinghong, but I did not come into contact with any of them.

19. In his study of three towns near Beijing, Pan Suiming (1999) notes seven different vertical layers for women working in the sex industry; massage or hair salon girls constitute the fifth layer. As such they have more freedom of movement, offer multiple sexual services, and thus also collect more money.

20. Owning a brothel is one of the crimes punishable by death under China's legal code.

21. I have chosen this pseudonym because he was a factory manager, because the term "manager" was used in early reform China in the late 1970s to denote respect, and because "Manager" provides readers with an easy point of recognition with the pseudonym "Zhou."

22. I want to thank Melissa Brown for reminding me of this notion of ethnicity in China.

CHAPTER 4

1. With this chapter title I have taken literary license and changed the translation of *qingchun fan* to reflect the subject matter of this chapter. For a more thorough explanation of this metaphor see the introduction.

2. The literature discussed here is by no means an exhaustive review, as prostitution has been discussed in many different venues, including numerous activist conventions, and in many different academic disciplines from social science to literary theory and public policy.

3. Studies on prostitution and transactional sex are too numerous to permit mentioning them all; however, debates over these particular social phenomena continue to be as vitriolic as ever. Another helpful source is Anne McClintock's (1993) article in a special issue of *Social Text* devoted to prostitution.

4. Elizabeth Remick is currently at work on this new research on how the prostitution tax funded many public works projects and filled public government coffers during the Republican Era (1911–49).

5. It should be noted that *xing gongzuozhe* is not exactly a direct translation of the Mandarin term for worker (*gongren*). However, since *gongren* is associated with the Maoist socialist era, the current term as it is used in Jinghong is closest to the western term of "sex worker."

6. In explaining the term *jinü*, I am following the lead of Gail Hershatter (1997). While "sex worker" has been translated into Chinese and is occasionally used in articles about AIDS and prostitution, it is a literal translation from English and a cumbersome one at that (*xingxingwei gongzuo fuwuzhe*). Linguistically there are numerous terms for prostitutes, but the most common is simply *jinü* or *jipo*. *Ji* in Mandarin means "prostitute"—the Chinese ideogram combines the two characters for woman and skill—and *nu* means girl or woman. *Po* in this context means "old woman" and comes from the term of endearment used to describe wives, *laopo*, in which *lao* means "old" and *po* means "mother's mother" or "grandma." Male customers are called *peike* or *piaoke*, "to ticket customers" or "to pay with regard to customers."

7. See Parish et al. (2002) for the most recent broad sociological study on STIs in China.

8. Cleo Odzer (1994) wrote a provocative ethnography of the Patpong district in Bangkok, a district known for its abundance of houses of prostitution and adult entertainment. I now realize it was a mistake to turn away from the first hair salon merely because the owner proposed marriage the first time we met. I now see it as a ridiculous play on affection and friendship, with no real intentions of proposing. I should have been less afraid and not worried about his assistant's insistence on the perfection of the match. Instead, I prematurely crossed that hair salon off my list of possible research sites.

9. Dr. Samir introduced me to this salon when he was working for a Save the Children project based in Kunming.

10. In 1997 a large billboard in Mengla actually advertised tours to watch Tai-Lüe women bathing. These bathing beauties were often the subject matter for picture postcards of the region.

11. See also minority tales from Yunnan in Lucien Miller's (1994) *South of the Clouds;* for stories about the Tai, see An Chunyang and Liu Bohua (1985).

12. In contrast to Taiwan, which legalized prostitution in 1988 and then outlawed it in the mid-1990s, mainland China has defined prostitution as illegal since liberation by the Communists in 1949. In more recent legal maneuvers, even second wives and lovers are being delegitimated by the state. Businessmen in the southern city of Guangzhou are being fined for having female escorts who function as business liaisons in other cities. The practice of having several wives is defined as undermining the Chinese family, which is at the heart of the Chinese "moral" state.

13. In a December 2000 report from the U.S. Embassy titled *AIDS in China: From Drugs to Blood to Sex,* Wang Yangguang of the Chinese Academy of Social Sciences Institute of Philosophy argues that neither the "strike-hard approach" nor the "red light district strategy" will be successful. He writes: "Rapid growth of China's sex industry is not simply a matter of the moral fall of women who sell themselves but the current rate of rapid economic growth, and the incredibly large buyer's market." His solution is to get two large government ministries, public health and security, involved to ensure condom use and regular medical care. However, Wang suggests this only for the women selling sex (Wang Yangguang 2000: 6). I think that since it is men who actually wear the condoms, they should also be part of the audience for these public health and security measures.

14. I take this to mean that many central government policies have a difficult time reaching all the way to China's borders with Southeast Asia. Policing a border is not unique to China, neither as a socialist country nor as a developing nation. When I lived in the town of Ornans, in the Jura Mountains bordering France and Switzerland, the border police often occupied the small bridge into town, plotting to arrest drug traffickers.

CHAPTER 5

1. Condoms are becoming more plentiful across China because of the introduction of international marketing techniques and of condom social marketing firms and chain stores (Poole 1998).

2. For a more detailed discussion of the scholarship on "sex work" and prostitution, see chapter 4.

3. There were rumors about the presence of gigolos (*mianshou*) in Jinghong. In a conversation with a Beijing businesswoman about my own experience with a harassing phone call (*saorao dianhua*), she explained that one Beijing official in Kunming received over one hundred phone solicitations from prostitutes one night at a major Kunming hotel. The official complained to the provincial tourist bureau, asking why it let this practice continue.

4. Cianna Stewart, a former outreach coordinator at the Asian Wellness Project (formerly the Asian AIDS Project), spoke to students in my course "Sexuality, Prostitution, and AIDS," about some of the prevention tactics she learned from the prostitutes working on the streets of San Francisco (June 1999).

5. The information in this section draws on several sources, including a French news agency press release on August 5, 1999, that was based on material originally printed in *China Daily,* an English-language Chinese newspaper. The other source is the article Baoying 2000.

6. The Chinese aphorism "holding up half the sky" (*banbian tian*) was a popular saying during the Maoist era. It represented the ideological commitment to promoting gender parity in Communist China. In the United States in the late 1970s, the aphorism was appropriated by liberal feminists but with the additional words "and the laundry too."

7. For additional sources and information on the eradication of STIs in 1950s and 1960s China, see M. Cohen 1996.

8. David Feingold (1998) suggests that there are high rates of trafficking in highland minority girls who come from rural villages in Southeast Asia into the seedier aspects of the Thai sex industry. I began my research in 1995 with this premise in mind, but while in Jinghong I found limited evidence for the trafficking of Tai women from Sipsongpanna into Thailand. For a discussion of how sex workers are often pawns in discussions of the epidemic in Cambodia, see Lisa Marten (2005), and for the Philippines, see Eric Ratliff (1999).

9. However, almost no accurate statistics are available on the period from 1964 to 1980, and even current statistics are suspect.

10. James Farrer (2002: 24) argues that money and foreign influence are the two bad guys of Chinese late socialism. He argues that from official points of view, AIDS is the metonymic agent of this invasion whereby money acts as the real viral carrier infecting, reproducing, and mutating into all of these new sexual perversions.

11. I want to thank Anne Williams for pointing out these concerns in her comments on an earlier version of this chapter presented at the first Yale-China Conference on Health Care in Contemporary China in June 2001.

12. The Chinese names for STIs were provided in consultation with Dr. Tong Huiqi, a psychiatrist from Shanghai working in Boston.

13. Condom manufacturers cater to a wide audience, with special attention paid to particular niche markets by using images of foreign white women as selling points for local condoms that are cheaper than actual foreign imports.

14. Beijing's Ailunsi Health Care Products Limited manufactures "strong man" condoms. In contrast to many domestically produced condoms, the package had an expiration date stamped on the box.

15. Elizabeth Miller (2002) explores how the discursive strategies of "foreign woman" and "prostitution" in containing the Japanese epidemic are closely linked to nationalist ideology in controlling and maintaining existing power relations.

16. A book of photographs circulated in the late 1980s that depicted Chinese women of all fifty-five minority groups. Han Chinese women are shown wandering around a park dressed in button-down gray and dark-blue Mao jackets; several are wearing glasses. The photograph would not be unusual except that it stands in stark contrast to the minority women, who are most often depicted in multicolored ethnic dress with big smiles on their faces.

17. My translation of a department store advertisement for "New Sexual Health Products" from Beijing's Yangtai qu fang chuang gongsi (literally, Yangtai Going to Bed Company).

18. Matthew Kohrman (1999) notes that 95 percent of men and women in China marry. Kohrman suggests that if marriage is tantamount to being a useful

and socially acceptable citizen, marriage is essential. Therefore, denying people with HIV a chance to get married has serious social consequences and marks them as polluted and, in many cases, would "out" them for their HIV status.

19. In these often illegal pseudoclinics, dipsticks measure the presence of protein levels in the urine—not a standard method for detection. If protein is present, patients are given antibiotics. However, an STI is not the only factor that can account for the presence of protein in urine.

CHAPTER 6

1. My translation of a line from a poem I found in Lijiang, Yunnan, in 1996. The author is unknown.

2. James Scott's (1976) notion of moral economy is based on his work among subsistence farmers in parts of Southeast Asia. He argues that peasants chose to keep a subsistence economy because to increase their crop yields and thus advance their livelihoods was to take unacceptable risks. These peasants' moral economy operates within an understanding that there exists a certain range of acquisition and retention of grain that must be present in order to survive.

3. Judith Farquhar (2002; Farquhar and Zhang 2005) argues that ethnographers of contemporary Chinese sexuality should consider moving away from Eurocentric interpretations according to which Chinese sexuality is perceived as following a strict lineal progression from feudalism through Maoism to emerge as something entirely new under market reforms.

4. The Aini are a smaller branch of the minority group called the Hani.

5. While these interviews were in progress, I wrote detailed notes; then, after the interviews were finished, I reclarified points with the informants. I decided a tape recorder actually prevented people from talking openly about sensitive topics. Some of the interviews were conducted over a period of time, while others were done in one day over several hours.

6. Mantinglu is a street named after a village; "Manjinglan" refers to the last remaining Tai village on the edges of Jinghong.

7. This local term means "to provide bribes," but literally, to *dianshui* is to throw droplets of water.

8. The red scarves were a symbol of Mao's young pioneers. To receive one was an important mark not only of one's scholarship but also of one's respect and pride for being Communist and Chinese.

9. For example, when I lived at a small guesthouse run by a local tobacco company, and the firm changed hands, one worker was allowed to stay on because she was a relative of the manager. Two other service workers *(fuwu yuan)* were asked to leave. One of them who had a relative in the company was therefore given a new job putting labels on bottles in their new mineral water factory in Jiangbei, but it was a job she detested compared to her old work at the guesthouse. She was the lucky one, as the other maid lost everything: with no familial connections, she was fired.

10. The concept of the iron rice bowl was instilled by Mao: under socialism everyone should always have enough to eat. Like iron, their rice bowls would never break or disintegrate *(tie fanwan)*.

11. I observed a medical worker giving a small child and then her mother an injection with the same syringe and same needle. The child looked very jaundiced. This occurred at a small clinic near the peasant's marketplace (*nongmao shichang*), a rundown area near the bus station. In this area there are lots of small private clinics that are dirty holes in the wall with a few drawers containing medicine, a white curtain that has a bed behind it for examinations, and some chairs out front for people waiting or receiving intravenous fluids (*dadiaozhen*). A Singaporean development aid doctor said that people are terribly dehydrated after working all day in the sun without drinking water, so, of course, a few cubic centimeters of glucose peps them up. But unclean needles are routes for iatrogenic infections and perhaps explain one of the reasons China has such epidemic rates of hepatitis B (thus the jaundiced child).

12. Although Sipsongpanna was once prosperous, especially in the early 1990s, the local economy as of 2002 had changed as a result of the increase in mainland Chinese who have the capital and freedom to venture outside China for vacations, or rather to travel to Sipsongpanna with agencies that are located outside the area. In the summer of 2002, the shift in the economy was noticeable: the number of state projects, such as building a bigger bridge over the Lancang, had increased, as had the visible presence of police officers and border guards, suggesting that they need to secure this border region from drug trafficking, disease, and the political instability of being so close to Laos. Laos was the third largest opium producer in the world in the late 1990s.

13. A bronze statue of Zhou Enlai wearing a Tai male headdress stands in the same park where the main Buddhist temple and school stand today in Manting Park.

14. There are a few records that document the Christian presence in Jinghong. A former German student of Tai and Mandarin found historical records including diaries and photographs in the library at MacGilvery University's Theological Union in Chiang-Mai, Thailand.

15. This building is a perfect metaphor for the historical changes to Sipsongpanna, as the structure went from being a church to a school of Mao Zedong thought and then to an abandoned building bought by a wealthy Zhejiang entrepreneur. The building is beautiful and has withstood time, as it was painstakingly built from river stones.

16. This name combines both the Tai name for the temple, *wan ba si*, with the Chinese word for Buddhist memorial, *fojiao jinian*, which puts forth the notion that it is a Buddhist tourist site for all to explore China's many minority cultures and their beliefs.

17. Susan McCarthy (2001), who conducted dissertation research on the Tai in Sipsongpanna, emphasized that in her conversations with local leaders in 1996 and 1997, they presented this period of history as somewhat elusive. In a personal communication, McCarthy noted that Dao Shi Shun had an opportunity to assume the monarchy; however, he declined in favor of another relative, Jiao Shun Xin, who was married to his niece. After the Communists took over, there was a power struggle and Jiao Shun Xin became the head of the autonomous county of Banna (*zhou zhang*) instead of being allowed to become the king (*zhaotian ling*).

EPILOGUE

1. I choose the question "What is to be done?" because it begins where I my-self began to learn Chinese as an undergraduate. In summer 1981, we read ele-mentary stories about comrade Lenin and learned the expression "what is to be done" (*zenmeban*). It seemed appropriate to bring a study of public health prac-tice and AIDS to a conclusion that takes into consideration AIDS as a devastat-ing disease that ravages much more than the individual biological body.

2. I do not mean to dismiss the fact that both Cambodia and Thailand have worked tirelessly to curb the spread of HIV/AIDS. Thailand has seen a fall in prevalence rates to 1.8 percent in 2004. As a result of condom campaigns in which the government worked closely with brothel owners, sex workers, and their clients, and by providing STI treatment, condom use has doubled to 80 percent (Bloom et al. 2004: 13).

3. There are several reasons for this demographic downsizing of the epi-demic. The Ministry of Health, in conjunction with the American Centers for Disease Control, collected data from several sources. Wider ranges of data were used, not just from high-prevalence areas. In 2005 the number of sentinel sur-veillance sites were expanded from 194 to 329, and more representative data were collected. The 2005 estimates were done at the prefectural rather than the provincial level. These new numbers are not without their critics, who claim the government is trying to cover up the extent of the epidemic and defeat its inter-national and national critics. Those on the front lines certainly do not see the epidemic slowing down. Some say that relying on prefectural-level data is highly suspect as local officials often hide the true prevalence and that those in suspect high-risk groups are not forthcoming about their HIV status, if they know it, due to stigma and discrimination. The biggest difference was the downsizing of the former commercial blood and plasma donors. One explanation is that most of those people have already died, thus leaving a smaller sample to begin with (see Yardley 2006).

4. The distribution of people living with HIV/AIDS in China at the end of 2005 is as follows: 44 percent are drug users, 19 percent are sex workers and their clients, and 17 percent are partners of HIV-positive individuals and any-one in the general population (both groups are strangely lumped under one "risk group"). The statistics in the January 2006 Ministry of Health, UNAIDS, and WHO report are biased in that they now report only 11 percent of infec-tions through blood transfusions, including the vast numbers of commercial blood and plasma donors in central China. However, since most of the people infected through blood have died, this statistic does not account for the group's high mortality rates—upwards of 50 percent, higher than any other risk cate-gory. Men who have sex with men (MSM) now account for 7 percent of all infections, and just over 1 percent are cases of mother-to-child transmission (MOH 2006: 2).

5. Youth peer education has been a popular activity among NGOs, partly because youth are an easy, accessible, and noncontroversial population with which to begin prevention education and because they are the future of China. Organizations such as Daytop operate private drug rehabilitation centers and

also provide basic care for people with HIV/AIDS who have limited resources. Christian NGOs such as World Vision and Salvation Army provide information, education, and communication materials (IEC). Other NGOs have cooperated and worked together to open centers, such as a Home AIDS Center that opened in April 2002, with funding from the Salvation Army, AusAID, and the Yunnan Red Cross. USAID began subcontracting to Family Health International for outreach to sex workers and their clients, to Futures Group for work on strengthening policies, and to Population Services International (PSI) for condom marketing research. Care International has been providing training for rural doctors since 2001. The government-sponsored NGOs (GONGOs) such as the Buddhist Association in Jinghong have been providing outreach education and materials in local languages including Sipsongpanna Tai. The Family Planning Associations have been working closely with clinics that serve women to provide IEC and care. The Central Government of the Ministry of Health plans to do large-scale voluntary counseling and testing but is having problems finding people interested. Other organizations, such as DKT International, work with the provincial family planning commission to supply quality contraceptives including condoms (Couzin 2004).

China AIDS Info, directed by Odilon Couzin (2005), has compiled a small directory of organizations working on HIV/AIDS in China. He has sorted the organizations into seven categories: people living with HIV/AIDS (PLWHA) support groups (20); NGOs, GONGOs, and other nonprofit groups (110); UN agencies and bilaterals (22); foundations and funding agencies (7); Chinese government departments and projects (15); the private sector (15); and Hong Kong, Taiwan, and Macau groups (8).

6. For more information and updates on these cases, see the website of Human Rights Watch.

7. Personal communication with Dr. Émile Fox, chief of UNAIDS in Beijing, August 8, 2000.

8. Cianna Stewart mentioned this when she gave a lecture in my Women's Studies course at the University of California, Berkeley, in June 1998.

9. Jay R. Schwartz (2000) went on a veritable sex tour in order to compile and publish a comprehensive guidebook to brothels in the state of Nevada. The note here was taken from his introduction.

10. Microbicides are gels or foams that a woman can insert into her vagina prior to sexual intercourse in order to kill viruses and bacteria (Barnett and Whiteside 2002: 330).

11. HIV/AIDS is increasingly a gendered epidemic. In parts of Africa women are overwhelmingly more infected than their male partners, and in China women are becoming a greater proportion of new infections. For this reason AIDS must be addressed as not only a health problem but as a crisis with repercussions for reproductive rights and freedoms (see Kaufman 2003). For an excellent account of sexual cultures and in particular the effects of HIV/AIDS on women, see Evelyne Micollier's (2004b) edited volume *Sexual Cultures in East Asia*.

12. I want to thank Matthew Kohrman (2005) for reminding me of this important point in his epilogue.

References

Abu-Lughod, Lila. 1991. "Writing Against Culture." In *Recapturing Anthropology: Working in the Present,* edited by R. G. Fox. Santa Fe: School of American Research Press.

———. 1993. *Writing Women's Worlds: Bedouin Stories.* Berkeley and Los Angeles: University of California Press.

Adams, Vincanne, and Stacey Leigh Pigg. 2005. *Sex in Development: Science, Sexuality, and Morality in Global Perspective.* Durham, N.C., and London: Duke University Press.

Agence France-Presse. 1999. "Sexually Transmitted Diseases Jump 37 percent in China." May 6.

———. 1999. "Chinese Bringing Prostitution to Tibet, Dharamsala Says." September 4.

Ai Feng Wang Song. 1995. *Daizu wenxue shi* [A Cultural History of the Dai]. Kunming: Yunnan Provincial Minority Press.

Ai Kham Ngeun. 2002. "Xishuangbanna: The Challenges of Cultural Survival and Preservation." Paper presented at Culture at the Crossroads: The Challenge of Preservation and Development in Sipsongpanna, Yunnan, Conference, Chiang Mai University, Chiang Mai, Thailand, July.

Aizhixing Research Group, 2006. "China Presents AIDS Prevention Policies without Using the Term *Human Rights.*" www.aizhi.net. February 6.

Allison, Anne. 1994. *Nightwork: Sexuality, Pleasure, and Corporate Masculinity in a Tokyo Hostess Club.* Chicago: University of Chicago Press.

Altman, Dennis. 2001. *Global Sex.* Chicago: University of Chicago Press.

Altman, Lawrence. 2003. "China Lags in Sharing SARS Clues, Officials Say." *New York Times,* August 5. D1, D6.

Anagnost, Ann. 1985. "Hegemony and the Improvisation of Resistance: Political Culture and Popular Practice in Contemporary China." Ph.D. dissertation, Anthropology Department, University of Michigan, Ann Arbor.

————. 1989. "Prosperity and Counterprosperity: The Moral Discourse on Wealth in Post-Mao China." In *Marxism and the Chinese Experience,* edited by A. Dirlik and M. Meisner. Armonk, N.Y.: M. E. Sharpe.

————. 1997. *National Past-Times: Narrative, Representation, and Power in Modern China.* Durham, N.C.: Duke University Press.

An Chunyang and Liu Bohua. 1985. *Where the Dai People Live.* Beijing: Foreign Languages Press.

Anderson, Benedict. 1992. *Imagined Communities: Reflections on the Origin and Spread of Nationalism.* Rev. ed. New York: Verso.

Anzaldúa, Gloria. 1999. *Borderlands = La Frontera.* 2nd ed. San Francisco: Aunt Lute Books.

Appadurai, Arjun. 1996. *Modernity at Large: Cultural Dimensions of Globalization.* Public Worlds, vol. 1. Minneapolis: University of Minnesota Press.

Aretxaga, Begoña. 2003. "Maddening States." *Annual Review of Anthropology* 32: 393–410.

Armijo-Hussein, Jacqueline. 1997. "Sayyid: 'Ajall Shams al-Din: A Muslim from Central Asia, Serving the Mongols in China and Bringing 'Civilization' to Yunnan." Ph.D. dissertation, Inner Asian Studies, Harvard University, Cambridge, Mass.

Armijo-Hussein, Jacqueline, and Allen Beesey. 1998. *Young People and Social Change in China: A Survey of Risk Factors for HIV/AIDS in Yunnan Province.* Report on the Yunnan HIV/AIDS Youth Survey conducted by the Australian Red Cross in collaboration with the Yunnan Red Cross. Kunming, China: Australian Red Cross.

Arnold, David. 1993. *Colonizing the Body: State Medicine and Epidemic Disease in Nineteenth-Century India.* Berkeley and Los Angeles: University of California Press.

Associated Press Wire. 2001. "Health Officials: Two-thirds of Chinese Have Potentially Deadly Hepatitis B." China AIDS Info, August 22, 2001. www .china-aids.org (accessed 2003).

Bao Jiemin. 1998. "Same Bed, Different Dreams: Intersections of Ethnicity, Gender, and Sexuality among Middle- and Upper-Class Immigrants in Bangkok." *Positions* 6(2): 475–502.

Baoying, Liu. 2000. "At the Convening of a Meeting of the State Council on the Prevention and Cure of STDS and AIDS, Li Lanqing Urged Every Level of Government and Its Leaders to Attach Great Importance in Working for the Prevention and Eradication of AIDS." *Renmin Ribao.* April 5.

Barnett, Tony, and Allan Whiteside. 2002. *AIDS in the Twenty-first Century: Disease and Globalization.* New York: Palgrave MacMillan.

Barth, Frederik. 1969. *Ethnic Groups and Boundaries: The Social Organization of Culture Difference.* Boston: Waveland Press.

Bayer, Richard. 1990. "AIDS and the Future of Reproductive Freedom." *Milibank Quarterly* 68, supplement (2).

Beijing Review. 1997. "Editorial on STDs and HIV/AIDS." February.

Bell, Daniel, and Gill Valentine. 1995. *Mapping Desire: Geographies of Sexualities.* New York: Routledge.

Benedict, Carol. 1996. *Bubonic Plague in Nineteenth-Century China.* Stanford, Calif.: Stanford University Press.

Berdahl, Daphne. 1999. *Where the World Ended: Re-unification and Identity in the German Borderland*. Berkeley and Los Angeles: University of California Press.

Beyrer, Chris. 1998. *The War in the Blood: Sex, Politics, and HIV/AIDS in Southeast Asia*. New York: Zed Books.

Beyrer, Chris, et al. 2000. "Overland Heroin Trafficking Routes in HIV-I Spread in South and Southeast Asia." *AIDS* 14(1): 75–83.

Biehl, João. 2001. "Technology and Affect: HIV/AIDS Testing in Brazil." *Culture, Medicine and Psychiatry* 25(1): 87–129.

———. 2005. *Vita: Life in a Zone of Social Abandonment*. Berkeley and Los Angeles: University of California Press.

Bishop, Ryan, and Lillian Robinson. 1998. *Night Market: Sexual Cultures and the Thai Economic Miracle*. New York: Routledge.

Bloom, David E., et al. 2004. *Asia's Economies and the Challenge of AIDS*. Manila, Philippines: Asia Development Bank.

Borchert, Thomas. 2005. "Of Temples and Tourists: The Effects of Tourist Political Economy on a Minority Buddhist Community in Southwest China." Paper presented at Association for Asian Studies Conference, Chicago, March 21–23.

Bourdieu, Pierre. 1977. *Outline of a Theory of Practice*. Translated by R. Nice. Cambridge: Cambridge University Press.

———. 1990. *The Logic of Practice*. Translated by R. Nice. Stanford, Calif.: Stanford University Press.

Brookes, Adam. 2001. "Bad Blood Spreads AIDS in China." *BBC News* (Beijing). May 30.

Brownell, Susan. 1995. *Training the Body for China: Sports in the Moral Order of the People's Republic*. Chicago: University of Chicago Press.

Burawoy, Michael, and Janos Lukacs. 1992. *The Radiant Past: Ideology and Reality in Hungary's Road to Capitalism*. Chicago: University of Chicago Press.

Burchell, Graham, Colin Gordon, and Peter Miller, eds. 1991. *The Foucault Effect: Studies in Governmental Rationality*. Chicago: University of Chicago Press.

Burt, Kate. August 23, 2005. "Whatever Happened to the Femidom?" *Guardian Weekly*, August 23: 14.

Butler, Judith. 1990. *Gender Trouble: Feminism and the Subversion of Identity*. New York: Routledge.

Cai Hua. 2001. *A Society without Fathers or Husbands: The Na of China*. Translated by A. Hustvedt. New York: Zone Books.

Campbell, Carole A. 1990. "Women and AIDS." *Social Science and Medicine* 30(4): 407–15.

Campbell, Catherine. 2003. *"Letting Them Die": Why HIV/AIDS Prevention Programs Fail*. Bloomington: Indiana University Press.

Canguilhem, Georges. 1991. *The Normal and the Pathological*. Translated by C. Fawcett. New York: Zone Books.

Carillo, Hector. 2002. *The Night Is Young: Sexuality in Mexico in the Time of AIDS*. Chicago: University of Chicago Press.

Castoriadis, Cornelius. 1987. *The Imaginary Institution of Society*. Cambridge, Mass.: MIT Press.

Celantano, David D., et al. 1996a. "Social Mobility, Human Sexuality and HIV in Northern Thailand." Study published in conjunction with Family Health International, AIDSCAP, USAID, National Institute of Health, the Armed Forces Research Institute in Medical Science, Bangkok, and the Henry Jackson Foundation. Bangkok.

———. 1996b. "Changes in the Sexual Behaviour and a Decline in HIV Infection among Young Men in Thailand." *New England Journal of Medicine* 395: 297–302.

Chan, John. 2001. "HIV/AIDS Epidemic in Rural China." *World Social Web Site*, 2001. www.wsws.org (accessed August 6, 2001).

Chen, Nancy. 2003. *Breathing Spaces: Qigong, Psychiatry, and Healing in China*. New York: Columbia University Press.

Chen, Robert T. 1988. *On Discussions Held between the Ministry of Public Health, the People's Republic of China, and the WHO Mission on AIDS Prevention and Control, May 17–June 2, 1988*. San Francisco: WHO Regional Office for the Western Pacific.

Chen Xiangsheng et al. 2000. "Epidemiologic Trends of Sexually Transmitted Diseases in China." *Sexually Transmitted Diseases*, March: 138–43.

Cheng Hehe et al. 1994. *HIV Infection in Yunnan Province, China, 1986–1993*. Kunming: Yunnan Provincial Health and Anti-Epidemic Center.

Cheng Hehe et al. 1996. "Yunnan sheng HIV ganran quyu xiang quansheng bosan [The Trend toward HIV Infection and Transmission throughout Yunnan Province]." *Zhongguo xingbing aizibing fangzhi* [Chinese Journal of Prevention and Control of STIs and HIV/AIDS] 2(2): 54–57.

Cheng Hehe, Zhang Jiapeng, Pan Songfeng, Jia Manhong, et al. 2000. "Yunnan aizibing ganran liuxing qushi fenxi he yuce [An Analysis and Prediction of the Trend of HIV Epidemic in Yunnan Province]." *Zhongguo xingbing aizibing fangzhi* [Chinese Journal of Prevention and Control of STDs and AIDS] 6(5): 257–60.

Cheng Sealing. 2005. "Popularizing Purity: Gender, Sexuality, and Nationalism in HIV/AIDS Prevention in South Korean Youths." *Asia Pacific Viewpoint* 46(1).

China AIDS Info. 2006. "Global Fund Round 5 China AIDS Program—Draft 2 Year Work Plan." www.china-aids.org.cn. March 22.

China Daily. 1996. "Yunnan Expands Disease Control along Borders." April 16.

Choi Kyung Hee et al. 2000. "HIV Risk among Patients Attending Sexually Transmitted Disease Clinics in China." *AIDS and Behavior* 4(1): 111–19.

———. 2003. "Emerging HIV-1 Epidemic in China in Men Who Have Sex with Men." *Lancet* 361: 2125.

Chow, Rey. 1987. "Ethnic Minorities in Chinese Films: Cinema and the Exotic." *East-West Film Journal* 1(2): 15–32.

———. 2002. *The Protestant Ethnic and the Spirit of Capitalism*. New York: Columbia University Press.

Chung, Juliette. 1999. "Struggle for National Survival: Chinese Eugenics in a Transnational Context, 1896–1945." Ph.D. dissertation, Department of History, University of Chicago.

Clifford, James, and George E. Marcus. 1986. *Writing Culture: The Poetics and Politics of Ethnography*. Berkeley and Los Angeles: University of California Press.

Cohen, Jean L., and Andrew Arato. 1992. *Civil Society and Political Theory*. Cambridge, Mass.: MIT Press.

Cohen, Lawrence. 1998. *No Aging in India: Alzheimer's, the Bad Family, and Other Modern Things*. Berkeley and Los Angeles: University of California Press.

Cohen, Myron. 2001. "HIV and Classical Sexually Transmitted Diseases: A Global Problem with Local Solutions." Paper presented at Health Care East and West: Moving into the 21st Century Conference, Boston, June 24–29.

Cohen, Myron et al. 1996. "Successful Eradication of Sexually Transmitted Diseases in the People's Republic of China: Implications for the 21st Century." *Journal of Infectious Diseases* 174 supplement (2): S223–S229.

———. 2000. "Sexually Transmitted Diseases in the People's Republic of China in Y2K: Back to the Future." *Sexually Transmitted Diseases,* March: 143–45.

Cornue, Virginia. 2003. *Sex, Tenderness, and Chinese Women*. Piscataway, N.J.: Rutgers University Press.

Couzin, Odilon. 2004. "Research on the History of AIDS NGOs in Yunnan." Unpublished report. Montreal, August 23.

———. 2005. *China HIV/AIDS Directory (Zhongguo aizibing minglu)*. Beijing: China AIDS Info.

Cowley, Geoffrey. 1996. "From Freedom to Fear: When AIDS Hits China." *Newsweek* 127(14): 49.

Dai Sijie. 2002. *Balzac and the Little Chinese Seamstress*. Edited by P. Rousselet. China/France: Seville Pictures.

Dalton, Harlon L. 1989. "AIDS in Blackface." *Daedalus* 118(3): 205–25.

Davis, Sara L. M. 1999. "Singers of Sipsongbanna: Folklore and Authenticity in Contemporary China." Ph.D. Dissertation, Asian and Middle Eastern Studies, University of Pennsylvania.

———. 2005. *Song and Silence: Ethnic Revival on China's Southwest Borders*. New York: Columbia University Press.

de Certeau, Michel. 1984. *The Practice of Everyday Life*. Translated by S. Rendall. Berkeley and Los Angeles: University of California Press.

Dean, Mitchell. 1999. *Governmentality: Power and Rule in Modern Society*. London: Sage Publications.

Dechamp, Jean-Francois, and Odilon Couzin. 2004. "International Property Rights, Generics and Access to Needed Drugs." Paper presented at the Third Asia Public Policy Workshop and Fourth W.H.R. Rivers Symposium: Social Development, Social Policy and HIV/AIDS in China, John F. Kennedy School of Government, May 6–8.

Delacosta, Frédérique, and Priscilla Alexander. 1987. *Sex Work: Writings by Women in the Sex Industry*. Pittsburgh: Cleis Press.

Deng Xian. 1990. *Zhongguo zhiqing meng* [Dreams of China's Sent-Down Youth]. Beijing: Guofang daxue chubanshe (Guofang University Press).

Di Ya, ed. 1989. *Zhongguo 1987 nian canjiren chouyang diaocha cailiao* [Data from China's 1987 Sample Survey of Disabled Persons]. Beijing: Office of the National Sample Survey of Persons with Disabilities.

Diamond, Norma. 1995. "Defining the Miao: Ming, Qing, and Contemporary Views." In *Cultural Encounters on China's Ethnic Frontiers*, edited by S. Harrell. Seattle: University of Washington Press.

Dikötter, Frank. 1992. *The Discourse on Race in Modern China.* Stanford, Calif.: Stanford University Press.

———. 1995. *Sex, Culture, and Modernity in China: Medical Science and the Construction of Sexual Identities in the Early Republican Period.* Honolulu: University of Hawaii Press.

Dodd, William Clifton. 1923. *The Tai Race: Elder Brother of the Chinese.* Cedar Rapids, Iowa: Torch.

Donzelot, Jacques. 1979. *The Policing of Families.* New York: Pantheon.

Dreyfus, Hubert L., and Paul Rabinow. 1982. *Michel Foucault: Beyond Structuralism and Hermeneutics.* Chicago: University of Chicago Press.

Du Shanshan. 2002. *Chopsticks Work in Pairs: Gender Unity and Gender Equality among the Lahu in Southwest China.* New York: Columbia University Press.

Eaton, David. 2002. "Emotion and Change in Sexual Culture: Responses to AIDS among Young Men of Congo." Ph.D. dissertation, Anthropology Department, University of California, Berkeley.

Ebron, Paulla. 2002. *Performing Africa.* Princeton, N.J.: Princeton University Press.

EChina Romance. 2001. "Sipsongbanna (Jinghong)." *Yunnan Attraction.* www.echinaromance.com.

Elias, Norbert. 1982. *The History of Manners.* The Civilizing Process, vol. 1. New York: Pantheon.

Entz, Achara, et al. 2001. "STD History, Self Treatment, and Healthcare Behaviors among Fisherman in the Gulf of Thailand and the Andaman Sea." *Sexually Transmitted Infections* 77: 436–40.

Epstein, Steven. 1996. *Impure Science: AIDS, Activism, and the Politics of Knowledge.* Berkeley and Los Angeles: University of California Press.

Erwin, Kathleen. 2000. "Heart-to-Heart, Phone-to-Phone: Family Values, Sexuality, and the Politics of Shanghai's Advice Hotlines." In *The Consumer Revolution in Urban China,* edited by Deborah S. Davis. Berkeley and Los Angeles: University of California Press.

Evans, Grant. 1996. "The Transformation of Jinghong Xishuangbanna, P.R.C." Unpublished Conference Proceedings, Department of Anthropology, Hong Kong University.

———. 2000. *Where China Meets Southeast Asia: Social and Cultural Change in the Border Regions,* edited by Grant Evans, Chris Hutton, and K. Khuneng. Singapore: ISEAS.

External Propaganda Office of Xishuangbanna Dai Autonomous Prefecture Party Committee and the Press Office of Xishuangbanna Prefecture Administration. 2003. www.xsbn.gov.cn; www.chacheng.cn.

Fabian, Johannes. 2000. *Out of Our Minds: Reason and Madness in Exploration of Central Africa.* Berkeley and Los Angeles: University of California Press.

Fairclough, Gordon. 1995. "AIDS: A Gathering Storm." *Far Eastern Economic Review* 158(38): 26–28.

Fan Zhiwei. 1990. *Xingbing fangyi shouce* [The Manual for the Prevention and Cure of STDs]. Edited by the Zhongguo renmin gongheguo weishengbu, weisheng fangyice (The People's Republic of China Ministry of Health, Health Prevention Section). Nanjing: Jiangsu kexue jishu chubanshe (Jiangsu Science and Technology Publishers).

Farmer, Paul. 1992. *AIDS and Accusation: Haiti and the Geography of Blame.* Berkeley and Los Angeles: University of California Press.

———. 1999. *Infections and Inequalities: The Modern Plague.* Berkeley and Los Angeles: University of California Press.

Farmer, Paul, and Arthur Kleinman. 1989. "AIDS as Human Suffering." *Daedalus* 118(2): 135–60.

Farmer, Paul, Margaret Connors, and Janie Simmons, eds. 1996. *Women, Poverty, and AIDS: Sex, Drugs, and Structural Violence.* Monroe, Maine: Common Courage Press.

Farquhar, Judith. 1991. "Objects, Processes, and Female Infertility in Chinese Medicine." *Medical Anthropology Quarterly* 5(4): 370–99.

———. 1994. *Knowing Practice: The Clinical Encounter of Chinese Medicine.* Boulder, Colo.: Westview Press.

———. 2002. *Appetites: Food and Sex in Post-Socialist China.* Durham, N.C.: Duke University Press.

Farquhar, Judith, and Zhang Qicheng. 2005. "Biopolitical Beijing: Pleasure, Sovereignty, and Self-Cultivation in China's Capital." *Cultural Anthropology* 20(3): 303–27.

Farrer, James. 2002. *Opening Up: Youth Sex Culture and Market Reform in Shanghai.* Chicago: University of Chicago Press.

Fee, Elizabeth, and Daniel Fox. 1988. *AIDS: The Burden of History.* Berkeley and Los Angeles: University of California Press.

———. 1992. *AIDS: The Making of a Chronic Disease.* Berkeley and Los Angeles: University of California Press.

Fei Xiaotong. 1980. "Ethnic Identification in China." *Social Science in China* 1: 94–107.

Feingold, David. 1998. "Sex, Drugs and the IMF: Some Implications of Structural Readjustment for the Trade in Heroin, Girls, and Women in the Upper Mekong Region." In "The New Cargo: The Global Business of Trafficking in Women." Special issue, *Refuge* 17 (November).

Feng Zhang. 2004. "Blood Reserve Growing in Quality, Quantity." *China Daily,* September 15.

Ferguson, James. 1996. *The Anti-Politics Machine.* 3rd ed. Minneapolis: University of Minnesota Press.

Fisher, William. 1997. "Doing Good? The Politics and Antipolitics of NGO Practices." *Annual Review of Anthropology* 26: 439–64.

Foreign Broadcast Information Service. June 10, 1992. "705 Cases of HIV-Infected Persons Discovered." Zhongguo Xinwen (China News Service), 22–23.

———. 1992. "Health Officials Report 968 AIDS Cases." *Xinhua,* December: 92–232.

———. 1999. American Associated Press Wire. *Qingnian Bao* [*Youth Daily*], April 18.

———. April 19, 2000. "Beijing Cracks Down on Prostitution, Gambling and Drug Trafficking." Xinhua (New China News Agency).

Foucault, Michel. 1977. *Discipline and Punish: The Birth of the Prison.* Translated by A. Sheridan. New York: Vintage.

———. 1980. *History of Sexuality.* Vol. 1: *An Introduction.* Translated by R. Hurley. New York: Vintage Books.

———. 1991. "Governmentality." In *The Foucault Effect: Studies in Governmental Rationality,* edited by G. Burchell, C. Gordon, and P. Miller. Chicago: University of Chicago Press.

———. 1997. *The Essential Works of Foucault, 1954–1984.* Translated by Robert Hurley et al. New York: New Press.

Fox, Émile. 1996. "Background, History and Present Situation of HIV/AIDS in the People's Republic of China." Newsletter, UNAIDS Country Programme Advisor, Beijing, China. April.

Frankenberg, Ronald. 1993. "Risk: Anthropological and Epidemiological Narratives of Prevention." In *Knowledge, Power, and Practice,* edited by Shirley Lindenbaum and Margaret Lock. Berkeley and Los Angeles: University of California Press.

Gao Ming. 2004. "Hennan aizi diaocha tanfang youren louwang youren jiamao [A Henan Survey Reveals That People Are Hiding from Getting Tested and Others Are Passing Themselves Off as Having AIDS]." *Xinjing Bao,* November 15.

Gao Yaojie. 2005. *Zhongguo aizibing diaocha* [The Investigation of AIDS in China]. Guilin: Guangxi shifan daxue chubanshe (Guangxi Normal University Press).

Geertz, Clifford. 1977. *The Interpretation of Cultures.* New York: Basic Books.

Gil, Vincent. 1993. "Sexual Culture and HIV/AIDS in the People's Republic of China." Paper presented at the 92nd annual meeting of the American Anthropology Association, Washington, D.C, November 17–21.

Giles, John, Albert Park, and Juwei Zhang. 2005. "What Is China's Unemployment Rate?" *China Economic Review* 16(2): 149–70.

Gilman, Sander L. 1988a. *Disease and Representation: Images of Illness from Madness to AIDS.* Ithaca, N.Y.: Cornell University Press.

———. 1988b. "AIDS and Syphilis: The Iconography of Disease." In *AIDS: Cultural Analysis Cultural Activism,* edited by Douglas Crimp. Cambridge, Mass.: MIT Press.

Gilmartin, Christina. 1994. *Engendering China: Women, Culture, and the State.* Harvard Contemporary China Series 10. Cambridge, Mass.: Harvard University Press.

Gladney, Dru C. 1991. *Muslim Chinese: Ethnic Nationalities in the People's Republic.* Cambridge, Mass.: Harvard University Press.

———. 1994. "Representing Nationality in China: Refiguring Majority/Minority Identities." *Journal of Asian Studies* 53(11): 92–123.

———. 2002. "Internal Colonialism and the Uyghur Nationality: Chinese Nationalism and Its Subaltern Subjects." *Cemoti: Cahiers d'Etudes sur la Mediterranee Orientale et le Monde Turco-Iranien* 35 (La Question de l'enchantement en Asie Centrale).

Good, Mary-Jo DelVecchio. 1995. "Cultural Studies of Biomedicine: An Agenda for Research." *Social Science and Medicine* 41(4): 461–73.

———. 2001. "Biotechnical Embrace." *Culture, Medicine and Psychiatry* 25(4): 395–410.

Goodman, David S. G. 1983. "Guizhou and the PRC: The Development of an Internal Colony." In *Internal Colonialism: Essays around a Theme*, edited by D. Drakakis-Smith. Edinburgh: Developing Areas Research Group, Institute of British Geographers.

Gorman, Michael. 1986. "The AIDS Epidemic in San Francisco: Epidemiological and Anthropological Perspectives." In *Anthropology and Epidemiology: Interdisciplinary Approaches to the Study of Health and Disease*, edited by C. R. Jones et al. Boston: Norwell.

Gould, Stephen Jay. 1996. *The Mismeasure of Man*. 2nd ed. New York: W. W. Norton.

Greenhalgh, Susan. 1994. "Controlling Births and Bodies in Village China." *American Ethnologist* 21(1): 3–20.

———. 2005. "Globalization and Population Governance in China." In *Global Assemblages: Technology, Politics, and Ethics as Anthropological Problems*, edited by Aihwa Ong and Stephen J. Collier. Oxford: Blackwell.

Gregory, Steven. 2003. "Men in Paradise: Sex Tourism and the Political Economy of Masculinity." In *Race, Nature, and the Politics of Difference*, edited by M. Donald, J. Kosek, and A. Padian. Durham, N.C.: Duke University Press.

Guldin, Greg Eliyu. 1994. *The Saga of Anthropology in China: From Malinowski to Moscow to Mao*. Armonk, N.Y.: M. E. Sharpe.

Gupta, Akhil. 1995. "Blurred Boundaries: The Discourse of Corruption, the Culture of Politics, and the Imagined State." *American Ethnologist* 2: 375–402.

Gupta, Akhil, and James Ferguson. 1992. "Beyond 'Culture': Space, Identity, and the Politics of Difference. *Cultural Anthropology* 7(1): 6–23.

———, eds. 1997. *Culture, Power, Place: Explorations in Critical Anthropology*. Durham, N.C.: Duke University Press.

Hacking, Ian. 1986. "The Archaeology of Foucault." In *Foucault: A Critical Reader*, edited by David Hoy. Cambridge: Cambridge University Press.

———. 1990. *The Taming of Chance*. Cambridge: Cambridge University Press.

Hall, Stuart. 1992. "Cultural Studies and Its Theoretical Legacies." In *Cultural Studies*, edited by L. Grossberg, C. Nelson, and P. Treichler. New York: Routledge.

Hammonds, Evelyn. 1987. "Race, Sex and AIDS: the Construction of 'Other.'" *Radical America* 20(6): 28–36.

Hansen, Metta Halskov. 1999. *Lessons in Being Chinese*. Seattle: University of Washington Press.

Hansen, Thomas Blom, and Finn Stepputat. 2001. *States of Imagination: Ethnographic Explorations of the Postcolonial State*. Durham, N.C.: Duke University Press.

Harrell, Stevan. 1990. "Ethnicity, Local Interests, and the State: Yi Communities in Southwest China." *Comparative Studies in Society and History* 32(3): 515–48.

———. 1991. "Anthropology and Ethnology in the PRC: The Intersection of Discourses." *China Exchange News* 19(2): 3–6.

————. 1995. "Introduction: Civilizing Projects and the Reaction to Them." In *Cultural Encounters on China's Ethnic Frontiers,* edited by S. Harrell. Seattle: University of Washington Press.

Harrell, Stevan (ed.). 1995. *Cultural Encounters on China's Ethnic Frontiers.* Seattle: University of Washington Press.

Hart, Angie. 1998. *Buying and Selling Power: Anthropological Reflections on Prostitution in Spain.* Boulder, Colo.: Westview Press.

He Zuoshun et al. 2000. "Yunnan sheng yijunren aizibing zhishi de xianshi diaocha [A Survey of the General Population's Knowledge about HIV/AIDS in Yunnan]." *Xiandai yufang yizhi* [Modern Preventative Medicine] 1(27): 512–14.

Henderson, Gail, and Myron Cohen. 1984. *The Chinese Hospital: A Socialist Work Unit.* New Haven, Conn.: Yale University Press.

Henriot, Christian. 1992. "Medicine, VD and Prostitution in Pre-Revolutionary China." *Social History of Medicine* 5: 95–120.

————. 2001. *Prostitution and Sexuality in Shanghai: A Social History, 1849–1949.* Cambridge: Cambridge University Press.

Herbert, Daniel, and Richard Parker, ed. 1993. *Sexuality, Politics and AIDS in Brazil: In Another World?* London: Falmer Press.

Herdt, Gilbert, and Shirley Lindenbaum. 1992. *The Time of AIDS: Social Analysis, Theory and Method.* Newbury Park, Calif.: Sage Publications.

Hershatter, Gail. 1997. *Dangerous Pleasures: Prostitution and Modernity in Twentieth-Century Shanghai.* Berkeley and Los Angeles: University of California Press.

————. 2005. "State of the Field: Women in China's Long Twentieth Century." *The Journal of Asian Studies* 63(4): 991–1065.

Hershatter, Gail, et al. 1996. *Remapping China: Fissures in Historical Terrain.* Stanford, Calif.: Stanford University Press.

Hinsch, Bret. 1990. *Passions of the Cut Sleeve: The Male Homosexual Tradition in China.* Berkeley and Los Angeles: University of California Press.

Holder, Chauna. 1995. "China's Newest Problem: AIDS." Unpublished position paper, DePauw University China Program.

Hong Kong Department of Health: Advisory Council on AIDS. 1996. "Gongchuang xin xiwang [Building New Hope Together]." Paper read at Xianggang aizibing huiyi (The [First] Hong Kong AIDS Conference), Hong Kong, November 8–9.

Honig, Emily. 1992. *Creating Chinese Ethnicity: Subei People in Shanghai 1850–1980.* New Haven, Conn.: Yale University Press.

Hood, Johanna. 2005. "Narrating HIV/AIDS in the PRC Media: Imagined Immunity, Distracting Others, and the Configuration of Race, Place and Disease." Master's thesis, School of Asian and Pacific Studies, Australia National University, Canberra.

Hsieh Shih-chung. 1995. "On the Dynamics of Tai/Dai-Lüe Ethnicity: An Ethnohistorical Analysis." In *Cultural Encounters on China's Ethnic Frontiers,* edited by S. Harrell. Seattle: University of Washington Press.

Huang Yingying et al. 2004. "HIV/AIDS Risk among Brothel-Based Female Sex Workers in China: Assessing the Terms, Content, and Knowledge of Sex

Work." *American Sexually Transmitted Diseases Association* 33(11): 695–700.

Human Rights Watch. 2005. *World Report: Country Report on China and Tibet*. New York: Human Rights Watch.

Hunter, Susan. 2005. *AIDS in Asia: A Continent in Peril*. New York: Palgrave MacMillan.

Hussein, Nagib. 1996. *AIDS in Asia Newsletter*. New York: World Bank. June.

Hyde, Sandra Teresa. 1999. "Sex, Drugs and Karaoke: Making HIV/AIDS in Southwest China." Ph.D. dissertation, Anthropology Department, University of California, Berkeley.

———. 2000. "Selling Sex and Sidestepping the State: Prostitutes, Condoms, and HIV/AIDS Prevention in Southwest China." *East Asia: An International Quarterly* 18(4): 108–36.

———. 2001. "Sex Tourism Practices on the Periphery: Eroticizing Ethnicity and Pathologizing Sex on the Lancang." In *Ethnographies of the Urban in 1990s China*, edited by N. Chen, C. Clark, S. Gottschang, and L. Jeffery. Durham, N.C.: Duke University Press.

———. 2002. "The Cultural Politics of HIV/AIDS and the Chinese State in Late-Twentieth Century Yunnan." *Tsantsa* [The Review of the Swiss Society of Ethnology] 7: 56–65.

———. 2003. "When Riding a Tiger It Is Difficult to Dismount: STIs and HIV/AIDS in Contemporary China." *Yale China Health Journal* 2(2): 72–82.

———. 2004. "Eating Spring Rice: Transactional Sex in the Age of Epidemics." *Harvard China Review*, Spring.

James, Clifford, and George E. Marcus. 1986. *Writing Culture*. Berkeley and Los Angeles: University of California Press.

Jeffrey, Leslie Ann. 2002. *Sex and Borders: Gender, National Identity, and Prostitution Policy in Thailand*. Vancouver: University of British Columbia Press.

Jeffreys, Elaine. 1997. "'Dangerous Amusements': Prostitution and Karaoke Halls in Contemporary China." *Asian Studies Review* 20(3): 43–54.

———. 2004. "China, Sex and Prostitution." In *Routledge Curzon Studies on China in Transition*, edited by D. S. G. Goodman. New York and London: Routledge Curzon.

Jia Manhong et al. 2003. "Yunnansheng shoulun jingmaixidu renqun aizibing ganran xingwei jiance jieguo fenxi [Data Analysis of the First Pools of AIDS Transmission through Intravenous Drug Users in Yunnan]." *Jibing jiance* [Disease Monitoring] 18(7): 249–52.

Jing Jun. 1996. *The Temple of My Memories: History, Power, and Morality in a Chinese Village*. Stanford, Calif.: Stanford University Press.

———. 2004. "Fear and Stigma: An Exploratory Study of AIDS Patient Narratives in China." Paper presented at the Third Asia Public Policy Workshop and Fourth W. H. R. Rivers Symposium: Social Development, Social Policy and HIV/AIDS in China, John F. Kennedy School of Government, Harvard University.

Jinghong Publicity Department (Jinghong shiwei xuanchuanbu). 2005. *Renkou minzu* [Ethnic Group Population]. Zhongguo Yunnansheng Jinghong shi-

zhengfu (Yunnan, China: Jinghong City Government), 2002. www.jhs.gov
.cn/jhgk/jhgk-02.shtm (accessed August 9, 2005).

Kaufman, Joan. 2003. "Reproductive Health Policy and Programs in China:
Opportunities for Responding to China's AIDS Epidemic." *Yale China
Health Journal* 2(2): 83–94.

———. 2005. "China and AIDS: Epidemic Update and Public Policy Responses." Paper presented at the Rising Peril of HIV/AIDS in China: Sex
Workers, Human Rights and the Challenges Facing Public Policy Conference, Luce Lecture Series, Skidmore College, Saratoga Springs, N.Y. March
24.

Kaufman, Joan, Anthony Saich, and Arthur Kleinman. 2004. "Social Policy and
HIV/AIDS in China." Paper presented at the Third Asia Public Policy Work-
shop and Fourth W. H. R. Rivers Symposium: Social Development, Social
Policy, and HIV/AIDS in China, John F. Kennedy School of Government,
Harvard University. May 6–8.

Kaufman, Joan, and Jing Jun. 2002. "China and AIDS—The Time to Act Is
Now." *Science* 296: 2339–40.

Kempadoo, Kamala, and Jo Doezema. 1998. *Global Sex Workers: Rights, Resistance, and Redefinition*. New York: Routledge.

Keyes, Charles. 1996. "Who Are the Dai-Lüe?" Paper presented at the Tai Studies Conference, Chiang Mai, Thailand.

King, Anthony. 1996. "Introduction: Cities, Texts and Paradigms." In *Representing the City: Ethnicity, Capital and Culture in the 21st-Century Me-
tropolis,* edited by A. King. New York: New York University Press.

Kipnis, Andrew B. 1997. *Producing Guanxi: Sentiment, Self, and Subculture in
a Northern China Village.* Durham, N.C.: Duke University Press.

Kleinman, Arthur. 1986. *Social Origins of Distress and Disease: Depression,
Neurasthenia, and Pain in Modern China.* New Haven, Conn.: Yale University Press.

———. 1994. "How Bodies Remember: Social Memory and Bodily Experience
of Criticism, Resistance, and Delegitimation following China's Cultural Revolution." *New Literary History* 25(3): 707–23.

Kleinman, Arthur, and James L. Watson, 2006. *SARS in China: A Prelude to
Pandemic?* Stanford, Calif.: Stanford University Press.

Kleinman, Arthur, Veena Das, and Margaret Lock, eds. 1997. *Social Suffering.*
Berkeley and Los Angeles: University of California Press.

Kohrman, Matthew. 1999. "Grooming *Quezi:* Marriage Exclusion and Identity
Formation among Disabled Men in Contemporary China." *American Ethnologist* 24(4): 890–909.

———. 2005. *Bodies of Difference: Experiences of Disabilities and Institutional Advocacy in the Making of Modern China.* Berkeley and Los Angeles:
University of California Press.

Krieger, Nancy. 1987. "The Epidemiology of AIDS in Africa." *Science for the
People* (January–February): 18–21.

Krieger, Nancy, and Rose Appleman. 1986. *The Politics of AIDS.* Oakland,
Calif.: Frontline.

Kristof, Nicolas, and Wudunn Sheryl. 1994. *China Wakes—The Struggle for the
Soul of Rising Power.* New York: Times Books.

Law, Lisa. 2000. *Sex Work in Southeast Asia: The Place of Desire in a Time of AIDS*. London: Routledge.

Lee Ching Kwan. 1998. *Gender and the South China Miracle: Two Worlds of Factory Women*. Berkeley and Los Angeles: University of California Press.

Lee, Stella. 2003. "Border Bolsters to Counter Rise in Illegal Sex Workers." *South China Morning Post*, January 25: 4.

Li Dexi. 1999. *Zhongguo minzu tongji nianlan* [China's Statistical Yearbook]. Beijing: Minzu chubanshe (Ethnic Publishing House).

———. 2003. *Zhongguo minzu gongzuo nianjin* [China's Yearbook of Ethnic Works]. Beijing: Zhongguo minzu gongzuo nianjin bianji weiyuanhui (Editorial Committee of China's Yearbook of Ethnic Works).

Li Hong et al. 2001. "Yunnansheng yufang kongzhi muying chuizhi chuanbo aizibingdu de yanjiu (Study of the Prevention of HIV Transmission from Mother to Child in Yunnan)." *Modern Preventive Medicine* 28(1): 68.

Li, Virginia, et al. 1992. "AIDS and Sexual Practices, Knowledge, Attitudes, Behaviors and Practices in China." *AIDS Education and Prevention*. 4(1): 1–5.

Li Xuezhong. 1996. *Yunnan gonganzhi* [Yunnan Public Security Gazette]. Kunming: Yunnan People's Publishing House.

Liao Susu et al. 1997. "Extremely Low Awareness of AIDS, Sexually Transmitted Diseases, and Condoms among Dai Ethnic Villagers in Yunnan Province, China." *AIDS*, September 11, supplement (1): S27–S34.

Lindquist, Johan. 2005. "Organizing AIDS in the Borderless World: A Case Study from the Indonesia-Malaysia-Singapore Growth Triangle." *Asia Pacific Viewpoint* 46(1): 49–63.

Ling, L. H. M. 1999. "Sex Machine: Global Hypermasculinity and Images of Asian Women in Modernity." *Positions* 7(2): 277–306.

Litzinger, Ralph. 1998. "Memory Work: Reconstitutions of the Ethnic in Post-Mao China." *Cultural Anthropology* 132: 224–55.

———. 2000a. *Other Chinas: The Yao and the Politics of National Belonging*. Durham, N.C.: Duke University Press.

———. 2000b. "Questions of Gender: Ethnic Minority Representation in Post-Mao China." *Bulletin of Concerned Asian Scholars* 32(4): 3–14.

Liu Baoying. 2000. "Li Lanqing zai guowuyuan zhaokai de fangzhi aizibing xingbing bandahui shang qiangdiao geji zhengfu he lingdao yao gaodu zhongshi aizibing yu kongzhi gongzuo [At the Convening Meeting of the State Council on the Prevention and Cure of STDs and AIDS, Li Lanqing Urged Every Level of Government and Its Leaders to Attach Great Importance in Working for the Prevention and Eradication of AIDS]." *Renmin Ribao*. April 5.

Liu Dajing. 2004. "*Wozhou lüyouye maishang xin taijie* [Tourism in Xishuangbanna Has Moved Forward to a New Level]." *Xishuangbanna Bao*. December 28.

Liu Xin. 2000. *In One's Own Shadow: An Ethnographic Account of the Condition of Post-reform Rural China*. Berkeley and Los Angeles: University of California Press.

Lufkin, Felicity. 1990. "Images of Minorities in the Art of People's Republic of China." Master's thesis, Department of East Asian Studies, University of California, Berkeley.

Lyttleton, Chris. 2000. *Endangered Relations: Negotiating Sex and AIDS in Thailand*. Amsterdam: Harwood Academic.

Lyttleton, Chris, and Amorntip Amarapibal. 2002. "Sister Cities and Easy Passage: HIV, Mobility and Economies of Desire in a Thai/Lao Border Zone." *Social Science and Medicine* 54: 505–18.

MacCannell, Donald. 1973. "Staged Authenticity: Arrangements of Social Space in Tourist Settings." *American Journal of Sociology* 79(3): 589–603.

MacPherson, Kerrie L. 1987. *A Wilderness of Marshes: The Origins of Public Health in Shanghai, 1843–1893*. Oxford: Oxford University Press.

Madsen, Richard. 1998. *China's Catholics: Tragedy and Hope in an Emerging Civil Society*. Berkeley and Los Angeles: University of California Press.

Malkki, Liisa. 1995. *Purity and Exile: Violence, Memory, and National Cosmology among Hutu Refugees in Tanzania*. Chicago: University of Chicago Press.

Manderson, Leonore, and Margaret Jolly. 1997. *Sites of Desire: Economies of Pleasure: Sexualities in Asia and the Pacific*. Chicago: University of Chicago Press.

Mann, Jonathan. 1992. "AIDS, the 2nd Decade: A Global Perspective." *Journal of Infectious Diseases* 165(2): 245–50.

Marcus, George E., and Michael Fischer, M.J. 1986. *Anthropology as Cultural Critique: An Experimental Moment in the Human Sciences*. Chicago: University of Chicago Press.

Margraf, Josef. 1999. "Guanzhu Xishuangbanna de shengwu yu wenhua duoyangxing" (GTZ Project Concerning Biological and Cultural Diversity in Xishuangbanna). In *Zhongguo shengwujuan chuliang* (China's Biosphere Reserves), translated by Yang Zhengbin. China: Editorial Division of China's Biosphere Reserves.

Marten, Lisa. 2005. "Commercial Sex Workers: Victims, Vectors, or Fighters of the HIV Epidemic in Cambodia." *Asia Pacific Viewpoint* 46(1): 21–34.

McCarthy, Susan Kathleen. 2001. "Whose Autonomy Is It Anyway? Minority Cultural Politics and National Identity in PRC." Ph.D. dissertation, Political Science Department, University of California, Berkeley.

McClintock, Anne. 1995. *Imperial Leather: Race, Gender and Sexuality in the Colonial Contest*. New York: Routledge.

McClintock, Anne (ed.). 1993. "A Special Issue on Sex Work and Sex Workers." *Social Text* (Winter): 1–83.

McKhann, Charles F. 1995. "The *Naxi* and the Nationalities Question." In *Cultural Encounters on China's Ethnic Frontiers*, edited by S. Harrell. Seattle: University of Washington Press.

Micollier, Evelyn. 2004a. "The Social Significance of Commercial Sex Work in China: Implicitly Shaping a Sexual Culture?" In *Sexual Culture in East Asia: Social Construction of Sexuality and Sexual Risk in a Time of AIDS*, edited by E. Micollier. London and New York: Routledge Curzon.

———. 2004b. *Sexual Culture in East Asia: Social Construction of Sexuality and Sexual Risk in a Time of AIDS*. London and New York: Routledge Curzon.

Miller, Elizabeth. 2002. "What's in a Condom? HIV and Sexual Politics in Japan." *Culture, Medicine and Psychiatry* 26(1): 1–32.

Miller, Lucien. 1994. *South of the Clouds: Tales from Yunnan*. Translated by G. Xu, L. Miller, and X. Kun. Seattle: University of Washington Press.

Min, Anchee. 1997. *Red Azalea*. New York: Pantheon Books.

Ming, Kevin D. 2005. "Cross-border 'Traffic': Stories of Dangerous Victims, Pure Whores, and HIV/AIDS in the Experiences of Mainland Female Sex Workers in Hong Kong." *Asia Pacific Viewpoint* 46(1): 35–48.

Ministry of Health, Joint United Nations Programme on HIV/AIDS, and World Health Organization. 2006. "2005 Update on the HIV/AIDS Epidemic and Response in China." Beijing: National Center for AIDS/STD Prevention and Control. January 24.

Mitchell, Timothy. 2002. *Rule of Experts: Egypt, Techno-Politics, Modernity*. Berkeley and Los Angeles: University of California Press.

MOH. *See* Ministry of Health, Joint United Nations Programme on HIV/AIDS, and World Health Organization.

Moore, Lisa Jean. 1998. "The Variability of Safer Sex Messages: What Do the CDC, Sex Manuals and Sex Workers Do When They Produce Safer Sex?" In *Prostitution: On Whores, Hustlers, and Johns Amherst*, edited by J. Elias, V. L. Bullough, V. Elias, and G. Brewer. New York: Prometheus Books.

Mueggler, Erik. 2001. *The Age of Wild Ghosts: Memory, Violence, and Place in Southwest China*. Berkeley and Los Angeles: University of California Press.

Nader, Laura. 1997. "Controlling Processes: Tracing the Dynamic Components of Power." *Current Anthropology* 38 (December 5).

National Bureau of Statistics of China. 2005. "2004 Nian Zhongguo nongcun pinkun zhuang jiance gongbao [2004 Report on the Poverty Level among Rural Villages in China]." China Statistical Information Network. www.stats.gov.cn.

Nee, Victor. 1992. "Organizational Dynamics of Market Transition: Hybrid Forms, Property Rights, and Mixed Economy in China." *Administrative Science Quarterly* 37: 1–27.

Nguyen, Vinh-Kim. 2001. "Epidemics, Interzones, and Biosocial Change: Retroviruses and Biologies of Globalization in West Africa." Ph.D. dissertation, Department of Anthropology, McGill University, Montreal.

———. 2005. "Antiretroviral Globalism: Biopolitics and Therapeutic Citizenship." In *Global Assemblages: Technology, Politics, and Ethics as Anthropological Problems*, edited by Aihwa Ong and Stephen J. Collier. Oxford: Blackwell.

Nie Jingbao. 2005. *Behind the Scenes: Chinese Voices on Abortion*. Lanham, Md.: Rowman and Littlefield.

O'Rouke, Dennis. 1994. *The Good Woman of Bangkok* (film). O'Rouke and Associates Filmmakers, Australia.

Oakes, Tim. 1995. "Tourism in Guizhou: The Legacy of Internal Colonialism." In *Tourism in China: Geographical, Political and Economic Perspectives*, edited by A. A. Lew and L. Yu. Boulder, Colo.: Westview Press.

———. 1998. *Tourism and Modernity in China*. New York: Routledge.

———. 1999. "Bating in the Far Village: Globalization, Transnational Capital, and the Cultural Politics of Modernity in China." *Positions* 7(2): 307–42.

Odzer, Cleo. 1994. *The Patpong Sisters: An American Woman's View of the Bangkok Sex World*. New York: Blue Moon Books, Arcade Publishing.

Office of the State Council Working Committee on AIDS, China. 2005. *Report on Progress on Implementing UNGASS Declaration of Commitment in China 2005*. December.

Ong, Aihwa, and Don Nonini (eds.). 1997. *Ungrounded Empires: The Cultural Politics of Modern Chinese Transnationalism*. New York: Routledge.

Ortner, Sherry. 1974. "Is Female to Male as Nature Is to Culture?" In *Women, Culture and Society*, edited by M. Z. Rosaldo and L. Lamphere. Stanford, Calif.: Stanford University Press.

Packard, Randall M., and Paul Epstein. 1991. "Epidemiologists, Social Scientists, and the Structure of Medical Research on AIDS in Africa." *Social Science and Medicine* 33(7): 771–94.

Pan Suiming. 1992. "Decipher the Myth of Prostitution." *Shanghai Shehui* (April 20): 55–56.

———. 1999. *Cunzai yu huangmiu: Zhongguo dixia xingchanye kaocha* [Existing in Falsehoods: An Investigation of China's Underground Sex Industry]. Beijing: Qunyan.

———. 2000. "Zhongguo xing chanye: Wo zhi zhisuo yu suoxiang [China's Sex Industry: What I Know and Think]." Paper presented at Shehui kexue yu Zhongguo xingbing aizibing fangzhi gongzuo yantaohui (Social Science for STI and HIV/AIDS Prevention and Care in China Symposium), Beijing.

Pandolfi, Mariella. 2003. "Contract of Mutual (In)difference: Governance and Humanitarian Apparatus in Albania and Kosovo." *Indiana Journal of Global Legal Studies* 10(1): 369–81.

Parish, William L. and Pan Suiming. 2004. "Sexual Partners in China: Risk Patterns for Infection by HIV and Possible Infections." Paper presented at the Third Asia Public Policy Workshop and Fourth W.H.R. Rivers Symposium: Social Development, Social Policy and HIV/AIDS in China, at John F. Kennedy School of Government, Harvard University.

Parish, William L., et al. 2002. "The Resurgent Epidemic of STDs in China: A Population-Based Study of Behavioral and Demographic Correlates and Implications for Public Health Policy." Paper presented at the Third Asia Public Policy Workshop and Fourth W. H. R. Rivers Symposium: Social Development, Social Policy and HIV/AIDS in China, John F. Kennedy School of Government, Harvard University, May 6–8.

Park, Alice. 2003. "China's Secret Plague." *Time Magazine*, December 15: 54–58, 60, 62.

Parker, Andrew, et al., eds. 1993. *Nationalisms and Sexualities*. New York: Routledge.

Parker, Richard. October 2001. "Sexuality, Culture and Power in HIV/AIDS Research." *Annual Review of Anthropology* 30: 163–79.

Parker, Richard, and Daniel Herbert. 1993. *Sexuality, Politics and AIDS in Brazil*. London: Falmer Press.

Patton, Cindy. 1990. *Inventing AIDS*. New York: Routledge.

———. 1996. *Fatal Advice: How Safe-Sex Education Went Wrong*. Durham, N.C.: Duke University Press.

————. 2002. *Globalizing AIDS*. Minneapolis: University of Minnesota Press.

Petryna, Adriana. 2002. *Life Exposed: Biological Citizens after Chernobyl.* Princeton, N.J.: Princeton University Press.

Pigg, Stacey Leigh. 2001. "Languages of Sex and AIDS in Nepal: Notes on the Social Production of Commensurability." *Cultural Anthropology* 16(4): 481–541.

————. 2002. "Expecting the Epidemic: A Social History of the Representation of Sexual Risk in Nepal." In "Women, AIDS, and Globalization," edited by Cindy Patton and Meredith Raimondo. Special issue, *Feminist Media Studies* 20(1): 97–125.

Piper, Nicola, and Brenda S. A. Yeoh. 2005. "Introduction: Meeting the Challenges of HIV/AIDS in Southeast and East Asia." *Asia Pacific Viewpoint* 46(1): 1–5.

Poole, Teresa. 1998. "China Starts Chain of Condom Shops: World's Largest Manufacturer Moves in to Spur Sales." *San Francisco Examiner*, Sunday, March 29.

Porter, Doug. 1995. "Wheeling and Dealing: HIV/AIDS and Development in Eastern Shan State Myanmar." In *UNDP HIV and Development Issue Papers*. New York: United Nations Development Program.

————. 1997. "A Plague on the Borders: HIV, Development, and Traveling Identities in the Golden Triangle." In *Sites of Desire, Economies of Pleasure: Sexualities in Asia and the Pacific,* edited by L. Manderson and M. Jolly. Chicago: University of Chicago Press.

Qin Hongping. 1995. "Lizu shiji, jiakuai fazhan Xishuangbanna lüyoushiye [Taking Advantage of the Present Situation to Revitalize Xishuangbanna's Tourism Industry]." *Xueshu lunwen ji* [A Collection of Research Papers from Xishuangbanna Education College]. Combined issues 2 & 3: 71–73.

Ratliff, Eric A. 1999. "Women as 'Sex Workers,' Men as 'Boyfriends': Shifting Identities in Philippine Go-go Bars and Their Significance in STD/AIDS Control." *Anthropology and Medicine* 6(1): 79–101.

Remick, Elizabeth Justine. 2003. "Prostitution Taxes and Local State-Building in Republican China." *Modern China* 29(1): 38–70.

————. 2004. *Building Local States: China during the Republican and Post-Mao Era.* Cambridge, Mass.: Harvard University Press.

Ren Hai. 1998. "The Displacement and Museum Representation of Aboriginal Cultures in Taiwan." *Positions* 6(2): 323–44.

————. 2005. "Consuming Ethnic Culture and the Formation of the Chinese Middle Class." Paper presented at Association for Asian Studies Annual Meeting, Chicago, March 7.

Renmin Ribao. 2000. Press release on "AIDS cases in China." Originally from a translation of an article in *Renmin Ribao,* French Press Agency.

Reuters. 2005. "China Could Have 10 Million HIV Cases by 2010." October 24.

Ries, Nancy. 1997. *Russian Talk: Culture and Conversation during Perestroika.* Ithaca, N.Y.: Cornell University Press.

Rofel, Lisa. 1992. "Rethinking Modernity: Space and Factory Discipline in China." *Cultural Anthropology* 7(1): 93–114.

————. 1999. *Other Modernities: Gendered Yearnings in China after Socialism.* Berkeley and Los Angeles: University of California Press.

Rose, Nicolas. 1999. *Governing the Soul: The Shaping of the Private Self.* 2nd ed. London: Free Association Books.

Rosenthal, Elizabeth. 2000. "In Rural China, a Steep Price of Poverty: Dying of AIDS." *New York Times,* October 28.

Ruan Fangyu. 1991. *Sex in China: Studies in Sexology in Chinese Culture.* New York and London: Plenum.

Rui Xia. 2005. "Asphalt Net Covers China's West." *Asia Times Online.* www.atimes.com (accessed September 15, 2005).

Ruxrungtham, Kiat, Tim Brown, and Praphan Phanuphak. 2004. "HIV/AIDS in Asia." *Lancet* 364: 69–82.

Sabatier, René. 1988. *Blaming Others: Prejudice, Race and Worldwide AIDS.* Santa Cruz, Calif.: New Society Publishers.

Said, Edward. 1978. *Orientalism.* New York: Vintage Books.

Saiget, Robert J. 2000. "China Urged to Take Fresh Look at Rampant Prostitution and AIDS." *Agence France-Presse,* June 22.

Sassen, Saskia. 2002. *The Global City: New York London Tokyo.* 1st ed. Princeton, N.J.: Princeton University Press.

Sautman, Barry. 2000. "Is Xinjiang an Internal Colony?" *Inner Asia* 2(1): 239–71.

Schein, Louisa. 1994. "The Consumption of Color, and the Politics of White Skin in Post-Mao China." *Social Text* 41: 141–64.

————. 1996. "The Other Goes to the Market: The State, the Nation, and Unruliness in Contemporary China." *Identities: Global Studies in Culture and Power* 2(3): 197–222.

————. 1997. "Gender and Internal Colonialism in China." *Modern China* 23(1): 69–78.

————. 1999. "Of Cargo and Satellites: Imagined Cosmopolitanism." *Postcolonial Studies* 2(3): 345–75.

————. 2000. *Minority Rules: The Miao and the Feminine in China's Cultural Politics.* Durham, N.C.: Duke University Press.

Scheper-Hughes, Nancy. 1994. "An Essay: AIDS and the Social Body." *Social Science and Medicine* 39(7): 99–1003.

Schoepf, Brooke Grundfest. 1992. "Women at Risk: Case Studies from Zaire." In *The Time of AIDS,* edited by G. Herdt and S. Lindenbaum. Newbury Park: Sage Publications.

Schwartz, Jay R. (ed.) 2000. *The Official Guide to the Best Cathouses in Nevada: Everything You Want to Know about Legal Prostitution in Nevada.* Boise, Idaho: Straight Arrow Publishing.

Scott, James C. 1976. *The Moral Economy of the Peasant: Rebellion and Subsistence in Southeast Asia.* New Haven, Conn.: Yale University Press.

————. 1985. *Weapons of the Weak: Everyday Forms of Peasant Resistance.* New Haven, Conn.: Yale University Press.

SEA-AIDS. 2006. "Disappearance and Detention of Hunger Strikers." sea-aids@eforums.healthdev.org (accessed March 1, 2006).

Setel, Philip. 1999. *A Plague of Paradoxes: AIDS, Culture and Demography in Northern Tanzania.* Chicago: University of Chicago Press.

Sethakul, Ratanaporn. 2000. "Community Rights of the Lüe in China, Laos, and Thailand." *Tai Culture: International Review on Tai Cultural Studies* 5(2): 69–103.

Settle, Edmund. 2003. *AIDS in China: An Annotated Chronology, 1985–2003.* Monterey, Calif.: China AIDS Survey.

Shan Guangnai. 1995. *Zhongguo changji: Guoqu yu xianzai* [Prostitutes in China: The Past and Present]. Beijing: Legal Press.

Shen Jie. 2004. "Recent Policy Developments in HIV/AIDS in China." Paper presented by Yu Dongbao at Social Policy and HIV/AIDS in China Conference, at John F. Kennedy School of Government, Harvard University, Cambridge, Mass., May 6–8.

Shilts, Randy. 1987. *And the Band Played On: Politics, People and the AIDS Epidemic.* New York: St. Martin's Press.

Shue, Vivienne. 1988. *The Reach of the State: Sketches of the Chinese Body Politic.* Stanford, Calif.: Stanford University Press.

———. 1999. "State Legitimation through Officially Sponsored Charity and Relief." Paper presented at the Center for Chinese Studies, University of California, Berkeley, Shorenstein Seminars on Contemporary East Asia, May 8–9.

Sigley, Gary. 1998. "Issue on Sex" (guest editor's introduction). *Chinese Sociology and Anthropology* 31(1): 3–13.

Simao Prefecture Party Committee. 2003. *Prefecture Statistics.* Simao: External Propaganda Office of the Simao Prefecture Party Committee and the Press Office of Simao Prefecture Administration. www.sm.yn.gov.cn (accessed July 2004).

Singer, Linda. 1993. *Erotic Welfare: Sexual Theory and Politics in the Age of Epidemic.* New York: Routledge.

Singer, Merrill (ed.). 1998. *The Political Economy of AIDS.* Amityville, N.Y.: Baywood.

Singer, Merrill, et al. 1990. "SIDA: The Economic, Social and Cultural Context of AIDS Among Latinos." *Medical Anthropology Quarterly* no. 1: 72–114.

Siu, Helen. 1989. *Agents and Victims in South China: Accomplices in Rural Revolution.* New Haven, Conn.: Yale University Press.

Skeldon, Ronald. 2000. "Population Mobility and HIV Vulnerability in Southeast Asia: An Assessment and Analysis." United Nations Development Program, 2000. www.hiv-development.org (accessed November 30, 2000).

Smith, Christopher J. 2005. "Social Geography of Sexually Transmitted Diseases in China: Exploring the Role of Migration and Urbanization." *Asia Pacific Viewpoint* 46(1): 65–80.

Smith, Christopher J., and Yang Xiushi. 2005. "Examining the Connection between Temporary Migration and the Spread of HIV/AIDS in China." *China Review* 5(1): 109–37.

Sobo, Elisa J. 1993. "Inner-city Women and AIDS: The Psychosocial Benefits of Unsafe Sex." *Cultural, Medicine and Psychiatry* 17(4): 455–85.

Solinger, Dorothy. 1998. *Contesting Citizenship in Urban China: Peasant Migrants, the State and the Logic of the Market.* Berkeley and Los Angeles: University of California Press.

Sommer, Matthew. 2000. *Sex, Law, and Society in Late Imperial China.* Stanford, Calif.: Stanford University Press.

State Council HIV/AIDS Working Committee and UN Theme Group on HIV/AIDS in China. 2004. *A Joint Assessment of HIV/AIDS Prevention, Treatment and Care in China*. Beijing.

Stewart, Cianna. 1999. "Lecture on the Wellness Project (Formerly the Asian AIDS Project) and AIDS Prevention among Sex Workers in San Francisco." Paper submitted in Sandra Teresa Hyde's Women Studies 111: Sexuality, Prostitution, and AIDS in Asia and the Pacific, Department of Women's Studies, University of California, Berkeley.

Stoler, Ann Laura. 1989. "Making Empire Respectable: The Politics of Race and Sexual Morality in 20th-Century Colonial Cultures." *American Ethnologist* 16(4): 634–60.

———. 1995. *Race and the Education of Desire: Foucault's History of Sexuality and the Colonial Order of Things*. Durham, N.C.: Duke University Press.

———. 1998. "Educating Desire in Colonial Southeast Asia: Foucault, Freud and Imperial Sexualities." In *Sites of Desire, Economies of Pleasure: Sexualities in Asia and the Pacific*, edited by L. Manderson and M. Jolly. Chicago: University of Chicago Press.

Sturgeon, Janet. 2004. "Border Practice, Boundaries, and the Control of Resource Access: A Case from China, Burma, and Thailand." *Development and Change* 35(3): 463–84.

———. 2005. *Border Landscapes: The Politics of Akha Land Use in China and Thailand*. Seattle: University of Washington Press.

Sun Tairen. 1995. *Sun Tairen Huaji* [Sun Tairen's Collection of Paintings]. Kunming: Yunnan meishu chubanshe (Yunnan Art Publishing House).

Sun Xinhua, Nan Junhua, and Guo Qili. 1994. "AIDS and HIV Infection in China." *AIDS* 8(supplement 2): S55–S59.

Swain, Margaret Byrne. 1990. "Commoditizing Ethnicity in Southwest China." *Cultural Survival* 14(1): 26–32.

Swain, Margaret Byrne, and Janet Henshall Momsen. 2002. *Gender/Tourism/Fun (Tourism Dynamics)*. Elmsford, New York: Cognizant Communications Corporation.

Taylor, Christopher. 1990. "Condoms and Cosmology: The Fractal Person and Sexual Risk in Rwanda." *Social Science and Medicine* 33(9).

Thailand Ministry of Public Health. 1995. "Political Leadership and Commitment to Fight against HIV/AIDS in Asia and the Pacific." Paper presented at Third International Conference on AIDS in Asia and the Pacific, and the Fifth National AIDS Seminar, Chiang Mai, Thailand, September 17–21.

Treichler, Paula. 1991. "How to Have Theory in an Epidemic: The Evolution of AIDS Treatment Activism." In *Technoculture*, edited by C. Penley and A. Ross. Minneapolis: University of Minnesota Press.

———. 1999. *How to Have Theory in an Epidemic: Cultural Chronicles of AIDS*. Durham, N.C.: Duke University Press.

Tropical Forest Ecosystem Management Project. 1999. "Biodiversity Utilization of Ethnic Minorities," in *Xishuangbanna de senlin yu ren* (Forests and People in Xishuangbanna). Beijing: GTZ-Office Beijing.

Tsai, Kellee. 2002. *Back-Alley Banking: Private Entrepreneurs in China.* Ithaca, N.Y.: Cornell University Press.

Tsing, Anna Lowenhaupt. 1993. *In the Realm of the Diamond Queen: Marginality in an Out-of-the-Way Place.* Princeton, N.J.: Princeton University Press.

Tu Qiao. 2000. *Shiji zhitong: Zhongguo songfen aizibingren wanquan jilu* [A Century's Sorrows: A Complete Record of a Person with AIDS from China]. Guangzhou, China: Southern Newspaper Publishing House (Nanfang Ribao chubanshe).

Tu Xiaowen. 1998. "Shanghai yaodian biyunyaoju de kejixing [Contraceptive Accessibility in Shanghai Drugstores]." *Zhongguo jihua shengyu xue zazhi* [Chinese Family Planning Journal] 6(12): 546–47.

Tuan Yifu. 1998. *Escapism.* Baltimore: Johns Hopkins University Press.

UNAIDS. 2001. "Population Mobility and AIDS," A Technical Update. Beijing.

———. 2002a. *HIV/AIDS: China's Titanic Peril—2001 Update on the HIV/AIDS Situation and Needs Assessment Report.* Beijing: UN Theme Group on HIV/AIDS in China. June.

———. 2002b. *Report on the Global AIDS Epidemic.* Geneva: UNAIDS. September.

———. 2003. *AIDS Epidemic Update: 2003.* Geneva: UN Theme Group on HIV/AIDS and World Health Organization. June.

———. 2004. *2004 Report on the Global AIDS Epidemic: 4th Global Report.* Geneva: UN Theme Group on HIV/AIDS. June.

UNAIDS and State Council AIDS Working Committee Office. 2004. *A Joint Assessment of HIV/AIDS Prevention, Treatment and Care in China.* Beijing: Ministry of Health of China, UN Theme Group on HIV/AIDS in China, and National Center for AIDS/STD Control and Prevention, China CDC. December 1.

Uretsky, Elanah. 2003. "Research Note: The Import of Research on Male Sexuality in China for Effective HIV/AIDS Prevention Programs." *Yale Journal of Chinese Health* no. 2: 45–54.

Van der Veen, Marjolein. 2001. "Rethinking Commodification and Prostitution: An Effort at Peacemaking in the Battles over Prostitution." *Rethinking Marxism* 13(2): 30–51.

Van Gennup, Arnold. 1960. *The Rites of Passage.* Translated by M. B. Vizedom and G. L. Caffee. Chicago: University of Chicago Press.

Verdery, Katherine. 1996. *What Was Socialism, and What Comes Next?* Princeton, N.J.: Princeton University Press.

Walby, Catherine. 1997. *AIDS and the Body Politic.* New York: Routledge.

Walsh, Eileen Rose. 2001. "The Mosuo: Beyond the Myth of Matriarchy, Gender Transformation and Economic Development." Ph.D. dissertation, Anthropology Department, Temple University, Philadelphia.

Walsh, Eileen Rose, and Margaret Byrne Swain. 2004. "Creating Modernity by Touring Paradise: Domestic Ethnic Tourism in Yunnan, China." Special issue, *Journal of Tourism and Recreation Research* 29(2).

Wan Yanhai. 2005. *Aizhi xingdong* (Love, Knowledge, Action). www.aizhi.net.

Wang Anyi. 1994. *Fuxi he muxi de shenhua* [Paternal and Maternal Deities]. Hangzhou: Zheijiang xinhua chubanshe (Zhejiang New China Publishing House).

Wang Chun. 1996. "An Epidemiological Analysis of HIV Infection among Women Who Cross [the] Border in Simao Prefecture, Yunnan Province." Simao Health & Anti-Epidemic Station.

Wang Lan et al. 2005. "Epidemiologic Study on Human Immunodeficiency Virus Infection among Children in Former Paid Plasma Donating Community in China." *Chinese Medical Journal* 118(9): 720–24.

Wang Lianfang. 1993. *Yunnan minzu gongzuo huiyi lu, Yunnan wenshi ziliao xuanze, di sishiwu zhang* [A Memoir and Record of Work among Yunnan's Minorities]. Yunnan Cultural History Data Collections, vol. 45. Kunming: Yunnan People's Publishing House.

Wang Lin Ganna. 2005. "Report on HIV/AIDS in Yunnan." *Zhongguo xinwen wang* (China's News Network). China News Society, Kunming. November 26.

Wang N. 1991. "First Reported Case of AIDS in China." *Chinese Medical Journal* 17(12): 671–73.

Wang Shunu. 1988. *Zhongguo changjishi* [The History of Prostitution in China]. Beijing: Sanlian Press.

Wang Yangguang. December 2000. *AIDS in China: From Drugs to Blood to Sex.* Beijing: United States Embassy.

Wasserstrom, Jeffrey, and Elizabeth Perry. 1992. *Popular Protest and Political Culture in China.* Boulder, Colo.: Westview Press.

Watney, Simon. 1987. *Policing Desire: Pornography, AIDS and the Media.* Minneapolis: University of Minnesota Press.

———. 1994. *Practices of Freedom: Selected Writings on HIV/AIDS.* Durham, N.C.: Duke University Press.

———. 1997. *Policing Desire: Pornography, AIDS, and the Media.* 3rd ed. London: Cassell.

Watts, Jonathan. 2003. "China Takes Drastic Action over SARS Threat." *Lancet* 361(9370): 1708.

———. 2004. "China's Shift in HIV/AIDS Policy Marks Turnaround on Health." *Lancet* 363: 1370–71.

Watts, Sheldon. 1997. *Epidemics and History: Disease, Power and Imperialism.* New Haven, Conn.: Yale University Press.

Wehrfritz, George. 1996. "Unbuttoning A Nation." *International Newsweek,* April 15: 8–11.

Weitzer, Ronald (ed.). 2000. *Sex for Sale: Prostitution, Pornography, and the Sex Industry.* New York: Routledge.

White, Luise. 1990. *The Comforts of Home: Prostitution in Colonial Nairobi.* Chicago: University of Chicago Press.

White, Sydney Davant. 1993. "Medical Discourses, Naxi Identities and the State: Transformations in Socialist China." Ph.D. dissertation, Anthropology department, University of California, Berkeley.

White, Tyrene. 1985. "Population Policy and Rural Reform in China, 1977–1984: Policy Implementation and Interdependency at the Local Level." Ph.D. dissertation, Ohio State University.

WHO. *See* World Health Organization.

Wijeyewardene, Gehan. 1990. "Thailand and the Tai: Versions of Ethnic Identity." In *Ethnic Groups across National Boundaries in Mainland Southeast Asia,* edited by G. Wijeyewardene. Singapore: Institute of Southeast Asian Studies.

Winichakul, Thongchai. 1994. *Mapping Siam: A History of the Geo-Body of a Nation.* Honolulu: University of Hawaii Press.

World Health Organization (WHO). 1989. *Broadcaster's Questions and Answers on AIDS.* Geneva: WHO.

Wu Zunyou et al. 1995. "Risk Factors for Intravenous Drug Use and Sharing of Equipment among Young Male Drug Users in Southwest China." Paper presented at the International Symposium on AIDS, Beijing, China.

Wuhan Ribao (Wuhan Daily). 2004. "Sexual Contact to Become Main Factor in Spread of HIV/AIDS." www.china-aids.org. February 11.

Xia Guomei. 2003. "Growing Population Mobility and HIV Intervention among Female Service Workers in China." Paper presented at Globalization, the State and Urban Transformation in China Conference, Hong Kong Baptist University, December 15.

———. 2004. *HIV/AIDS in China.* Beijing: Foreign Languages Press.

———. 2005. *Zhongguo aizibing shehui yufang moshi yanjiu* [*Research in the Social Prevention Mode of HIV/AIDS in China*]. Shanghai: Shanghai shehui kexueyuan aizibing shehui zhengce yanjiu zhongxin (SASS Research Center for HIV/AIDS Public Policy).

Xia Zhongli. 1996. "Cong maiyin piaochang renyuan zhong jiance chu 6 lie HIV/AIDS de baogao [Six Cases of HIV/AIDS Detected among Prostitutes and Their Clients]." *Zhongguo xingbing aizibing dangzhi* [Chinese Journal of Prevention and Control of STDs and AIDS] 2(2): 63–65.

Xinhua [New China News Agency]. 2004. "Yunnan sheng tichu dayichang jindu he fangzhi aizibing de renmin zhanzheng [Yunnan Attempts to Fight a Mass People's War on AIDS]." December 2.

Xishuangbanna-Daizu Zizhizhou Tongjiju (Xishuangbanna-Dai Minority Prefecture Bureau of Statistics). 2005. *2004 Nian guomin jingji he shehui fazhan gongbao* [2004 National Economy and Social Development Labor Report]. Yunnan: Xishuangbanna-Daizu Zizhizhou Renmin Zhengfu (People's Government of Xishuangbanna-Dai Minority Autonomous Prefecture).

Yan Yunxiang. 1996. *The Flow of Gifts: Reciprocity and Social Networks in a Chinese Village.* Stanford, Calif.: Stanford University Press.

Yang, Mayfair Meigui. 1994. *Gifts, Favors and Banquets: The Art of Social Relationships in China.* Ithaca, N.Y.: Cornell University Press.

Yang Rongge et al. 2002. "On-going Generation of Multiple Forms of HIV-1 Intersubtype Recombinants in the Yunnan Province of China." *AIDS* 16(10): 1401–07.

Yang Rongge et al. 2003. "Identification and Characterization of a New Class of Human Immunodeficiency Virus Type 1 Recombinants Comprised of Two Circulating Recombinant Forms, CRF07_BC and CRF08_BC, in China." *Journal of Virology* 77(1): 685–95.

Yang Xiushi. 2003. "Community Characteristics of HIV/AIDS and STD Prevalence in Southwestern China." Paper presented at Globalization, the State and Urban Transformation in China Conference, Hong Kong Baptist University, December 16.

———. 2005. "Does Where We Live Matter? Community Characteristics and HIV and Sexually Transmitted Disease Prevalence in Southwestern China." *International Journal of STD & AIDS* 16(1): 31–37.

Yardley, Jim. 2005. "Chinese City Emerges as Model in Nation's Effort to Reverse Once Abysmal AIDS Record." *New York Times*. www.nytimes.com/2005/06/15/international/asia.html. June 16.

———. 2006. "New Estimate in China Finds Fewer AIDS Cases." *New York Times*. www.nytimes.com/2006/01/26/international/asia/26aids.html. January 26.

Yin Shaoting. 1986. "Shuo zhang [Speaking of Miasma]." *Yunnan difangzhi tongxun* [The Communication Annals of Places in Yunnan] 4: 69–74.

YRHRA. See Yunnan Reproductive Health Research Association.

Yu Huifen. 2001. "Yunnan sheng 1999 nian HIV/AIDS jiance baogao [Report on HIV/AIDS Surveillance in Yunnan Province in 1999]." *Zhongguo xingbing aizibing fangzhi* [Chinese Journal of Prevention and Control of STIs and HIV/AIDS] 7(2): 74–76.

Yu Xiaofang et al. 2003. "Sequence Note: Characterization of HIV Type-1 Heterosexual Transmission in Yunnan, China." *AIDS Research and Human Retroviruses* 19(11): 1051–55.

Yuan Jianhua et al. 2002. "Yunnan sheng HIV/AIDS fangce [HIV/AIDS Projections for Yunnan]." *Zhongguo xingbing aizibing fangzhi* [Chinese Journal of STD/AIDS Prevention and Control] 8(2): 78–81.

Yunnan Anti-Epidemic Station. 1995. *HIV Infection in Yunnan Province, China, 1986–1993*. Kunming, Yunnan.

Yunnan Provincial Bureau of Statistics. 2005a. *2004 Nian Yunnan xian guomin jingji he shehui fazhan tongji gongbao* [The 2004 Report on the National Economy and Social Development of Yunnan Province]. China Statistical Information Network 2005. www.stats.gov.yn (accessed June 20, 2005).

———. 2005b. *2004 Nian Yunnansheng guomin jingji he shehui fazhan tongji gongbao* [2004 Statistical Labor Report of Yunnan Provincial Economic and Social Development]. Yunnan, China.

Yunnan Reproductive Health Research Association. 2001. *Literature Review: Condom Use in China*. Kunming, Yunnan: YRHRA.

Yunnan Ribao [Yunnan Daily]. 2004. "*Yunnan AIDS Prevention and Control Law to Take Effect*." China AIDS Info. February 5, 2004. www.china-aids.org (accessed February 18, 2004).

Zhang Feng. 2004. "Suppliers of Blood under Investigation." *China Daily*, July 30.

Zhang Konglai. 2001. "Trends in Sexually Transmitted Diseases and HIV/AIDS." Paper presented at Health Care East and West: Moving into the 21st Century Conference, Boston, June 24–29.

Zhang Li. 2001. *Strangers in the City: Reconfiguration of Space, Power, and Social Networks within China's Floating Population*. Stanford, Calif.: Stanford University Press.

Zhang Luanxin. 1985. *Qingchun Ji* [Sacrificed Youth]. Beijing Film Academy Youth Film Studio, directed by Z. Luanxin. China Film.

Zhang Min, Li Weidong, and Zhang Xun. 2005. "Yunnansheng jiaqiang rujing waijierenyuan aizibing jianguan [Yunnan Strengthens AIDS Surveillance Amongst Foreign Visitors at Immigration Control Ports]." *Yunnan Ribao*, June 18.

Zhang Wenjian, ed. 2000. *Jiankang jiaoyu congshu: Xingbing* (The Health Education Series on Sexually Transmitted Infections). Jiankang Jiaoyu Congshu [Health Education Series]. Beijing: Chinese Traditional Medicine Publishing House.

Zhang Xianliang. 1991. *Getting Used to Dying [Xiguan si wang]*. Translated by M. Avery. New York: Harper Collins.

Zhang Xiaobo and Ravi Kanbur. 2005. "Spatial Inequality in Education and Health Care in China." *China Economic Review* 6(2): 189–204.

Zhang Xiaobo et al. 2002. "Yunnan sheng 2001 nian HIV/AIDS jiance jieguo fenxi" (Analysis of the Surveillance Results of HIV/AIDS in Yunnan in 2001). *Jibing jiance* (Disease Surveillance) 17(9): 327–31.

Zhang Zhen. 2003. "Mediating Time: The 'Rice Bowl of Youth' in Fin de Siècle Urban China." In *Globalization*, edited by Arjun Appardurai. Durham, NC: Duke University Press.

Zhang Zizhuo. 2004. "Yunnan AIDS Prevention and Control Law to Take Effect in March." *Yunnan Daily*, February 5.

Zheng Lan. 1981. *Travels through Xishuangbanna: China's Subtropical Home of Many Nationalities*. Beijing: Foreign Languages Press.

Zheng Xiaoyun and Yu Tao. 1995. "Muyu shengshui de nüxing [Women Bathed in Holy Water]." In *Yunnan minzu nüxing wenhua ceshu* [Nationalities in Yunnan: Women's Culture Series]. Kunming: Yunnan jiaoyu chubanshe (Yunnan Education Publishing House).

Zheng Xiwan. 1991. "A Preliminary Study on the Behavior of 225 Drug Abusers and the Risk Factors of HIV Infection in Ruili County, Yunnan Province." *Chinese Medical Journal* 12(1): 12–14.

———. 1993. "Cohort Study of HIV Infection among Drug Users in Ruili City and Longchuang County, Yunnan Province, China." *Chinese Journal of Epidemiology* 14(1): 3–5.

Zhongguo Hongshizihui (Chinese Red Cross). 1997. *Baohu ziji, pengyou bei jiating, yufang aizibing, aizibing yufang qingnian tongban jiaoyu peixun shouce* [To Prevent AIDS, Take Care of Yourself, Your Friends and Family, Youth Peer Education Training Manual for the Prevention of AIDS]. Beijing and Kunming: UNICEF and UNAIDS.

Zhou Yan. 2005. "China Exclusive: Anti-AIDS Campaign Spotlights Sex Workers." Xinhua News Wire. China AIDS Info 2005. www.china-aids.org. May 4.

Zito, Angela, and Tani Barlow. 1994. *Body, Subject and Power*. Chicago: University of Chicago Press.

Index

Text:	10/13 Sabon
Display:	Sabon
Compositor:	Sheridan Books, Inc.
Indexer:	Sharon Sweeney
Cartographer/Illustrator:	Bill Nelson